THIRD EDITION

FIT TO BE WELL

Essential Concepts

Alton L. Thygerson, EdD, FAWM | Steven M. Thygerson, PhD, MSPH

College of Life Sciences
Brigham Young University

College of Life Sciences
Brigham Young University

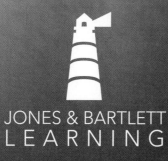

JONES & BARTLETT
LEARNING

World Headquarters

Jones & Bartlett Learning
5 Wall Street
Burlington, MA 01803
978-443-5000
info@jblearning.com
www.jblearning.com

Jones & Bartlett Learning books and products are available through most bookstores and online booksellers. To contact Jones & Bartlett Learning directly, call 800-832-0034, fax 978-443-8000, or visit our website, www.jblearning.com.

Substantial discounts on bulk quantities of Jones & Bartlett Learning publications are available to corporations, professional associations, and other qualified organizations. For details and specific discount information, contact the special sales department at Jones & Bartlett Learning via the above contact information or send an email to specialsales@jblearning.com.

The authors, editor, and publisher have made every effort to provide accurate information. However, they are not responsible for errors, omissions, or for any outcomes related to the use of the contents of this book and take no responsibility for the use of the products and procedures described. Treatments and side effects described in this book may not be applicable to all people; likewise, some people may require a dose or experience a side effect that is not described herein. Drugs and medical devices are discussed that may have limited availability controlled by the Food and Drug Administration (FDA) for use only in a research study or clinical trial. Research, clinical practice, and government regulations often change the accepted standard in this field. When consideration is being given to use of any drug in the clinical setting, the health care provider or reader is responsible for determining FDA status of the drug, reading the package insert, and reviewing prescribing information for the most up-to-date recommendations on dose, precautions, and contraindications, and determining the appropriate usage for the product. This is especially important in the case of drugs that are new or seldom used.

Production Credits

Chief Executive Officer: Ty Field
President: James Homer
SVP, Editor-in-Chief: Michael Johnson
SVP, Chief Technology Officer: Dean Fossella
SVP, Chief Marketing Officer: Alison M. Pendergast
Publisher: Cathleen Sether
Executive Acquisitions Editor: Shoshanna Goldberg
Editorial Assistant: Agnes Burt
Production Manager: Julie Champagne Bolduc
Production Assistant: Emma Krosschell
Marketing Manager: Jody Yeskey
V.P., Manufacturing and Inventory Control: Therese Connell
Composition: Circle Graphics
Cover Design: Scott Moden
Rights and Permissions Manager: Katherine Crighton
Permissions and Photo Research Assistant: Amy Rathburn
Cover Image: © Andres Rodriguez/Fotolia.com
Printing and Binding: Courier Kendallville
Cover Printing: Courier Kendallville

Some images in this book feature models. These models do not necessarily endorse, represent, or participate in the activities represented in the images.

Fit to Be Well: Essential Concepts is an independent publication and has not been authorized, sponsored, or otherwise approved by the owners of the trademarks referenced in this product.

To order this product, use ISBN: 978-1-4496-6140-3

Library of Congress Cataloging-in-Publication Data
Thygerson, Alton L.
    Fit to be well : essential concepts / Alton L. Thygerson, Steven M. Thygerson. — 3rd ed.
        p. cm.
    Includes bibliographical references and index.
    ISBN: 978-1-4496-4048-4
    1. Health.   2. Physical fitness.   I. Thygerson, Steven M.   II. Title.
    RA776.T539 2013
    613—dc22
                                                        2011041834

6048

Printed in the United States of America
16 15 14 13   10 9 8 7 6 5 4 3

Contents

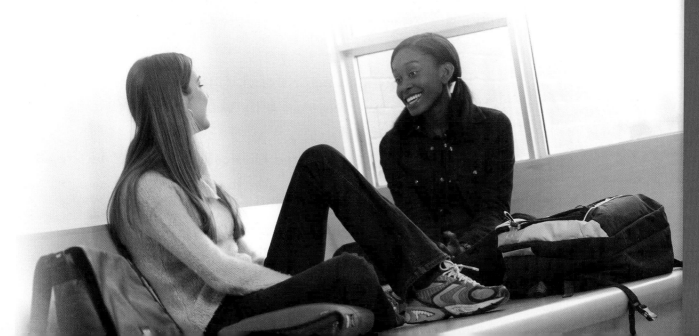

CHAPTER (3) Changing to a Healthy Lifestyle 28

CHAPTER (4) Preparing for Physical Activity and Exercise 44

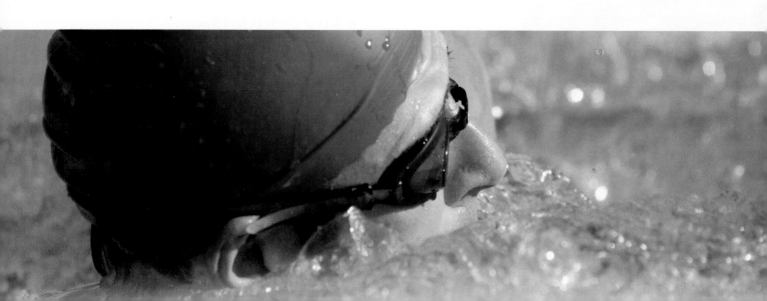

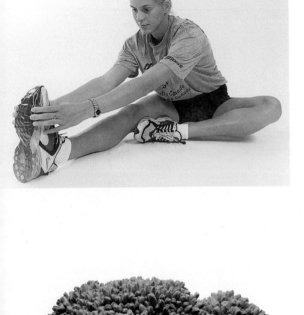

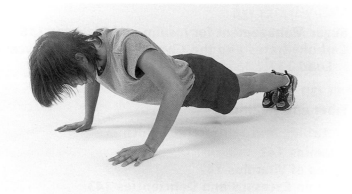

CHAPTER (**8**) Nutrition 126

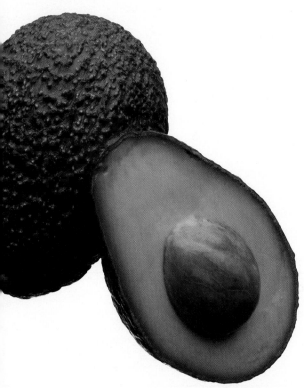

CHAPTER Body Composition and Body Fitness 176

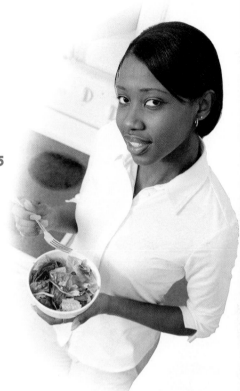

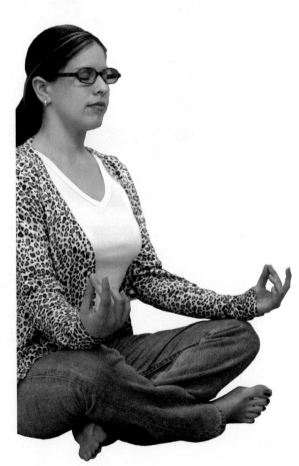

The purpose of this book is, first, to introduce you to the extraordinary world of physical fitness and, second, to change your life.

In a time of high-tech advances, we have lost sight of the fact that the greatest high-tech invention of all time is the human body. What happens to our bodies as we move through life is the result of our lifestyle.

As priceless as good health is, it is freely available to us if we live the right way. The child does not have to be taught to play, but the adult must learn how to exercise. As we age and our lives become busier, we lose that childhood instinct to run and jump, to skip, and to walk briskly. But it is movement in assorted styles and speeds on a regular basis that is critical in maintaining our high-tech machinery.

The good news is that it is never too late to start exercising, eating properly, and managing stress, regardless of your age or physical condition. This book can help you make the lifestyle changes that will sustain your health and make your life a better one.

Attempting to reach the goal of good health and wellness through physical fitness can be compared with preparing to take a journey. If you were driving from Los Angeles to New York City, you would first obtain a road map to determine the best route to follow. The journey to good health and wellness is very similar, but most people are not familiar with or do not know where to obtain a road map leading to good health and wellness.

This book is your road map. It takes you from your current level of fitness to increased cardiorespiratory endurance, strength, and flexibility, and helps you maintain a healthy weight and learn to relax.

Fit to Be Well: Essential Concepts, Third Edition offers a simple, workable approach to a healthy lifestyle.

Notes to Students and Instructors

No other fitness book is like this one.

The content of this book is organized in a succinct, easy-to-navigate manner, with emphasis placed on important concepts and applications. The advantages of this approach include:

- Decreased reading time
- Faster access to information
- Improved learning
- Less expense
- High reader satisfaction
- Creative uses of information (e.g., uses "chunking" to put content into manageable units for better learning)
- Content that is concise and straightforward, with information that a person "needs" to know rather than content that is simply "nice" to know
- Evidence-based medical sources that provide the content and latest recommendations

Special Features

Special features to improve learning include:

What's the word boxes throughout the text contain target terms and offer simple, clear definitions for terms of interest.

The Inside Track feature provides quick and easy guides to important information.

Medical News You Can Use consists of concise summaries from a range of recent medical journals and reports. They simplify the technical language to provide a rich source of information. They serve not only as interesting reading, but more importantly, also support many of this book's key concepts.

Tipping Point gives helpful hints and tips that explain to students how to manage their own fitness and healthy lifestyle program.

Knowledge Check provides multiple-choice questions at the end of each chapter, which test students' knowledge of the information covered in the text.

Modern Modifications sections in each chapter provide a list of simple suggestions related to that chapter's topic. Each of these suggestions is specifically intended to be easily absorbed into students' daily routines. The strategies are realistic and take into consideration "real-life" obstacles.

Critical Thinking sections give students a chance to apply what they learned in each chapter. Questions and scenarios about the work that they will do and the goals they want to achieve will bring about some critical thoughts. This will help students assimilate what they learn and apply it to their daily lives.

Going Above and Beyond provides a perfect opportunity for students to take their research one step further. Complete bibliographies and Web sites are included so that students can learn more about topics of interest to them.

Time Outs explore topics of interest to students such as energy production, fad diets, and ethnic diets.

Topics New to the *Third Edition*

- Life expectancy
- Exercising in the heat, in the cold, at high altitudes, and in areas with high air pollution
- Cross-training and interval-training
- How to overcome excuses for not exercising
- Emphasizes the FITT formula for designing an effective exercise program
- New chapter on the health benefits from physical activity and exercise adapted from *Physical Activity Guidelines for Americans*
- Emphasis on the Heart Rate Reserve (HRR) to calculate your intensity training range
- Walking techniques, how to gauge walking speeds, and pedometers
- Emphasis on waist-to-height ratio (WHtR) as a much better measure of obesity; also included: BMI, waist-to-hip ratio, and waist circumference for assessing obesity
- Content from the latest *Dietary Guidelines for Americans* with its emphasis on weight control and which foods to increase and to reduce
- MyPlate guidelines replace the heavily criticized MyPyramid recommendations
- Content from the latest *Physical Activity for Americans*
- *Healthy People 2020* topics and objectives
- *New labs:*
  - Online Diet Analysis
  - Fast-Food Analysis
  - Food Labels
  - Grocery Store Scavenger Hunt

Supplements

Instructor Resources

Comprehensive teaching resources are available as free downloads. These helpful teaching aids include an Instructor's Manual, PowerPoint Presentations, and a Test Bank.

Student Resources

Text-Specific Website http://go.jblearning.com/thygerson3e

Students can use the website to access animated flashcards, practice quizzes, crossword puzzles, an interactive glossary, and Web links that help reinforce key concepts in the text. This interactive website is accessible to students through the redeemable access code provided in every new text.

Lab Manual

A student lab manual is included at the end of the text at no additional cost to students! By adding self-assessments and related labs to each of the chapters, this text becomes an interactive guide to building and implementing a fitness program that will work with a student's individual needs and schedules.

Any book requires a great deal of effort, and not just on the part of the authors. This book is no exception to that rule.

We are fortunate to have a publisher who believed in this unique project and who encouraged us to write this textbook. We are very grateful to Shoshanna Goldberg, Executive Acquisitions Editor, for pushing the project along the way, and Agnes Burt, Editorial Assistant, for helping to make it a better book. A strong appreciation goes to the Jones & Bartlett Learning production staff, Julie Bolduc, Production Manager, and Amy Rathburn, Permissions and Photo Research Assistant; Joanne Revak at Circle Graphics, for producing a book of high quality; and the layout team at Circle Graphics for putting it all together.

We would also like to thank Karl Larson for his thorough analysis of the text, and the many reviewers of the *Second Edition*, whose suggestions and insight provided invaluable direction for the development of the *Third Edition*:

Heather R. Adams-Blair, PhD, Eastern Kentucky University

Tony D. Airhart, MS, Collin College

Curtiss Brown, MS, CSCS, Solano Community College

Jeff Burnett, EdD, Fort Hays State University

David L. Collins, MEd, ATC, LAT, East Texas Baptist University

Joyce Donatelli, Wilson College

John Finley, MEd, ATC, Goldey-Beacom College

Janet S. Hamilton, MA, RCEP, CSCS, Clayton State University

Kathy A. Mann, PT, MS, Kellogg Community College

Matthew Miltenberger, MS, ATC, CSCS, East Stroudsburg University

Lara B. Norton, EdS, East Georgia College

Melissa A. Parks, PhD, Louisiana State University at Alexandria

Christine M. Rockey, MS, Coastal Carolina University

Todd Sandberg, MS, ATC, AT/L, Whitworth University

Deonna Shake, BSED, MED ACU, Abilene Christian University

Scott C. Swanson, PhD, Ohio Northern University

Virginia E. Thomas, MA, CSCS, University of Portland

Jason B. White, MS, Ohio University

Jeff White, MEd, Gordon College

Carolyn Willingham, Phillips Community College

Andrea P. Willis, Abraham Baldwin College

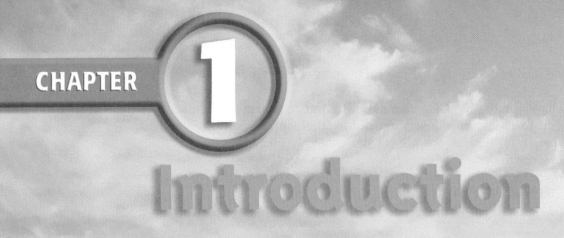

CHAPTER 1

Introduction

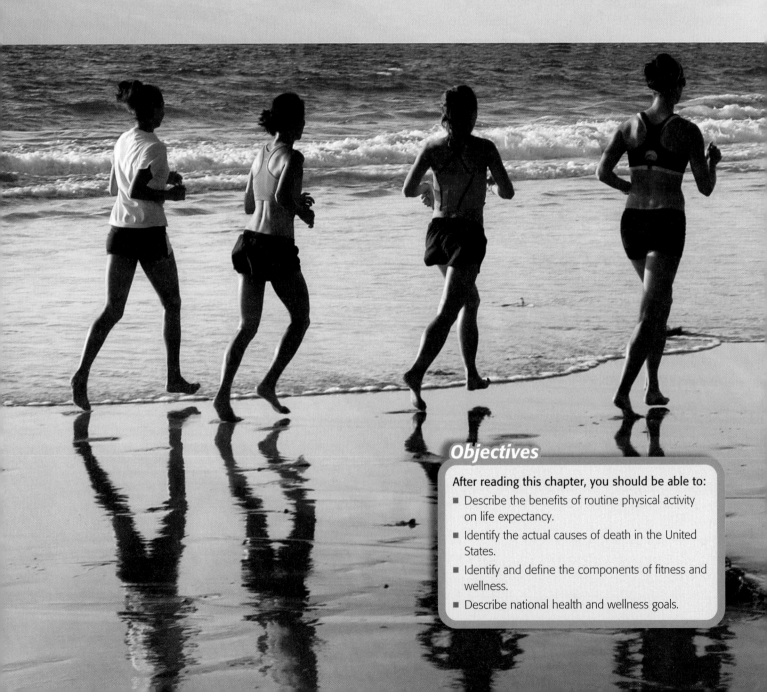

Objectives

After reading this chapter, you should be able to:

- Describe the benefits of routine physical activity on life expectancy.
- Identify the actual causes of death in the United States.
- Identify and define the components of fitness and wellness.
- Describe national health and wellness goals.

"He who has health, has hope; and he who has hope, has everything."

—Carlyle

How Long Can We Expect to Live?

Life expectancy in the United States in 2009 was the highest in recorded history, reaching 78.2 years (or about 78 years and 10 weeks). Since 2000, life expectancy has increased by 1.8% (or about 17 months) for the general population. Females continue to have the longer life expectancy (80.6 years), compared with males at 75.7 years.

Life expectancies rose dramatically in the past century. The average life span of anyone in an industrialized nation has increased since 1900 by over 30 years due to improvements in public health, vaccinations, and disease prevention. For example, fewer people have been affected by epidemics of infectious diseases that can be vaccinated against, such as smallpox. Penicillin, discovered in 1928, eliminated bacterial infections as a major cause of death (see **Figure 1.1**).

It is not likely that life expectancies will continue to rise as they have during the past century. The approximately 10 million cells in your body have a limited life span, meaning they can only divide a certain number of times before they begin to age and stop reproducing. This phenomenon, known as the Hayflick limit, is named after its discoverer, Dr. Leonard Hayflick. The human life-span limit is believed to be close to 125 years, although very few of us reach that age. Incidentally, Frenchwoman Jeanne Calment, who died in 1997 at the age of 122 years, 164 days, has the longest confirmed life span.

Various reasons explain why more of us do not make it even to 100 years. Nearly all of us experience life-shortening diseases (e.g., heart disease, cancer). While it may not be possible to change our cells' preprogramming, prevention or better treatment of these diseases allow us to come closer to our Hayflick limit. Some experts actually believe that United States' life expectancy will fall dramatically by at least 2 to 5 years in the near future because of obesity. These experts believe that future generations will have shorter and less healthy lives than their parents for the first time in modern history, unless changes are made (Olshansky 2005).

In the United States, the average person lives into his or her seventies. Your chronological age is your actual age in years from your birth date. However, what really matters is your biological age, which is an estimate of your well-being and general health compared to those of others of your age. For example, people with health problems at 50 are considered to be biologically older than a healthy and vigorous 70-year-old. The lesson here is for you to take control of your health sooner rather than later.

In the United States, women live about 5 years longer than men. For women, the most accurate predictor of their genetic effect is chronological age at menopause. The average age of menopause for American women is 52 years, but in general, the later her menopause occurs, the longer a woman will live. For those who have not reached that time in their lives, their mother's age at menopause will give an estimate of an expected menopause and an estimated genetic age.

Certain biomarkers of biological aging can let you know whether you are doing better or worse than your chronological age. These

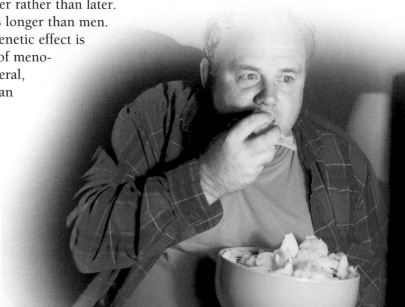

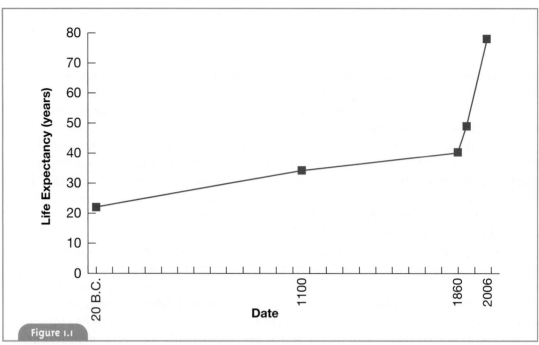

Figure 1.1

Life expectancy since Julius Caesar. (*Sources:* Reproduced with permission from Flanigan R. J., and Flanigan Sawyer K., *Longevity Made Simple*, First edition. Williams Clark Publishing, 2007. Data from U.S. Centers for Disease Control and Prevention; Lydia Bronte, *The Longevity Factor*, HarperCollins Publishers, 1993; Human Mortality Database, University of California, Berkeley [USA]; and Max Planck Institute for Demographic Research [Germany].)

Medical News You Can Use

Healthy Living Really Does Postpone Death

Four health risk behaviors—lack of physical activity, poor nutrition, tobacco use, and excessive alcohol consumption—are responsible for much of the illness and death related to chronic diseases. Seven out of 10 deaths among Americans each year are from chronic diseases. Heart disease, cancer, and stroke account for more than 50% of all deaths each year.

A Centers for Disease Control study finds that people can live longer if they practice one or more healthy lifestyle behaviors—not smoking, eating a healthy diet, getting regular physical activity, and limiting alcohol consumption. Not smoking provides the most protection from dying early from all causes.

People who engaged in all four healthy behaviors were 63% less likely to die early from cancer, 65% less likely to die early from cardiovascular disease, and 57% less likely to die early from other causes compared to people who did not engage in any of the healthy behaviors.

Source: Data from Ford E.S., et al., Low-risk lifestyle behaviors and all-cause mortality. *American Journal of Public Health* 2011. 101(10): 1922–1929.

markers primarily come from blood testing at a physician's office, but you can test several of these on your own:

- Blood pressure
- Blood glucose and cholesterol levels
- Field test for cardiorespiratory fitness (e.g., walking test)
- Muscular strength
- Bone mineral density
- Skin elasticity
- Cognitive abilities, including memory
- Blood markers for systemic inflammation

It is difficult to obtain a definite calculation of your biological age. However, if you can answer questions about different health factors, including cholesterol levels, blood pressure, exercise habits, and more, try one of several free online calculators:

- Life Expectancy Calculator available at http://www.livingto100.com
- Real Age Test available at www.realage.com

It is unknown how valid the tests are, but taking either or both of the online tests may point out some ways to change your lifestyle that can improve your health and wellness.

Most of us desire a long life; however, let us be mindful of the admonition given by the French essayist, Michel de Montaigne: "The usefulness of living lies not in duration but in what you make of it. Some have lived long and lived little."

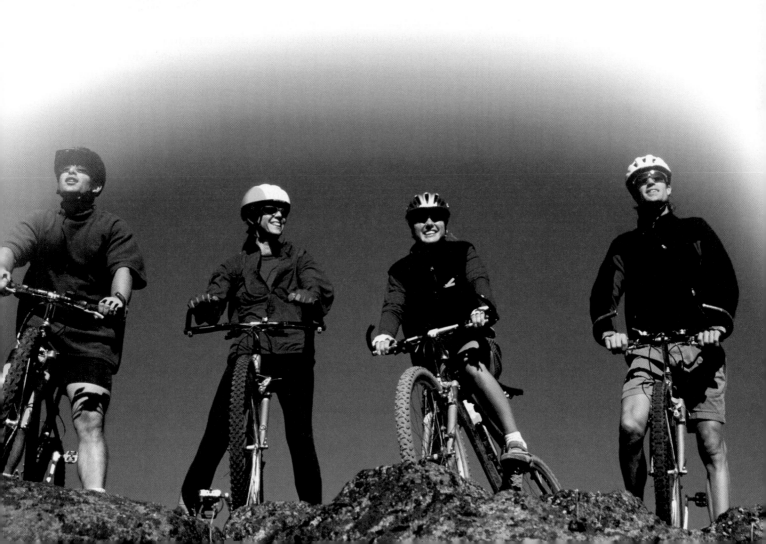

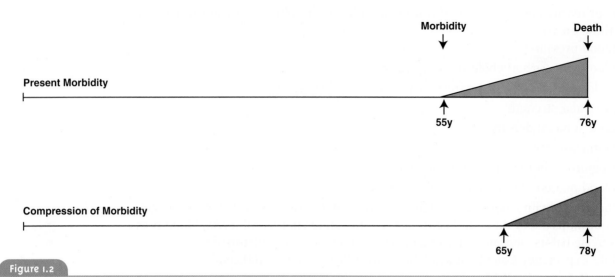

Figure 1.2

Compression of morbidity. Effects of good health habits. Death and serious medical problems occur earlier in life and medical problems have a longer period in those not practicing a healthy lifestyle. Serious medical problems occur much later in life and have a shorter period in those practicing a healthy lifestyle. (*Source:* Adapted from Fries, J. F. Measuring and monitoring success in compressing morbidity. *Annals of Internal Medicine* 2003; 139:455–459.)

Compression of Morbidity

As people live longer, some fear that they will spend additional years suffering poor health, disability, or dementia. In contrast, studies focusing on the concept known as compression of morbidity suggest that people can have both a longer life and a healthier old age. To do so, it is necessary to engage in healthy, preventive practices (see **Lab 1-1**).

Figure 1.2 shows two time lines for life-ending morbidity and longevity. The first line graph shows that today disability begins to be detectable around age 55 in the average individual, and death occurs on average around 76 years of age. Most disability occurs between these points, and the seriousness of the disability increases with time. The second line graph shows that a healthier lifestyle can extend your life, and if you become terminally ill, your life (and illness) will be shorter.

You want to minimize the number of years spent suffering, and maximize the total number of years living. Ideally, we want a long, healthy life, with a rapid decline leading to death.

Through a healthy lifestyle you can live longer. Although undesirable medical events will still occur near the end of your life, events leading to death will be delayed between 7 and 13 years, and time between that event and when death occurs is shortened.

You are the most important person taking care of your health. The key to taking responsibility for yourself is learning what works for you and then implementing what you have learned into your daily life. Some people view fitness-related goals as impossible dreams. The truth, however, is that everyone is capable of obtaining a healthy lifestyle. Keep in mind that every change you make is significant, no matter how big or small.

What Are the Leading Causes of Death?

There are more than 100,000 diseases. However, nearly 60% of the U.S. population dies from just three causes: heart disease, cancer, and stroke. The top 10 causes account for almost 80% of all deaths. Not one of the diseases below the top 10 accounts for even 1% of deaths. Therefore, to live a long and healthy life, the data suggest, that we focus primarily on preventing the top 10 diseases and not the 100,000 others.

Refer to **Figure 1.3** , 10 Leading Causes of Death. Note that the far-right column lists the leading causes of death for all ages.

Rank	<1	1–4	5–9	10–14	15–24	25–34	35–44	45–54	55–64	65+	Total
				Age Groups							
1	Congenital Anomalies 5,785	Unintentional Injury 1,588	Unintentional Injury 965	Unintentional Injury 1,229	Unintentional Injury 15,897	Unintentional Injury 14,977	Unintentional Injury 16,931	Malignant Neoplasms 50,167	Malignant Neoplasms 103,171	Heart Disease 496,095	Heart Disease 616,067
2	Short Gestation 4,857	Congenital Anomalies 546	Malignant Neoplasms 480	Malignant Neoplasms 479	Homicide 5,551	Suicide 5,278	Malignant Neoplasms 13,288	Heart Disease 37,434	Heart Disease 65,527	Malignant Neoplasms 389,730	Malignant Neoplasms 562,875
3	SIDS 2,453	Homicide 398	Congenital Anomalies 196	Homicide 213	Suicide 4,140	Homicide 4,758	Heart Disease 11,839	Unintentional Injury 20,315	Chronic Low. Respiratory Disease 12,777	Cerebro-vascular 115,961	Cerebro-vascular 135,952
4	Maternal Pregnancy Comp. 1,769	Malignant Neoplasms 364	Homicide 133	Suicide 180	Malignant Neoplasms 1,653	Malignant Neoplasms 3,463	Suicide 6,722	Liver Disease 8,212	Unintentional Injury 12,193	Chronic Low. Respiratory Disease 109,562	Chronic Low. Respiratory Disease 127,924
5	Unintentional Injury 1,285	Heart Disease 173	Heart Disease 110	Congenital Anomalies 178	Heart Disease 1,084	Heart Disease 3,223	HIV 3,572	Suicide 7,778	Diabetes Mellitus 11,304	Alzheimer's Disease 73,797	Unintentional Injury 123,706
6	Placenta Cord Membranes 1,135	Influenza & Pneumonia 109	Chronic Low. Respiratory Disease 54	Heart Disease 131	Congenital Anomalies 402	HIV 1,091	Homicide 3,052	Cerebro-vascular 6,385	Cerebro-vascular 10,500	Diabetes Mellitus 51,528	Alzheimer's Disease 74,632
7	Bacterial Sepsis 820	Septicemia 78	Influenza & Pneumonia 48	Chronic Low. Respiratory Disease 64	Cerebro-vascular 195	Diabetes Mellitus 610	Liver Disease 2,570	Diabetes Mellitus 5,753	Liver Disease 8,004	Influenza & Pneumonia 45,941	Diabetes Mellitus 71,382
8	Respiratory Distress 789	Perinatal Period 70	Benign Neoplasms 41	Influenza & Pneumonia 55	Diabetes Mellitus 168	Cerebro-vascular 505	Cerebro-vascular 2,133	HIV 4,156	Suicide 5,069	Nephritis 38,484	Influenza & Pneumonia 52,717
9	Circulatory System Disease 624	Benign Neoplasms 59	Cerebro-vascular 38	Cerebro-vascular 45	Influenza & Pneumonia 163	Congenital Anomalies 417	Diabetes Mellitus 1,984	Chronic Low. Respiratory Disease 4,153	Nephritis 4,440	Unintentional Injury 38,292	Nephritis 46,448
10	Neonatal Hemorrhage 597	Chronic Low. Respiratory Disease 57	Septicemia 36	Benign Neoplasms 43	Three Tied* 160	Liver Disease 384	Septicemia 910	Viral Hepatitis 2,815	Septicemia 4,231	Septicemia 26,362	Septicemia 34,828

*The three causes are: Complicated Pregnancy, HIV, Septicemia.
Source: National Vital Statistics System, National Center for Health Statistics, CDC.
Produced by: Office of Statistics and Programming, National Center for Injury Prevention and Control, CDC.

Figure 1.3

Ten leading causes of death by age group, United States – 2007. (*Source:* Modified from *Ten Leading Causes of Death and Injury* 2007. Courtesy of the National Center for Injury Prevention and Control/CDC.)

What Are the Actual Causes of Death?

What actually kills us? Many people and even health professionals have come up with the answer of heart disease, followed by cancer and stroke—the top three leading causes of death.

Epidemiologists thought that it did not help, when someone died of a heart attack, to conclude merely that the cause was disease of the heart. They wanted to know what caused the disease of the heart in the first place, and what caused cancer or the stroke. They determined that more than half the instances of these diseases were attributable to a handful of largely preventable behaviors: smoking, poor diet, physical inactivity, and alcohol consumption. Our lifestyle, not our genes, largely determines if and when we suffer from one or more of the top causes of death. See Table 1.1.

Table 1.1 — Actual Causes of Death in the United States

Rank	Actual Cause	Percentage of Deaths
1	Tobacco use	18.1
2	Obesity (inactivity/poor diet)	16.6
3	Alcohol consumption	3.5
4	Microbial agents (flu, pneumonia)	3.1
5	Toxic agents	2.3
6	Motor vehicles	1.8
7	Firearms	1.2
8	Sexual behavior	0.8
9	Illicit drug use	0.7
10	Other	<.05

Source: Data from Mokdad A. et al., Actual causes of death in the United States, 2000. *Journal of the American Medical Association* 2004; 291(10):1238–1245.

Medical News You Can Use

Heart Disease Prevention May Save Billions Annually in United States

Prevention is the key to slowing the soaring health care costs of heart disease in the United States. The costs reached $450 billion in 2010. Prevention of heart disease by managing programs to reduce cholesterol, blood pressure, and tobacco use would be a wise long-term investment in the nation's health and economy. Additionally, researchers calculated that every $1 spent on the construction of walking or biking paths would cut medical costs by $3. Slashing daily salt intake by Americans would help reduce the rate of high blood pressure by 25%. That could potentially save $26 billion in health care costs each year. The American Heart Association concluded by showing that the savings would not only be monetary but would also lengthen and improve the quality of life that people enjoy. These changes would also have an effect on generations to come.

Source: Data from Weintraub W.S., et al., Value of primordial and primary prevention for cardiovascular disease. *Circulation* 2011; 124:967–990.

Although there are no surefire recipes for good health, the mixture of regular exercise and healthy eating comes close. Tobacco and physical inactivity, combined with unhealthy diets, are running neck-and-neck at the top of the list of actual causes of death. Americans are sitting around and eating themselves to death.

With the benefits of regular exercise or physical activity capable of doing everyone a world of good, it is mind-boggling that only a minority of Americans get enough exercise or leisure-time physical activity. Studies that have followed the health of large groups of people for many years, as well as short-term studies, all point in the same direction: *A sedentary (inactive) lifestyle increases the chances of becoming overweight and developing a number of chronic diseases.*

Exercise or physical activity helps many of the body's systems function better and keeps a host of diseases at bay.

A U.S. Surgeon General's report analyzed the 10 leading causes of death and suggested that up to half of U.S. deaths were attributable to unhealthy behavior or lifestyle; 20% to environmental factors; 20% to human biological/genetic factors; and 10% to inadequacies in health care (see Figure 1.4).

Behavior remains the dominant cause of premature death and disability. Today, chronic diseases—such as cardiovascular disease (primarily heart disease and stroke), cancer, and type 2 diabetes—are among the most prevalent, costly, and preventable of all health problems and account for seven out of every 10 deaths in the United States. Chronic diseases are mostly preventable but can be difficult to change because the risk factors associated with developing chronic conditions are linked primarily to lifestyle behaviors.

Definitions

To prepare properly for physical activity and exercise, let us start by examining two key words—"fit" and "well"—plus a few others from our everyday conversations.

Fitness, as defined by the U.S. Department of Health and Human Services (DHHS), is "the ability to carry out daily tasks with vigor and alertness, without undue fatigue, and with ample energy to enjoy leisure-time pursuits and respond to emergencies. Physical fitness includes a number of components consisting of cardiorespiratory endurance; skeletal muscle endurance, strength and power; flexibility; and body composition."

Those four components of fitness provide the basis of a balanced workout program. They are made up of structured activities aimed at increasing specific elements of fitness. Each is a health-related component of physical fitness. The DHHS defines these components of physical fitness as follows:

- **Cardiorespiratory fitness (endurance)** is the ability of the circulatory and respiratory systems to supply oxygen during sustained physical activity.
- **Muscle-strengthening activity (strength training, resistance training, or muscular strength and endurance exercises)** is physical activity, including exercise, that increases skeletal muscle strength, power, endurance, and mass.
- **Flexibility** is the range of motion possible at a joint. Flexibility is specific to each joint and depends on a number of variables, including but not limited to the tightness of specific ligaments and tendons. Flexibility exercises enhance the ability of a joint to move through its full range of motion.
- **Body composition** refers to body weight and the relative amounts of muscle, fat, bone, and other vital tissues of the body. Most often, body composition addresses only fat and lean body mass (or fat-free mass).

The second key word is "well." Fitness leads to being well. **Wellness**, defined by the National Wellness Institute, is "an active process of becoming aware of and making choices toward a more successful existence." Some have described wellness as "the constant, conscious pursuit of living life to its fullest potential." It involves the whole person and is more than physical fitness. Wellness includes physical fitness, but it is multidimensional. A popular model adopted by many university, corporate, and public health programs encompasses these dimensions:

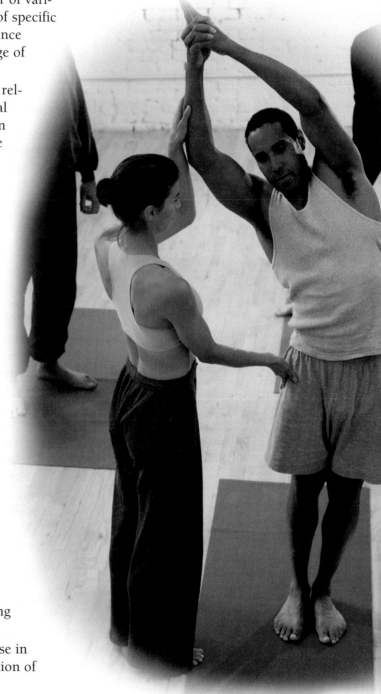

- **Physical:** encourages regular physical activity for cardiorespiratory, muscular, and flexibility fitness as well as knowledge about nutrition, and discourages the use of harmful substances.
- **Social:** encourages contributing to the common welfare of one's community and the pursuit of harmony in one's family.
- **Intellectual:** encourages creative, stimulating mental activities.
- **Emotional:** emphasizes an awareness and acceptance of one's feelings, enthusiasm about oneself and life, ability to deal with stress, and maintaining good relationships with others.
- **Spiritual:** encourages seeking meaning and purpose in human existence and developing a deep appreciation of life.

1

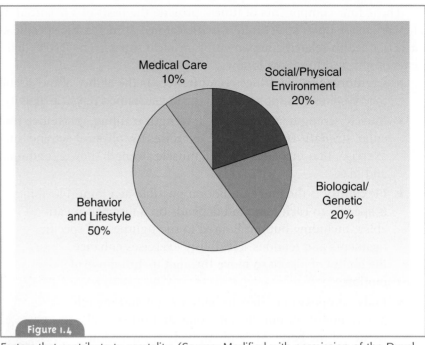

Figure 1.4

Factors that contribute to mortality. (*Source:* Modified with permission of the Duval County Center of Health Statistics, Florida Department of Health. Data from *Healthy People: The Surgeon General's Report on Health Promotion and Disease Prevention* 1979.)

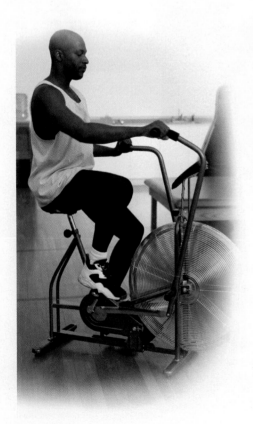

Some experts add environmental, occupational, and/or financial dimensions to the list.

The terms "wellness" and "health" often confuse people. The DHHS defines **health** as "the human condition with physical, social and psychological dimensions, each characterized on a continuum with positive and negative poles. Positive health is associated with a capacity to enjoy life and to withstand challenges; it is not merely the absence of disease. Negative health is associated with illness, and in the extreme, with premature death."

Finally, two other terms have been defined by DHHS: physical activity and exercise.

Physical activity is "any bodily movement produced by the contraction of skeletal muscle that increases energy expenditure above a basal level."

Physical activity includes any activity that gets you up and moving throughout the day. These activities could include grocery shopping, mowing the lawn, taking the dog for a walk, or shoveling snow from the driveway. While they may not be specifically intended to increase your muscular or cardiorespiratory endurance, daily physical activities are just as important as structured exercise.

Exercise is defined as "a subcategory of physical activity that is planned, structured, repetitive, and purposive in the sense that the improvement or maintenance of one or more compo-

Medical News You Can Use

Buying Weight Loss

Money trumps health benefits (e.g., lower risk of high blood pressure, stroke, heart attack) when it comes to losing weight. People were more likely to stick to weight-loss programs if they were offered cash incentives compared with delayed good health benefits. Scientists discovered that those offered cash incentives (no more than $100) over a 16-week program dropped an average of 4 lbs more than those who were not paid for losing pounds.

Source: Data from Volpp K.G., et al., Financial incentive–based approaches for weight loss—A randomized trial. *Journal of the American Medical Association* 2008; 300(22):2631–2637.

nents of physical fitness is the objective. 'Exercise' and 'exercise training' frequently are used interchangeably and generally refer to physical activity performed during leisure time with the primary purpose of improving or maintaining physical fitness, physical performance, or health."

Who Are the Physically Active?

The National Center for Health Statistics (CDC 2010) reported the following (see **Figure 1.5**, which shows data for men and women combined):

- Four in 10 adults (39.7%) engage in no leisure-time physical activity.
- More than one in five adults (21.9%) engage in light-moderate leisure-time physical activity at least five times per week.
- From 30% to 35% of adults reported participation in moderate- or vigorous-intensity activity sufficient to meet physical activity recommendations.

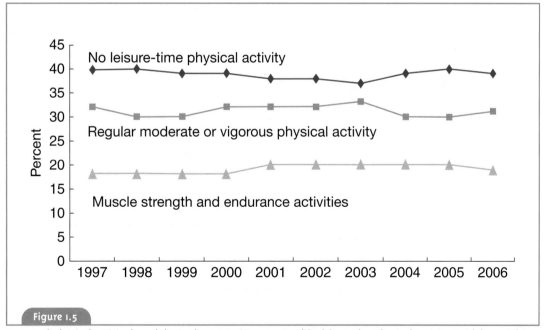

Figure 1.5

Reported physical activity by adults in the USA. (*Source:* Modified from the Physical Activity Guidelines Advisory Committee Report. Data from 1997–2006 *The Healthy People 2010 Database. Courtesy of the U.S. Department of Health & Human Services.*)

1

- About one in eight adults (11.1%) engage in vigorous leisure-time physical activity five times per week.
- About one-fourth of adults engage in at least some leisure-time strengthening activity.

The data also show the characteristics of those most likely to engage in leisure-time physical activity, as follows:

- Men
- Young adults (see Figure 1.6)
- Educated (those with graduate degrees were twice as likely as those with less than a high school diploma; see Figure 1.7)
- Higher income
- Married adults
- Live in the West (see Figure 1.8)

National Health and Wellness Goals

Healthy People 2020

For the past three decades, the DHHS has issued a national agenda aimed at improving the health of all Americans across each 10-year span. Under each of these Healthy People initiatives, DHHS established health benchmarks and monitored how well people were reaching them over time.

The DHHS launched *Healthy People 2020,* a comprehensive, nationwide health promotion and disease prevention agenda. *Healthy People 2020* serves as a road map for improving the health of all people in the United States.

Healthy People 2020 identifies the leading health topics and objectives intended to accomplish an increase in life span and quality of life as well as to decrease disparities in

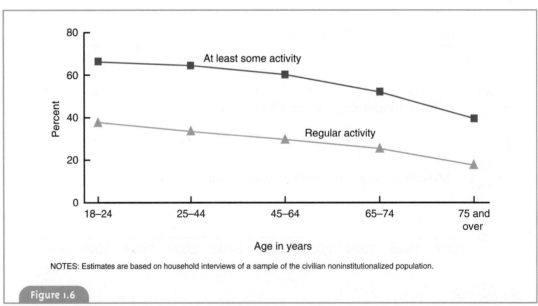

NOTES: Estimates are based on household interviews of a sample of the civilian noninstitutionalized population.

Figure 1.6

Percentage of adults who engaged in leisure activity, by level of activity and age. (*Source:* Data from *Health Behaviors of Adults: United States, 2005–2007*. National Center for Health Statistics. Vital and Health Stat Series No. 10 (245). 2010.)

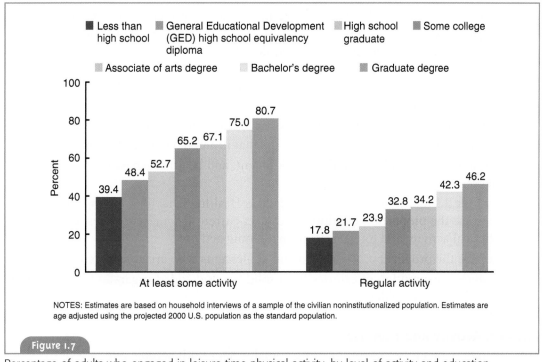

Percentage of adults who engaged in leisure time physical activity, by level of activity and education. (*Source:* Data from *Health Behaviors of Adults: United States, 2005–2007*. National Center for Health Statistics. Vital and Health Stat Series No. 10 (245). 2010.)

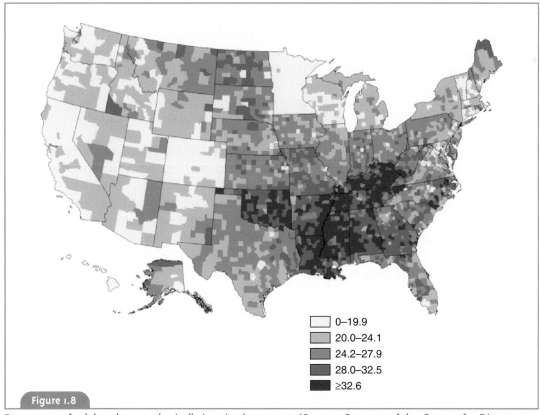

Percentage of adults who are physically inactive by county. (*Source:* Courtesy of the Centers for Disease Control and Prevention.)

health status among Americans. The document will help everyone to understand more easily the importance of health promotion and disease prevention and to encourage wide participation in improving health in the next decade.

The overarching goals of *Healthy People 2020* are to:

- Attain high-quality, longer lives free of preventable disease, disability, injury, and premature death;
- Achieve health equity, eliminate disparities, and improve the health of all groups;
- Create social and physical environments that promote good health for all; and
- Promote quality of life, healthy development, and healthy behaviors across all life stages.

One of the 12 topics in *Healthy People 2020* is Healthy Behaviors. Its objectives are:

- Increase the proportion of adults who meet current federal guidelines for aerobic physical activity and for muscle-strengthening activity.
- Reduce the proportion of children and adolescents who are considered obese.
- Reduce consumption of calories from solid fats and added sugars in the population aged 2 years and older.

Physical Activity and Exercise

More than 80% of adults do not meet the guidelines for both aerobic and muscle-strengthening activities found in *Healthy People 2020*. The Physical Activity objectives for *Healthy People 2020* reflect the strong state of the science supporting the health benefits of regular physical activity in moderate and vigorous physical activities and muscle-strengthening activities.

Nutrition and Weight Status

The Nutrition and Weight Status objectives for *Healthy People 2020* reflect strong science supporting the health benefits of eating a healthful diet and maintaining a healthy body weight. The objectives also emphasize that efforts to change diet and weight should address individual behaviors.

Dietary Guidelines for Americans

By law, *Dietary Guidelines for Americans* is reviewed, updated if necessary, and published every 5 years. The U.S. Department of Agriculture and the U.S. Department of Health and Human Services jointly create each edition.

Dietary Guidelines for Americans, 2010 was released at a time of rising concern about the health of the American population. Poor diet and physical inactivity are the most important factors contributing to an epidemic of overweight and obesity affecting men, women, and children. Even in the absence of overweight, poor diet and physical inactivity are associated with major causes of morbidity and mortality in the United States.

The intent of the *Dietary Guidelines* is to summarize and synthesize knowledge about individual nutrients and food components into an interrelated set of recommendations for healthy eating that can be adopted by the public. The guidelines encompass two over-arching concepts:

- Maintain calorie balance over time to achieve and sustain a healthy weight.
- Focus on consuming nutrient-dense foods and beverages.

Physical Activity Guidelines for Americans

Being physically active is one of the most important steps that Americans of all ages can take to improve their health. The 2008 *Physical Activity Guidelines for Americans* provides science-based guidance to help Americans improve their health through appropriate physical activity.

The DHHS issues the *Physical Activity Guidelines*. The content complements the *Dietary Guidelines for Americans*. Together, the two documents provide guidance on the importance of being physically active and eating a healthy diet to promote good health and reduce the risk of chronic diseases.

American College of Sports Medicine

The American College of Sports Medicine (ACSM) is the largest, most respected sports medicine and exercise science organization in the world. It is a nongovernmental organization that looks for and finds better methods to allow individuals to live longer and more productive lives. It develops guidelines on quantity and quality of exercise for adults.

Reflect >>>> Reinforce >>>> Reinvigorate

Knowledge Check

Answers in Appendix D

1. Life expectancy in the United States in 2009 has reached:
   A. 80 years
   B. 75.5 years
   C. 78.2 years
   D. 82.1 years

2. Your biological age refers to:
   A. Your actual age in years from your birth date
   B. Your life span in years
   C. The average age you are expected to live
   D. An estimate of your well-being compared to others of your age

3. What most accurately predicts a women's genetic effect on age?
   A. Age at menarche
   B. Age at menopause
   C. Age of your mother at death
   D. Weight at birth

4. Bill has started paying attention to his own biomarkers indicating his biological age. Which of the following is not a biomarker of Bill's biological age?
   A. Skin elasticity
   B. Blood pressure
   C. Bone mineral density
   D. Fitness tests

5. Sarah's father died suddenly at the age of 70. He was a smoker, was overweight, and watched a lot of television. What were the most likely causes of Sarah's father's death?
   A. Toxic agents, alcohol consumption
   B. Tobacco use, physical inactivity/poor diet
   C. Tobacco use, motor vehicle crash
   D. Inactivity/poor diet, firearms

6. Because of her current lifestyle, Janice does not believe she will live to be 100 years old. What factors in her lifestyle may affect her life span?
   A. Physical inactivity
   B. Poor diet
   C. Smoking
   D. All of the above

7. Mike lives in the state of Mississippi. According the the CDC, this region has the highest percentage of adults who are:
   A. More than 80 years old
   B. Under 20 years of age
   C. Physically inactive
   D. Chronically fatigued

8. "The ability to carry out daily tasks with vigor and alertness, without undue fatigue, and with ample energy to enjoy leisure-time pursuits and respond to emergencies..." is the definition of what term?
   A. Wellness
   B. Health
   C. Physical well-being
   D. Fitness

Modern Modifications

The chapters in this text illustrate a wide variety of the important aspects of a healthy lifestyle. In each chapter there will be a section in which you will be given a chance to:

Take a moment to look at your lifestyle in the terms of the topic discussed. What would you like to change in that area of your life?

Go through and pick one of the suggestions provided. These suggestions are meant to be easily absorbed into your daily routine and offer immediate opportunities for change.

Congratulate yourself. You are one step closer to a happier healthier lifestyle. Even small changes can make a big difference!

Critical Thinking

1. Does your current lifestyle meet the definitions of fitness and wellness? Do you consider yourself physically active? Why?
2. What are some behaviors you can change that will provide you with a longer, healthier life?

Going Above and Beyond

Centers for Disease Control and Prevention: Leading causes of death. Centers for Disease Control and Prevention.
http://www.cdc.gov/injury/wisqars/pdf/Death_by_Age_2007-a.pdf OR
http://www.cdc.gov/injury/wisqars/LeadingCauses.html
National Center for Health Statistics
http://www.cdc.gov/nchs/data/series/sr_10/sr10_245.pdf
Healthy People 2020.
http://www.healthypeople.gov/2020/default.aspx
Dietary Guidelines for Americans.
http://www.cnpp.usda.gov/dietaryguidelines.htm
Physical Activity Guidelines.
http://www.cdc.gov/physicalactivity/everyone/guidelines/index.html
Life Expectancy Calculator.
http://www.livingto100.com
Real Age Test.
www.realage.com

References and Suggested Readings

Mokdad A., Marks J., Stroup D., and Gerberding J. Actual causes of death in the United States, 2000. *Journal of the American Medical Association* 2004; 291:1238–1245.

Myers J., Prakash M., Froelicher V., Do D., Partington S., and Atwood J. E. Exercise capacity and mortality among men referred for exercise testing. *New England Journal of Medicine* 2002; 346:793–801.

U.S. Department of Health and Human Services (DHHS). *Healthy People 2010: Understanding and Improving Health.* Washington, DC: DHHS, 2000.

U.S. DHHS, Centers for Disease Control and Prevention (CDC). *Physical Activity and Health: A Report of the Surgeon General.* Atlanta, GA: DHHS, 2010.

Olshansky S. J., et al. A potential decline in life expectancy in the United States in the 21st century. *New England Journal of Medicine* 2005; 352:1138–1145.

Objectives

After reading this chapter, you should be able to:

- Describe the relationship between physical activity and health.
- Identify health-related concerns of inactivity.

Table 2.1	The Health Benefits of Physical Activity—Major Research Findings

- Regular physical activity reduces the risk of many adverse health outcomes.
- Some physical activity is better than none.
- For most health outcomes, additional benefits occur as the amount of physical activity increases through higher intensity, greater frequency, and/or longer duration.
- Most health benefits occur with at least 150 minutes a week of moderate-intensity physical activity, such as brisk walking. Additional benefits occur with more physical activity.
- Both aerobic (endurance) and muscle-strengthening (resistance) physical activity are beneficial.
- Health benefits occur for children and adolescents, young and middle-aged adults, older adults, and those in every studied racial and ethnic group.
- The health benefits of physical activity occur for people with disabilities.
- The benefits of physical activity far outweigh the possibility of adverse outcomes.

Source: Data from Warburton D., Nicol C.W., Bredin S., Health benefits of physical activity: the evidence. *Canadian Medical Association Journal* 2006; 174(6):801–809.

All people should be regularly physically active to improve overall health and fitness and to prevent many adverse health outcomes. Generally healthy people, people at risk of developing chronic diseases, and people with current chronic conditions or disabilities can all benefit from regular physical activity. This chapter gives an overview of research findings on physical activity and health. **Table 2.1** provides a summary of these benefits.

Physical activity affects many health conditions; the specific amounts and types of activity that benefit each condition vary. One consistent finding from research studies is that once the health benefits from physical activity begin to accrue, additional amounts of activity provide additional benefits.

Although some health benefits seem to begin with as little as 60 minutes (1 hour) a week, research shows that 150 minutes (2 hours and 30 minutes) a week of moderate-intensity aerobic activity, such as brisk walking, consistently reduces the risk of many chronic diseases and other adverse health outcomes.

Medical News You Can Use

Little Exercise Beats None

Even a little physical activity performed on a regular basis may reduce the risk of heart disease. The more exercise people do, the more benefit in reducing risk. Key findings of the study by Harvard School of Public Health researchers found:

- As little as 2.5 hours of moderate-intensity physical activity per week (150 minutes) can lower a person's overall risk of heart disease by 14%.

- The risk of developing coronary heart disease gets progressively lower the more physical activity a person does. While 150 minutes is beneficial, 300 minutes weekly will achieve even better results.

This study corroborates federal guidelines—even a little bit of exercise is good, but more is better. Researchers noticed a significant gender difference that showed that exercise had a greater effect in reducing heart disease risk in women than in men.

Source: Data from Sattelmair J., et al. Dose response between physical activity and risk of coronary heart disease: a meta-analysis. *Circulation* 2011; 124(7):789–795.

Examining the Relationship Between Physical Activity and Health

In many studies covering a range of issues, researchers have focused on exercise as well as on the more broadly defined concept of physical activity. Exercise is a form of physical activity that is planned, structured, repetitive, and performed with the goal of improving health or fitness. So, although all exercise is physical activity, not all physical activity is exercise.

Studies have examined the role of physical activity in many groups—men and women, children, teens, adults, older adults, people with disabilities, and women during pregnancy and the postpartum period. These studies have focused on the role that physical activity plays in many health outcomes, including:

- premature (early) death;
- diseases such as coronary heart disease, stroke, some cancers, type 2 diabetes, osteoporosis, and depression;
- risk factors for disease, such as high blood pressure and high blood cholesterol;
- physical fitness, such as aerobic capacity, and muscle strength and endurance;
- functional capacity (the ability to engage in activities needed for daily living);
- mental health, such as depression and cognitive function; and
- injuries or sudden heart attacks.

These studies have also prompted questions regarding what type and how much physical activity is needed for various health benefits. To answer this question, investigators have studied three main kinds of physical activity: aerobic, muscle strengthening, and bone strengthening, addressed in later chapters.

The Health Benefits of Physical Activity

Studies clearly demonstrate that participating in regular physical activity provides many health benefits. These benefits are summarized in (Table 2.2). Many conditions affected by physical activity occur with increasing age, such as heart disease and cancer. Reducing risk of these conditions may require years of participation in regular physical activity. However, other benefits, such as increased **cardiorespiratory fitness**, increased muscular strength, and decreased depressive symptoms and blood pressure, require only a few weeks or months of participation in physical activity.

The health benefits of physical activity are seen in children and adolescents, young and middle-aged adults, older adults, women and men, people of different races and ethnicities, and people with disabilities and chronic conditions. The health benefits of physical activity are generally independent of body weight. Adults of all sizes and shapes gain health and fitness benefits by being habitually physically active. The benefits of physical activity also outweigh the risk of injury and sudden heart attacks, two concerns that prevent many people from becoming physically active.

The following sections provide more detail on what is known from research studies about the specific health benefits of physical activity and how much physical activity is needed to get the health benefits.

Table 2.2	Health Benefits Associated with Regular Physical Activity

Children and Adolescents

Strong evidence
- Improved cardiorespiratory and muscular fitness
- Improved bone health
- Improved cardiovascular and metabolic health biomarkers
- Favorable body composition

Moderate evidence
- Reduced symptoms of depression

Adults and Older Adults

Strong evidence
- Lower risk of early death
- Lower risk of coronary heart disease
- Lower risk of stroke
- Lower risk of high blood pressure
- Lower risk of adverse blood lipid profile
- Lower risk of type 2 diabetes
- Lower risk of metabolic syndrome
- Lower risk of colon cancer
- Lower risk of breast cancer
- Prevention of weight gain
- Weight loss, particularly when combined with reduced calorie intake
- Improved cardiorespiratory and muscular fitness
- Prevention of falls
- Reduced depression
- Better cognitive function (for older adults)

Moderate to strong evidence
- Better functional health (for older adults)
- Reduced abdominal obesity

Moderate evidence
- Lower risk of hip fracture
- Lower risk of lung cancer
- Lower risk of endometrial cancer
- Weight maintenance after weight loss
- Increased bone density
- Improved sleep quality

Source: Data from the *2008 Physical Activity Guidelines for Americans.* Courtesy of the U.S. Department of Health and Human Services.

Reduced Risk of Premature Death

Strong scientific evidence shows that physical activity reduces the risk of premature death (dying earlier than the average age-at-death for a specific population group) from the leading causes of death, such as heart disease and some cancers, as well as from other causes of death. This effect is remarkable in two ways:

- First, only a few lifestyle choices have as large an effect on mortality as physical activity. It has been estimated that people who are physically active for approximately 7 hours a week have a 40% lower risk of dying early than those who are active for less than 30 minutes a week.

2

Medical News You Can Use

Can Exercise Make Us Smarter?

There are many published physical benefits of regular exercise. But what effects does exercise have on our cognitive function? Mental performance such as reaction time, perception and interpretation of visual images, and executive control processes has shown measureable improvements with moderately intense aerobic exercise. The most positive influences have been seen in executive control processes such as:

- planning;
- scheduling;
- coordination of people, places, events, etc.;
- working memory; and
- inhibition.

These positive effects of exercising are related to increase in blood flow to the brain and stimulation of nerve cells. Moderate exercise gives you a double benefit for your time spent. Not only will your fitness be improved, but your ability to concentrate and perform mental tasks will improve as well.

Source: Data from Focus On Fitness - Can exercise make us smarter?, Issue No. 3, Harvard Health Publications, Harvard Medical School, 2011.

■ Second, it is not necessary to do high amounts of physical activity or vigorous-intensity activity to reduce the risk of premature death. Studies show substantially lower risk when people do 150 minutes of at least moderate-intensity aerobic physical activity a week.

Research clearly demonstrates the importance of avoiding inactivity. Even low amounts of physical activity reduce the risk of dying prematurely. The most dramatic difference in risk is seen between those who are inactive (30 minutes a week) and those with low levels of activity (90 minutes, or 1 hour and 30 minutes, a week). The relative risk of dying prematurely continues to be lower with higher levels of reported moderate- or vigorous-intensity, leisure-time physical activity.

All adults can gain this health benefit of physical activity. Age, race, and ethnicity do not matter. Men and women younger than 65 years as well as older adults have lower

Medical News You Can Use

Exercise Fights Middle-Age Spread

A 20-year study of more than 3,500 men and women found that high activity levels led to less excess weight (5.7 fewer pounds gained each year in men and 13.4 fewer pounds gained each year in women) when compared to adults with low activity levels. The key is to start an exercise program before middle age. Sticking with the national guidelines of 30 minutes of moderate exercise each day had a significant effect over the two decades of the study.

Source: Data from Hankinson A.L., et al., Maintaining a high physical activity level over 20 years and weight gain. *Journal of the American Medical Association* 2010; 304(23):2603–2610.

---

rates of early death when they are physically active than when they are inactive. Physically active people of all body weights (normal weight, overweight, obese) also have lower rates of early death than do inactive people.

Cardiorespiratory Health

The benefits of physical activity on cardiorespiratory health are some of the most extensively documented of all the health benefits. Cardiorespiratory health involves the health of the heart, lungs, and blood vessels.

Heart diseases and stroke are two of the leading causes of death in the United States. Risk factors that increase the likelihood of cardiovascular diseases include smoking, high blood pressure (called hypertension), type 2 diabetes, and high levels of certain blood lipids (such as low-density lipoprotein, or LDL, cholesterol). Low cardiorespiratory fitness is also a risk factor for heart disease.

People who do moderate- or vigorous-intensity aerobic physical activity have a significantly lower risk of cardiovascular disease than do inactive people. Regularly active adults have lower rates of heart disease and stroke, lower blood pressure, better blood lipid profiles, and better fitness. Significant reductions in risk of cardiovascular disease are observed at activity levels equivalent to 150 minutes a week of moderate-intensity physical activity. Even greater benefits are seen with 200 minutes (3 hours and 20 minutes) a week. The evidence is strong that greater amounts of physical activity result in even further reductions in the risk of cardiovascular disease.

Everyone can gain the cardiovascular health benefits of physical activity. The amount of physical activity that provides favorable cardiorespiratory health and fitness outcomes is similar for adults of various ages, including older people, as well as for adults of various races and ethnicities. Aerobic exercise also improves cardiorespiratory fitness in individuals with some disabilities, including people who have lost the use of one or both legs and those with multiple sclerosis, stroke, spinal cord injury, and cognitive disabilities.

Moderate-intensity physical activity is safe for generally healthy women during pregnancy. It increases cardiorespiratory fitness without increasing the risk of early pregnancy loss, preterm delivery, or low birth weight. Physical activity during the postpartum period also improves cardiorespiratory fitness.

Metabolic Health

Regular physical activity strongly reduces the risk of developing type 2 diabetes as well as the metabolic syndrome. The metabolic syndrome is a condition in which people have some combination of high blood pressure, a large waistline (abdominal obesity), an adverse blood lipid profile (low levels of high-density lipoprotein [HDL] cholesterol, raised triglycerides), and impaired glucose tolerance.

People who regularly engage in at least moderate-intensity aerobic activity have a significantly lower risk of developing type 2 diabetes than do inactive people. Although some experts debate the usefulness of defining the metabolic syndrome, good evidence exists that physical activity reduces the risk of having this condition, as defined in various ways. Lower rates of these conditions are seen with 120 to 150 minutes (2 hours to 2 hours and 30 minutes) a week of at least moderate-intensity aerobic activity. As with cardiovascular health, additional levels of physical activity lower the risk even further. In addition, physical activity helps control blood glucose levels in persons who already have type 2 diabetes.

Medical News You Can Use

Exercise May Block Colds

It appears that being fit by exercising at least 5 days a week is associated with a reduction in upper respiratory tract infections. Those who exercised regularly had 43% fewer days with an upper respiratory tract infection compared to those who exercised no more than 1 day a week. Recirculation of immunoglobulins and neutrophils and natural killer cells is increased with each aerobic exercise session. Additionally, stress hormones that may suppress immunity are not elevated during moderate exercise. In addition to the reduced number of days with an upper respiratory tract infection, the severity of such infections was reduced as well.

Source: Data from Nieman D., Upper respiratory tract infection is reduced in physically fit and active adults. *British Journal of Sports Medicine* 2011; 45(12):987–992.

Physical activity also improves metabolic health in youth. Studies find this effect when young people participate in at least 3 days of vigorous aerobic activity a week. More physical activity is associated with improved metabolic health, but research has yet to determine the exact amount of improvement.

Weight and Energy Balance

Overweight and obesity occur when fewer calories are expended, including calories burned through physical activity, than are taken in through food and beverages. Physical activity and caloric intake both must be considered when trying to control body weight. Because of this role in energy balance, physical activity is a critical factor in determining whether a person can maintain a healthy body weight, lose excess body weight, or maintain successful weight loss. People vary a great deal in how much physical activity they need to achieve and maintain a healthy weight. Some need more physical activity than others to maintain a healthy body weight, to lose weight, or to keep weight off once it has been lost.

Strong scientific evidence shows that physical activity helps people maintain a stable weight over time. However, the optimal amount of physical activity needed to maintain weight is unclear. People vary greatly in how much physical activity results in weight stability. Many people need more than the equivalent of 150 minutes of moderate-intensity activity a week to maintain their weight.

Medical News You Can Use

Walking the Dog Benefits You, Too

Walking helps control blood pressure and red blood cell distribution width, according to the Society for Vascular Surgery. A U.S. National Institutes of Health-funded study of 2000 adults found that those who regularly walked their dogs were more physically active and less likely to be obese than those who did not walk their dogs. Dogs can offer still other health benefits. For example, studies have found that petting a dog reduces people's blood pressure and heart rate. About 77.5 million dogs live in 39% of U.S. households, according to the Humane Society of the United States.

Source: Data from Society for Vascular Surgery, News Release, June 6, 2011.

Reproduced from *2008 Physical Activity Guidelines for Americans.* Courtesy of the U.S. Department of Health and Human Services, and the Centers for Disease Control and Prevention.

Over short periods of time, such as a year, research shows that it is possible to achieve weight stability by doing the equivalent of 150 to 300 minutes (5 hours) a week of moderate-intensity walking at about a 4-mile-an-hour pace. Muscle-strengthening activities may help promote weight maintenance, although not to the same degree as aerobic activity.

People who want to lose a substantial (more than 5% of body weight) amount of weight and people who are trying to keep a significant amount of weight off once it has been lost need a high amount of physical activity, unless they also reduce their caloric intake. Many people need to do more than 300 minutes of moderate-intensity activity a week to meet weight–control goals.

Regular physical activity also helps control the percentage of body fat in children and adolescents. Exercise training studies with overweight and obese youth have shown that they can reduce their body fat by participating in physical activity that is at least of moderate intensity for 3 to 5 days a week, at 30 to 60 minutes each time.

Musculoskeletal Health

Bones, muscles, and joints support the body and help it move. Healthy bones, joints, and muscles are critical to the ability to do daily activities without physical limitations.

Preserving bone, joint, and muscle health is essential with increasing age. Studies show that the frequent decline in bone density that happens during aging can be slowed with regular physical activity. These effects are seen in people who participate in aerobic, muscle-strengthening, and bone-strengthening physical activity programs of moderate or vigorous intensity. The range of total physical activity for these benefits varies widely. Important changes seem to begin at 90 minutes a week and continue up to 300 minutes a week.

Hip fracture is a serious health condition that can have life-changing negative effects for many older people. Physically active people, especially women, have a lower risk of hip fracture than do inactive people. Research studies on physical activity to prevent hip fracture show that participating in 120 to 300 minutes a week of physical activity that is of at least moderate intensity is associated with a reduced risk. It is unclear, however, whether activity also lowers risk of fractures of the spine or other important areas of the skeleton.

Building strong, healthy bones is also important for children and adolescents. Along with having a healthy diet that includes adequate calcium and vitamin D, physical activity is critical for bone development in children and adolescents. Bone-strengthening physical activity done 3 or more days a week increases bone-mineral content and bone density in youth.

Regular physical activity also helps people with arthritis or other rheumatic conditions affecting the joints. Participation in 130 to 150 minutes (2 hours and 10 minutes to 2 hours and 30 minutes) a week of moderate-intensity, low-impact physical activity improves pain management, function, and quality of life. Researchers do not yet know whether participation in physical activity, particularly at low to moderate intensity, reduces the risk of osteoarthritis. Very high levels of physical activity, however, may have extra risks. People who participate in very high levels of physical activity, such as elite or professional athletes, have a higher risk of hip and knee osteoarthritis, mostly due to the risk of injury involved in competing in some sports.

Progressive muscle-strengthening activities increase or preserve muscle mass, strength, and power. Higher amounts (through greater frequency or higher weights) improve muscle function to a greater degree. Improvements occur in younger and older adults. Resistance exercises also improve muscular strength in persons with such conditions as stroke, multiple sclerosis, cerebral palsy, spinal cord injury, and cognitive disability. Though it does not increase muscle mass in the same way that muscle-strengthening activities do, aerobic activity may also help slow the loss of muscle with aging.

Functional Ability and Fall Prevention

Functional ability is the capacity of a person to perform tasks or behaviors that enable him or her to carry out everyday activities, such as climbing stairs or walking on a sidewalk. Functional ability is key to a person's ability to fulfill basic life roles, such as personal care, grocery shopping, or playing with the grandchildren. Loss of functional ability is referred to as functional limitation.

Middle-aged and older adults who are physically active have lower risk of functional limitations than do inactive adults. It appears that greater physical activity levels can further reduce risk of functional limitations.

Older adults who already have functional limitations also benefit from regular physical activity. Typically, studies of physical activity in adults with functional limitations tested a combination of aerobic and muscle strengthening activities, making it difficult to assess the relative importance of each type of activity. However, both types of activity appear to provide benefit.

In older adults at risk of falls, strong evidence shows that regular physical activity is safe and reduces this risk. Reduction in falls is seen among participants in programs that include balance and moderate-intensity muscle-strengthening activities for 90 minutes a week plus moderate-intensity walking for about an hour a week. It is not known whether different combinations of type, amount, or frequency of activity can reduce falls to a greater degree. Tai chi exercises also may help prevent falls.

Lower Cancer Risk

Physically active people have a significantly lower risk of colon cancer than do inactive people, and physically active women have a significantly lower risk of breast cancer. Research shows that a range of moderate-intensity physical activity—between 210 and 420 minutes a week (3 hours and 30 minutes to 7 hours)—is needed to significantly reduce the risk of colon and breast cancer; currently, 150 minutes a week does not provide a major benefit. It also appears that greater amounts of physical activity lower risks of these cancers even further, although exactly how much lower is not clear.

Although not definitive, some research suggests that the risk of endometrial cancer in women and lung cancers in men and women also may be lower among those who are regularly active compared to those who are inactive.

Finally, cancer survivors have a better quality of life and improved physical fitness if they are physically active, compared to survivors who are inactive.

Medical News You Can Use

More Exercise Means Better Heart Health

People who exercise for the recommended 150 minutes of moderately intense physical activity weekly had a 14% reduction in the risk of coronary heart disease compared with individuals who reported no physical activity; benefits were even greater for those who exercise at least 300 minutes per week.

Source: Data from Sattelmair J., et al. Dose response between physical activity and risk of coronary heart disease: a meta-analysis. *Circulation* 2011; 124(7):789–795.

Mental Health

Physically active adults have lower risk of depression and cognitive decline (declines with aging in thinking, learning, and judgment skills). Physical activity also may improve the quality of sleep. Whether physical activity reduces distress or anxiety is currently unclear.

Mental health benefits have been found in people who do aerobic or a combination of aerobic and muscle-strengthening activities 3 to 5 days a week for 30 to 60 minutes at a time. Some research has shown that even lower levels of physical activity also may provide some benefits.

Regular physical activity appears to reduce symptoms of anxiety and depression for children and adolescents. Whether physical activity improves self-esteem is not clear.

Lower Risk of Adverse Events

Some people hesitate to become active or to increase their level of physical activity because they fear getting injured or having a heart attack. Studies of generally healthy people clearly show that moderate-intensity physical activity, such as brisk walking, has a low risk of such adverse events.

The risk of musculoskeletal injury increases with the total amount of physical activity. For example, a person who regularly runs 40 miles a week has a higher risk of injury than a person who runs 10 miles each week. However, people who are physically active may have fewer injuries from other causes, such as motor vehicle collisions or work-related injuries. Depending on the type and amount of activity that physically active people do, their overall injury rate may be lower than the overall injury rate for inactive people.

Participation in contact or collision sports, such as soccer or football, has a higher risk of injury than participation in noncontact physical activity, such as swimming or walking. However, when performing the same activity, people who are less fit are more likely to be injured than people who are more fit.

Cardiac events, such as a heart attack or sudden death during physical activity, are rare. However, the risk of such cardiac events does increase when a person suddenly becomes much more active than usual. The greatest risk occurs when an adult who is usually inactive engages in vigorous-intensity activity (such as shoveling snow). People who are regularly physically active have the lowest risk of cardiac events both while being active and overall.

The bottom line is that the health benefits of physical activity far outweigh the risks of adverse events for almost everyone.

Reflect >>>> Reinforce >>>> Reinvigorate

Knowledge Check

Answers in Appendix D

1. Gary is interested in beginning a physical activity program. He has 30 minutes each afternoon to dedicate to physical activity. He is not sure 30 minutes each day is enough. How many minutes each week should he dedicate to physical activity?

   A. 30
   B. 90
   C. 150
   D. 240

2. Gary's doctor is concerned about Gary's high blood pressure and high blood cholesterol. In terms of disease, these measures are considered:

   A. Diseases
   B. Cognitive functions
   C. Safety factors
   D. Risk factors

3. There are several types of physical activity Gary could include in his routine. However, which of the following have been the most studied of the physical activities?

   A. Anaerobic, mental health, bone strengthening
   B. Aerobic, muscle-strengthening, bone strengthening
   C. Physical fitness, brisk walking, running
   D. Static, low intensity, high intensity

4. Jakob has not been physically active for years. What are the two main concerns that prevent individuals like Jakob from beginning physical activity?

   A. Fear of exertion, 'couch potato' lifestyle
   B. Age, gender
   C. Time to exercise, premature death
   D. Risk of injury, sudden heart attacks

5. Jesse has been engaged in regular physical activity for one year. His goal is to lose 20 pounds. After one year, he is still struggling to reach his goal. What else should Jesse consider when trying to control his body weight?

   A. Caloric intake
   B. Body dimension
   C. Age
   D. Increase time of exercise

6. Physical activity has many health benefits for older adults. One of the benefits is a lower risk of which type of fracture?

   A. Skull
   B. Hip
   C. Tibia/fibula
   D. Rib

---

7. Research shows that physically active adults have lower risk of wich mental disorder?
   A. Distress
   B. Anxiety
   C. Bipolar disorders
   D. Depression
8. According to research, reduction in cancer risks is not associated with regular physical activity.
   A. True
   B. False

Modern Modifications

Only a few lifestyle choices have as large an impact on your health as physical activity. People who are physically active for about 7 hours a week have a 40 percent lower risk of dying early than those who are active for less than 30 minutes a week.

You don't have to do high amounts of activity or vigorous-intensity activity to reduce your risk of premature death. You can put yourself at lower risk of dying early by doing at least 150 minutes a week of moderate-intensity aerobic activity.

Critical Thinking

1. What health benefits of physical exercise are most important to you? How can you prioritize you lifestyle to focus on those health benefits and physical activity?
2. What information about health benefits could you provide to a friend who is considering beginning a regular physical activity routine?

Going Above and Beyond

Physical Activity Guidelines for Americans
http://www.cdc.gov/physicalactivity/everyone/guidelines/index.html
CDC Physical Activity Information
http://www.cdc.gov/nccdphp/dnpa/physical/index.htm
Health A to Z
http://www.healthatoz.com

CHAPTER 3

Changing to a Healthy Lifestyle

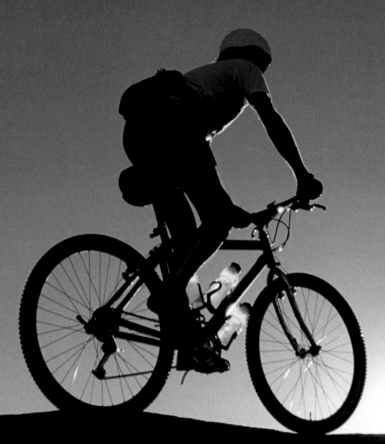

Objectives

After reading this chapter, you should be able to:

- Describe the benefits of changing to a healthier lifestyle.
- Describe the Stages of Change model used in changing to a healthy lifestyle.
- Design a personal contract for changing a health-related behavior.

Prochaska and colleagues developed the Transtheoretical Model of Change, better known as the Stages of Change model, which can help us to change a problem behavior (Prochaska, Norcross, and DiClemente, 1994). This model says that people move through a series of stages of change (some call it a readiness to change). Its authors describe behavior change as a process, not an event. Change does not happen overnight—it could take weeks, months, or even years.

In adopting healthy behaviors (e.g., regular physical activity) or eliminating unhealthy ones (e.g., eating saturated fat), people progress through five stages related to their readiness for change. At each stage, different intervention strategies help them progress to the next stage. The five distinct stages are:

1. Precontemplation
2. Contemplation
3. Preparation
4. Action
5. Maintenance

Progression through the stages of change is cyclical rather than linear. Rarely does a person successfully go through the stages sequentially without encountering setbacks. Most people will recycle through the stages several times before being successful (Prochaska, Norcross, and DiClemente, 1994). **Figure 3.1** represents the stages of change in a graphical cyclic manner.

After identifying the stage of change you are in using **Figure 3.2** and **Lab 3-1**, the next step is to determine the appropriate processes of change to be used for the particular stage. These processes have also been referred to as techniques or strategies.

Figure 3.1

Stages of change. (*Source:* Courtesy of the Centers for Disease Control and Prevention.)

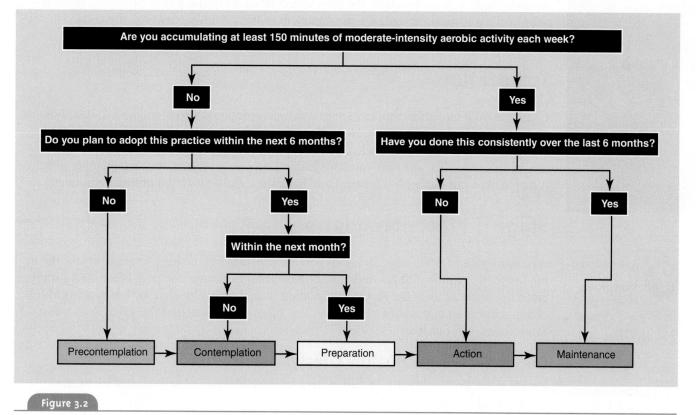

Figure 3.2

Assessing your stage or readiness to change.

3

Medical News You Can Use

Sitting a Risk Factor for Death

People who spent at least 6 hours of their daily leisure time sitting died sooner than people who sat less than 3 hours, according to a 14-year study. Those who sit a lot and exercise little are at even greater risk of death. Researchers found that sitting for that length of time by itself was detrimental to health. Sitting increased the risk of cancer death, but the main death risk linked to sitting was heart disease. Sedentary individuals should be encouraged to stand up and walk around. Reaching optimal levels of physical exercise should also be encouraged.

Source: Data from Patel A.V. et al., Leisure time spent sitting in relation to total mortality in a prospective cohort of U.S. Adults. *American Journal of Epidemiology* 2010; 172(4):419–429.

Refer to **Table 3.1** for the major processes of change. These are activities and experiences that individuals engage in when they attempt to change a behavior. **Figure 3.3** matches the processes of changes and the stages of change.

The key to successful change is to determine what stage you are in, and then to decide what processes (strategies) to use. There is no set time frame for each stage; you may spend more time in one stage than another. Change is a process that is unique to the individual and situation.

In addition to the stages and processes, the Stages of Change model features several other unique insights.

Weighing Pros and Cons

At each stage, a person weighs the pros and cons of adopting a new behavior. To help people move toward change, it is necessary to make the pros outweigh the cons. This is especially true in the precontemplation and contemplation stages.

Temptation

Change is difficult and a combination of cravings, emotional stress, and social situations can lead a person back to old habits. Not only is this possible, but it should also be expected. Should you slip or have a setback, do not think of this as a failure, but learn from it. What caused this setback? Now that you have learned this, avoid it next time! Remember: Change is a cycle that can move both forward and backward. Either way, the process continues!

Stage 1: Precontemplation

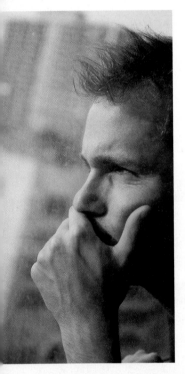

Precontemplation is the stage in which you are considering making a change in your life in the foreseeable future. Others in this stage have tried to change the past, failed, and simply given up. Many of us know that it is important to make healthy choices, but in a world full of temptations and unhealthy alternatives it is often difficult to find the strength to make those changes in our lives.

Difficulty Living a Healthy Lifestyle

People often find it difficult to adhere to a healthy lifestyle of self-control because of:

- Firmly established habits
- Immediate gratification—people often want instant results or pleasure

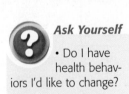

Ask Yourself

- Do I have health behaviors I'd like to change?

- Do I participate in activities that do not promote health?

- Do I practice behaviors passed down through my family?

Table 3.1 — Processes That Promote Change

Processes of Change	Stages of Change	Examples of Techniques
Consciousness-raising: increased awareness	Precontemplation Contemplation	Read news stories or a book; watch a TV program; talk with a friend or doctor
Social liberation: societal support for the healthy behavior change	Precontemplation Contemplation Preparation Action	Availability of a health club; restaurants offering low-fat/low-carb foods
Helping relationships: support system of family, friends, and co-workers	All five stages	Discuss your plans with others; join with another who is working on the behavior
Emotional arousal: emotional experience related to the unhealthy behavior	Contemplation Preparation	Personal testimony of someone who has solved a similar behavioral problem; seeing someone suffering the harmful consequences of his or her unhealthy behavior
Self-reevaluation: understanding that your behavior is how you are known	Contemplation Preparation	See yourself as fit
Commitment: making a firm commitment to change and believing that it can be done	Preparation Action Maintenance	Make a New Year's resolution; tell others about your intentions
Reward: increasing the rewards for positive behavioral change and decreasing the rewards for unhealthy behavior	Action Maintenance	Reward the behavior change (e.g., buying new clothes, movie ticket)
Countering: substituting healthy behavior for an unhealthy behavior	Action Maintenance	Take a walk instead of watching TV
Environmental control: avoiding triggers or using cues	Action Maintenance	Avoid dessert parties; leave encouraging messages on a calendar or stuck to the mirror or refrigerator

Source: Adapted from Prochaska J.O., Redding C.A., and Evers K., The Transtheoretical Model and Stages of Change, in *Health Behavior and Health Education: Theory, Research, and Practice*, Glanz K., Lewis F.M., and Rimer B.K. (eds.), San Francisco: Jossey-Bass, 1996.

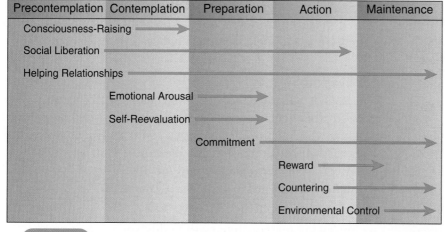

Figure 3.3

Select appropriate processes to promote change. (*Source:* Adapted from Prochaska J.O., et al., *Changing for Good*, First edition. Quill, 2002.)

- Delayed negative health consequences of an unhealthy lifestyle—it may take years or even decades before the effects are seen
- Invincibility—"it won't happen to me" belief in which it is assumed that poor health happens to others but not me; prefer dealing with life by taking risks or playing the odds that they will not contract a disease or get injured
- Too much scientific information, which sometimes overwhelms or confuses
- Fear of failure—often based on past failed attempts
- Feeling a loss of control over one's life
- Too many choices from which to pick for type of exercise, food, and weight control

Stage 2: Contemplation

The contemplation stage occurs when you are aware that a problem exists and are seriously thinking about overcoming it, but have not yet made a commitment to take action. This is a time of reflection. Finding the reasons to change, the motivation to reach a goal, and the strength to make a plan work requires a lot of soul-searching. This stage can take a good amount of time and should not be rushed. As important as it is to make a healthy change in your life, take the time to find what truly motivates you and your behavior. This stage is the key to a successful course of action.

What Helps Change a Lifestyle?

Factors that influence an individual to change may include:

- Increasing knowledge—this can influence one's behavior, but often may not be enough to influence people to change. The maxim "Why do we do what we do, when we know what we know?" illustrates that knowledge often is insufficient to affect behavior.
- Motivation, having a reason—a person may want to change to avoid sickness, to look and feel better, to live longer, or because of pressure from a spouse, child, or friend.
- Readiness—motivation is required, but may involve physical capabilities as well. Another maxim—"You can lead a horse to water, but you can't make it drink"—may reflect a lack of motivation or perhaps the physical inability to act for a variety reasons.
- Landmark events—resolutions to change often occur at the start of a new year, during a personal health crisis, on a birthday, upon the birth of a child, or the death of someone close to you.
- Self-management techniques—the ability to employ them helps individuals to make lifestyle changes.

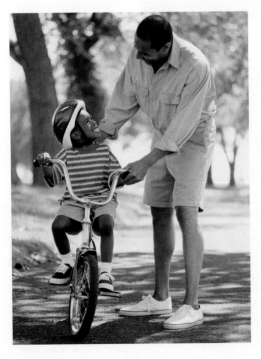

Motivation

Motivation is what drives us to make changes. No matter how big or how small the change may be, we must be inspired to make choices. Finding what inspires or motivates you is an essential step in making a successful adjustment in your lifestyle.

Motivations for change could include:

- Improving self-image and/or self-esteem
- Being a role model for someone else
- Improving relationships with family and peers
- Reducing stress
- Reducing risk of disease

Locus of Control

Life involves many struggles for control. Sometimes external factors can control aspects of your life for a moment. At other times the power is in your hands. The key to change is locating what controls a certain behavior. A locus of control is the figurative place where a person locates the source of responsibility in his or her life. It can be external or internal.

An external locus of control could be:

- Believing others' actions determine your actions
- Environmental factors—weather, location, and so on
- Another person or social group
- Blaming outside influences for your behavior

An internal locus of control might be:

- Self-expectations
- Internal thoughts ("I can do this")
- How open one is to change

To create a successful change in your life, you must be the one who takes the responsibility for your actions while developing methods for overcoming external barriers. Individuals with an internal locus of control are more likely to see their behavior as something they can adapt or change. If you believe it is within your abilities, you may experience greater success!

Stage 3: Preparation

The preparation phase combines intention and behavior. Here you will monitor your current behavior, analyze and identify patterns in your activity, and then set a goal. The most important concept in this stage is honesty. It is easy to try to make your behavior fit a certain pattern or profile. Sometimes the truth isn't what we want to see, but it is imperative to set realistic goals and to achieve real changes. When in the preparation stage, individuals are intending to take action within the next 30 days.

Self-Monitoring

Self-monitoring means observing and recording one's own behavior. This process is necessary to:

- Make you aware of the size and seriousness of a problem
- Provide a benchmark to compare your original behavior (the point at which you began to try to change) with your later behavior

Behaviors need recording as they occur, not days later. Self-monitoring devices to measure the frequency of a behavior include:

- A health notebook, journal, or diary to record the occurrence of a behavior
- Counters to collect data (e.g., pedometers, golf counters)
- Graph paper (horizontal axis represents time—usually days—and vertical axis represents the amount of the behavior to be changed—body weight, exercise, number of hours of sleep) **Table 3.2**

Analysis

Once you have gathered your data, sit back and review your record. You are looking for patterns or clues about why and how you engage in the unhealthy behavior you wish to change. You should look at the following:

Ask Yourself

- If I were going to change a behavior, which ones would I need to learn more about before I could change?

- Where would I find this information?

What's the word. . .

locus of control The figurative place where a person locates the source of responsibility for the events in his or her life.

Ask Yourself

- Why do I want to make this change?

- For whom am I changing? If we choose to change for our own well-being instead of trying to garner the attention of others, we are more likely to maintain the progress.

| Table 3.2 | **Self-Managed Behavior Change Graph** |

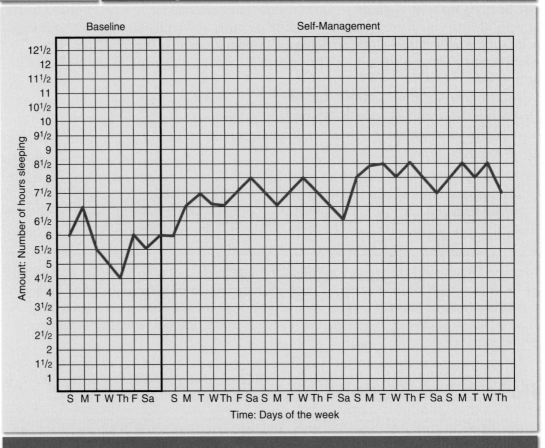

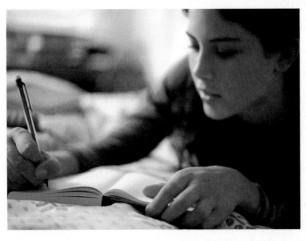

- **Time.** When during the day or week do you find yourself resorting to the activity? Is it linked with another activity (e.g., smoking after a meal or with a beer)?
- **Place.** Is there a specific place that you tend to be during the activity (e.g., making unhealthy diet choices on the way to class)?
- **Reason.** Can you link the behavior with a mood or an event that might trigger it (e.g., indulging in comfort food before an exam)?

Sometimes these aspects may not be immediately clear. Take a few days to look over your log. Remember that you are analyzing your behavior, not you as an individual. Keep a positive outlook—this behavior may be less than perfect, but you are making strides to change it, and that is more than the majority can say!

Goal Setting

At this point, you have determined the where, when, and why for your behavior in question. The next step is to set a goal. Don't rush through this step. You may think that the goal is obvious, but certain factors must be taken into consideration for this goal to be effective. It must be:

Medical News You Can Use

Prolonged TV Watching Affects Risk of Death, Diabetes, and Cardiovascular Disease

A review of studies on prolonged amounts of television viewing showed that the risk of type 2 diabetes increased by 20%, the risk of cardiovascular disease increased by 15%, and the risk of all-cause mortality increased by 13%. The authors of the study commented that watching TV is worse than other sedentary activities, such as driving, reading, and working at a computer, because it is a very passive activity. Watching television is associated with unhealthy eating behavior. People tend to eat when watching TV and tend to eat junk food and sugary beverages. One way to combat the passive nature of watching television is to increase physical activity while watching. This could include using a treadmill or other exercise equipment. Exercises like pushups, sit-ups, and pull-ups are simple activities that can be done when watching television.

Source: Data from Grontved A., Hu F.B., Television viewing and risk of type 2 diabetes, cardiovascular disease, and all-cause mortality: a meta-analysis. *Journal of the American Medical Society* 2011. 305(23):2448–55.

- **Realistic.** While it is good to aim high, watch out for making your goal a bit too ambitious. If you set an unrealistic goal, you will become frustrated along the way and lose your motivation quickly. Aim for a moderate expectation—one that will challenge you but is within your ability. Remember that you can always set a higher goal once you reach this one.

- **Quantitative.** Many times people set goals that are very abstract (i.e., wanting to lose weight). That is a fine ambition, but it is not an effective goal. You want your goal to be quantitative so that you can track your progress. A more effective goal would be to lose 10 pounds, or to stretch for 30 minutes three times a week. Try to define your goal in some type of measurable unit: minutes, pounds, number of servings, percentages, quantities, and so on.

- **Broken down in steps.** If you start out thinking that you are aiming toward this one big goal from the beginning, you will find that it is easy to get discouraged during the first few weeks. You need to choose a goal that can be broken down into smaller intermediate steps—mini goals—along the way. For example, if the goal is to stop drinking soda, perhaps the mini goals could be to cut back to three sodas per day, then two, then one, and so on. Make sure your mini goals are quantitative.

- **Tracked on a timeline.** Having the ambition to live a healthy lifestyle is different than trying to achieve your goal. The ambition can be carried with you for as long as you want. The goal, however, must have an end date. By using a timeline it is easier to keep your progress on track. The end date is not the end of the healthy behavior. After you have completed your goal within the time frame you chose, be sure to continue practicing the healthy habits until they stick!

- **Important to you.** If you do not feel that this goal is important or worthwhile, it will not be a success. It does not matter how many people tell you that your goal is great, you have to believe in it yourself. If you don't, go back and revise the goal until it fits with your expectations and your motivation.

Having a plan and a contract will help further your success as you begin to reach toward your goal. See a personal contract in **Figure 3.4** and **Lab 3-2**.

PERSONAL CONTRACT

Start Date: _____ Finish Date: _____

The Goal: _____

Motivation (benefits): _____

Identify your current stage of change: _____

Match your current stage of change and other stages you anticipate progressing through with the appropriate processes of change (see Figure 3.3):

_____   _____

_____   _____

What specific techniques will you use for each of the processes identified above (see Table 1.1)?	
Processes	Specific techniques
Stage of change on the finish date:	

Mini goals	Date	Reward
_____	_____	_____
_____	_____	_____
_____	_____	_____

I, _____, agree to work toward a healthier lifestyle and in doing so shall comply with the terms and dates of this contract.

Signature: _____ Date: _____

Witness: _____ Date: _____

Figure 3.4

A personal contract to bind yourself to your chosen course of action.

The Inside Track

Graduated Regimen Implementation

Starting a new behavior or stopping a behavior all at once is difficult.

Graduated programs can shape desired behaviors. Example: slowly start exercising.

The Plan

The plan is where you break your goal down into manageable steps. Your plan should include:

- What you will need. Do you need a newly stocked cabinet with healthier food? Do you need a gym membership? What equipment will you need for each of your steps?
- What is your timeline? When will you start this plan? When is your ending date for your goal?
- The steps you will take. Your goal should be broken down into smaller mini goals, each with its own timeline.

The Contract

Write a contract binding yourself to the chosen course of action. Your contract should include:

- ■ **Start date** Write the date that you will begin your plan.
- ■ **Finish date** Write the date when you will have completed your goal.
- ■ **The goal** Be specific and concise.
- ■ **Motivation (benefits)** Determine what is in it for you.
- ■ **Identify your current stage of change.**
- ■ **Identify the processes (strategies) of change** Use Figure 3.3 for each possible stage of change.
- ■ **For each process of change to be used, identify a specific technique.** See Table 3.1.
- ■ **Identify the stage of change when you finish.**
- ■ **Mini goals with rewards** What are the intervals along the way that will indicate you are making progress?
- ■ **Your signature** Sign your name as a sign of your commitment to your plan.
- ■ **Witness signature** Have a close friend or family member sign your contract as well.

Stage 4: Action

The action stage is where you begin to move toward a healthier behavior. You have your motivation, your internal locus of control, and your goal. You are ready to make this change! Action involves the most observable behavioral changes and requires the greatest commitments of time and energy.

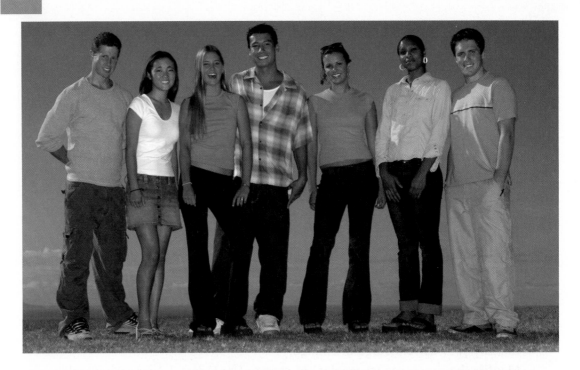

Sometimes your energy during the action phase can dwindle down, leaving the success of your plan vulnerable to barriers.

The five main barriers to successful change are:

- Social impact
- Stress
- Postponing
- Justification
- Denying responsibility

Social Impact

There can be both positive and negative social impacts on your plan to change a behavior.

Positive social impacts may be in the form of:

- Structured support groups
- Cheerleading by friends and family
- Role models—people around you whom you respect and admire

Negative social impacts may include:

- Feeling like the odd one out
- Peer pressure
- Attending functions that tempt you to break your contract

Let those around you know that you are trying to change this specific behavior. They may be able to offer tips and suggestions to help you along. More importantly, if you explain your goals to them, they are more likely to respect your decision and less likely to pressure you into relapsing into old behavior patterns.

Stress

One of the biggest barriers to changing lifestyle behaviors is stress. Stress can occur anywhere in our daily lives and without the correct management techniques it can lead you away from your goal. Eating comfort food, drinking, and engaging in other reckless behavior are common ways that many people deal with stress—none of which are effective or healthy. Learning effective coping techniques can make it easier for you to stay on track

What's the word...

stress The physical and emotional tension that comes from situations the body perceives as threatening.

Tipping Point

Dealing with Negative Social Impact

- Realize that this is your individual goal. Not everyone around you will have the same intentions as you.
- Stay committed to your goal. Review your contract before you go out to remind yourself how important this change is to you.
- Try to choose healthy alternatives whenever possible.
- Be a role model to others. By sticking with your plan and committing yourself to a healthier lifestyle, you may motivate others to do the same!
- Have a friend who wants you to push the limits of your goal? Assign that person as your personal coach or cheerleader. By making him or her feel like a responsible party in your plan, that individual may very well take on a role of support rather than peer pressure!

with your plan of action and help you to create a better sense of wellness overall. You will cover stress and its impact on your health more completely in Chapter 8.

When life throws curve balls at you, try these helpful tips to calm down and get back on track:

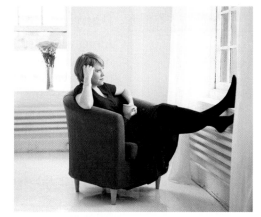

- Close your eyes and count to 10. Take deep breaths between each number.
- Have a CD on hand with calming music. Put it on and focus on the music for 5 minutes.
- Keep a journal. Record how you feel; sometimes just getting your thoughts on paper can help release tension.
- Go for a short brisk walk. The change of scenery and fresh air can renew your mood.
- Stop, stretch your muscles, and breathe deeply.

See Chapter 10 for more information on how to manage stress.

Postponement

After that initial surge of motivation in the beginning of the action phase, it can get difficult to muster the energy to continue to make the healthy choices. Many times the steps to reaching your goal get pushed aside or postponed until a later point in time. It is best to stop the procrastination as soon as you feel yourself slipping into that mindset.

When you realize that you are postponing a step in your plan:

- Stop and identify out loud that you are procrastinating.
- Try to pin down why you are avoiding that particular step. For example, is cold weather causing you to avoid going to the gym? Or is that healthy dish too time-consuming to make?
- Once you have identified why you are postponing a particular step, try to revise that step to fit better with your life. For example, buy a few exercise DVDs for working out at home when the weather is bad. Or, find simpler recipes that still offer the same nutritional value.

Justification

Many times when we procrastinate we justify or rationalize our actions. We make excuses for why we have not completed the task. It is important to catch yourself if you find that

What's the word...

procrastination
Pushing a task to a later point in time.

rationalization
Making excuses for not carrying out a task.

3

you are justifying not meeting your goal or one of your steps. Your plan may quickly become a slippery slope where nothing is accomplished, but everything is rationalized. When you feel yourself making excuses:

- Say your excuse out loud and listen—is it credible?
- Write down those times when you push your task off and explain why you did so. If you find yourself falling off course with your goal, these logs will provide a good resource describing when and why you aren't meeting each step.
- Understand that there will be times when you can't complete a step that second. Make sure that you are justifying the valid procrastinations, not the ones made out of low motivation.

Denying Responsibility

Along with justification can come **blaming**. Blaming occurs when you displace the responsibility for missing a step or not completing a goal onto someone else (external locus of control). Because of *him/her/them* or what *they* did, the goal was not met. This is an easy trap to fall into because it is convenient and gives the appearance that you are not at fault. No matter how good blaming looks on paper, it will not help you reach your goal. You will still be left with an unfinished plan. It is important to accept responsibility for your own actions.

Stage 5: Maintenance

After at least 6 months in the action stage, the person may move into the fifth stage: maintenance. This phase is when you keep up the new healthier habits that have replaced the old habits without much worry of returning to the old behavior. Change is main-

Medical News You Can Use

How to Lose 1 Pound: Exercise or Diet?

Suppose you do 30 minutes of brisk walking 5 days per week. If walking a mile expends 10 calories, and if you walk at 3 miles per hour, you burn an extra 150 calories per day (1 pound of fat is equivalent to about 3,500 calories), it could take 3 weeks to lose 1 pound. This can be disappointing, and most people won't stick with it.

For the average person, caloric intake—rather than calorie burning from exercise—appears to be the most important factor in weight loss. Even if calorie intake trumps exercise, this does not mean exercise does not play a key role in helping people stay trim.

Source: Data from Ballantyne C., Does Exercise Really Make You Healthier?, *Scientific American*, January 2 2009. Accessed October 2011 at: http://www.scientificamerican.com/article.cfm?id=does-exercise-really-make.

tained more easily now. There may be an initial excitement associated with making a change in which your motivation and commitment will both be high and the outlook toward your goal is positive.

Many of the activities used in the maintenance phase are the same as you'll use if you are in the action phase, just with small adaptations. For instance:

- **Rewards** You still need to set reward dates; however, they are more distant and the rewards should become smaller as the behavior becomes more natural.

- **Environmental control** Once the first set of influences is overcome, new challenges can be established.

Issues to Face in Maintenance

Relapse

Relapse can occur at any stage of the change process. It can be triggered by many things: an extra stressful day or week, an unexpected event, low levels of motivation. If you find yourself relapsing along the way, try to identify a reason. Are you losing motivation? Is your plan unrealistic? Do you not have the right equipment or facilities?

This is a process; nothing is set in stone. You have the freedom to go back and revise your goal at any time. Don't be afraid to reevaluate your plan. If something is not working for you, find alternatives that will still help you change the behavior. Most importantly: Do not give up! A relapse is normal—it doesn't mean that you will never complete your goals. It is a minor setback that can be overcome.

Acceptance

Acceptance is the finish line. The old unhealthy behavior has been fully replaced at this point. Not only have you completed your goal, but you have also integrated healthy habits into your daily routine. Be aware that this stage may not come quickly. Achieving your goal and dealing with relapses may take a long while, but your healthy new lifestyle is definitely worth it.

Conclusion

Lifestyle change is a process that involves many steps and a lot of persistence. Although not recommended, it is possible to have multiple changes taking place at once. The chapters in this text provide a wealth of information on many different aspects of healthy living. By incorporating each topic into your daily life, you will be working toward a more rounded sense of wellness.

Reflect >>>> Reinforce >>>> Reinvigorate

Knowledge Check

Answers in Appendix D

1. What is the first stage of change?
   A. Preparation
   B. Precontemplation
   C. Action

2. An effective plan for changing a behavior should have:
   A. The steps to be taken
   B. How long it will last
   C. List of items needed
   D. All of the above

3. Which factors influence a person to change?
   A. Obtaining more knowledge
   B. The ability to use self-management skills
   C. Having a reason
   D. All of the above

For each of the following, identify which stage of change the person is in, two strategies that may move the person to the next stage, one significant barrier the person may face, and a method to overcome that barrier.

4. Experiencing an episode or time frame when current behavior goes back to previously discontinued behavior is called:
   A. Maintenance
   B. Relapse
   C. Action
   D. Acceptance

5. When an individual makes excuses for not taking action on an issue, he or she is said to be:
   A. In denial
   B. Preparing
   C. Procrastinating
   D. In action

6. Lateisha has researched the benefits of becoming active. She has developed a scheme to move forward and is scheduled to begin taking steps in 2 weeks. What stage is Lateisha in?
   A. Contemplation
   B. Preparation
   C. Action
   D. Maintenance

7. The individual behavior responsible for more deaths than any other behavior is:
   A. Alcohol consumption
   B. Use of illegal drugs
   C. Irresponsible sexual behavior
   D. Tobacco use

8. The strategy that substitutes a healthy behavior for an unhealthy one is called:
   A. Reinforcement
   B. Self-evaluation
   C. Countering
   D. Emotional arousal

Modern Modifications

Take a moment to weigh the pros and cons of maintaining and regular physical activity program. What are the pros? What are the cons? Write these down.

Are there costs associated with your physical activity program such as fitness club membership, new clothing, or new equipment? How do the benefits outweigh the costs? Are there ways to reduce the cost of your physical activity program? Can you walk in your neighborhood or nearby park? Can you buy used equipment or discounted equipment? Does your company offer discounts for fitness club membership?

Critical Thinking

Take a moment to analyze these situations:

1. Angela had been involved in ballet for many years, and she now wants to begin dancing again. She knows she lacks the flexibility to do so, but is willing to work on it—she just isn't sure how.

2. Max has been smoking since he was 12 (he is now 22). He looks forward to that first drag in the morning and is unconcerned with all the "hype" about cancer. Everyone in his family smokes and no one has ever gotten cancer!

Going Above and Beyond

MedlinePlus: Exercise and Physical Fitness

http://www.nlm.nih.gov/medlineplus/exercisephysicalfitness.html

Physician and Sports Medicine

http://www.physsportsmed.org

Morbidity and Mortality Weekly Report

http://www.cdc.gov/mmwr

Transtheoretical Model

www.uri.edu/research/cprc/transtheoretical.htm

References and Suggested Readings

Marcus B., et al. Assessing motivational readiness and decision-making for exercise. *Health Psychology* 1992; 22:257–261.

Prochaska J. O. Strong and weak principles for progressing from precontemplation to action on the basis of twelve problem behaviors. *Health Psychology* 1994; 13:47–51.

Prochaska J. O. and Markus B. H. The Transtheoretical Model: Applications to Exercise, in *Advances in Exercise Adherence*, Dishman R. K. (ed.), Champaign, IL: Human Kinetics, 1994.

Prochaska J. O., Norcross J. C., and DiClemente C. O. *Changing for Good.* New York: HarperCollins Publishers, 1994. Reprinted by Quill, 2002.

Prochaska J. O. and Velicer W. F. The transtheoretical model of health behavior change. *American Journal of Health Promotion* 1997; 12:38–48.

U.S. DHHS. *Healthy People 2020.* Washington, DC: DHHS, 2010.

———. *Physical Activity and Health: A Report of the Surgeon General.* Atlanta, GA: DHHS, 1996.

Zimmerman G. L., et al. A "Stages of Change" approach to helping patients change behavior. *American Family Physician*, March 1, 2000: American Academy of Family Physicians.

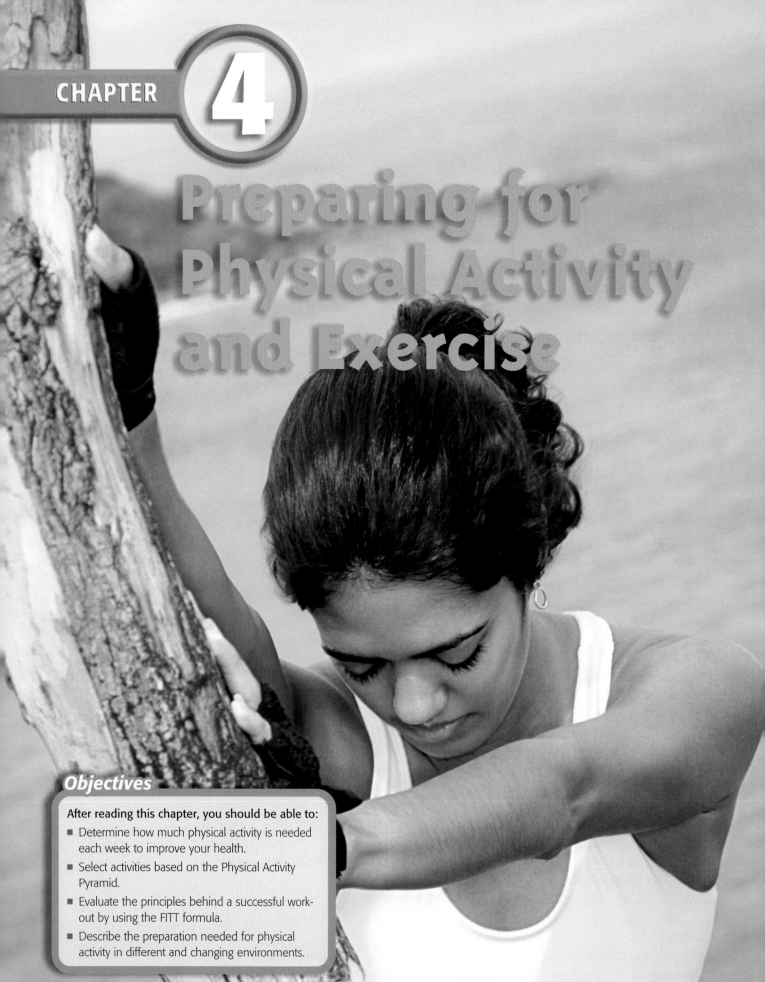

Objectives

After reading this chapter, you should be able to:

- Determine how much physical activity is needed each week to improve your health.
- Select activities based on the Physical Activity Pyramid.
- Evaluate the principles behind a successful workout by using the FITT formula.
- Describe the preparation needed for physical activity in different and changing environments.

Before Starting an Exercise Program

Check your health status.

Moderate physical activity, like walking the dog, gardening, or working around the house, is not dangerous for most people, and no medical clearance is needed for it.

People with chronic diseases, such as a heart condition, arthritis, diabetes, or high blood pressure, should talk to their physician about what types and amounts of physical activity are appropriate.

Complete the Physical Activity Readiness Questionnaire (PAR-Q) in (Lab 4-1). If you answered "yes" to any of the checklist items, discuss your answers with a physician before having your fitness assessed or starting an exercise program.

The American Heart Association suggests that you see a physician before exercising if:

- you have a heart condition;
- you take medicine for your heart and/or blood pressure;
- you get pains in your chest, left side of your neck, or your left shoulder or arm when you exercise;
- your chest has been hurting for about a month;
- you tend to get dizzy, lose consciousness, and fall;
- you get breathless with mild exertion;
- you have bone or joint problems that a physician told you could be worsened by exercise;
- you have an overweight or obesity problem;
- you have a medical condition, such as insulin-dependent diabetes, that requires special attention in an exercise program; or
- you are middle-aged or older (40 years for men; 50 years for women).

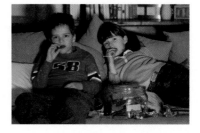

How Much Physical Activity Do I Need?

Physical activity is anything that gets your body moving. According to the *Physical Activity Guidelines for Americans,* you need to do two types of physical activity each week to improve your health—aerobic and muscle-strengthening.

We know 150 minutes (Table 4.1) each week sounds like a lot of time, but you do not have to do it all at once. Not only is it best to **spread your activity out during the week,** but you can **break it up into smaller chunks of time during the day.** As long as you are doing your activity at a moderate or vigorous effort for **at least 10 minutes at a time.**

If you go beyond 300 minutes a week of moderate-intensity activity, or 150 minutes a week of vigorous-intensity activity, you will gain even more health benefits (Table 4.2).

The Physical Activity Pyramid (Figure 4.1) graphically displays the recommendations of the *2008 Physical Activity for Americans.*

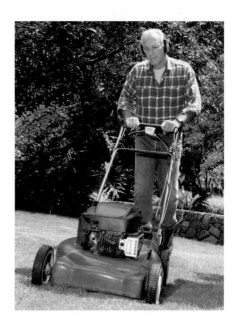

FITT Formula

After warming up in preparing to exercise, the FITT formula is an easy way to remember the essential facts for a good and effective exercise workout. Later chapters apply the FITT formula directly to the various components of

Table 4.1	**For Important Health Benefits**

Adults need at least:

2 hours and 30 minutes (150 minutes) of moderate-intensity aerobic activity (e.g., brisk walking) every week **and**
muscle-strengthening activities on 2 or more days a week that work all major muscle groups (legs, hips, back, abdomen, chest, shoulders, and arms).

OR

1 hour and 15 minutes (75 minutes) of vigorous-intensity aerobic activity (e.g., jogging or running) every week **and**
muscle-strengthening activities on 2 or more days a week that work all major muscle groups (legs, hips, back, abdomen, chest, shoulders, and arms).

OR

An equivalent mix of moderate- and vigorous-intensity aerobic activity **and**
muscle-strengthening activities on 2 or more days a week that work all major muscle groups (legs, hips, back, abdomen, chest, shoulders, and arms).

Source: Centers for Disease Control and Prevention. Accessed at: http://www.cdc.gov/physicalactivity/everyone/guidelines/adults.html

What's the word. . .

frequency How often; the number of times an exercise or group of exercises is performed within a certain time frame.

intensity How hard; the amount of energy exerted while performing an exercise.

time How long; the duration of an exercise or group of exercises.

type The classification of exercise.

exercise (e.g., cardiorespiratory, muscular strength and endurance, and flexibility). The FITT formula sums up the essential elements of a good workout as follows:

- **Frequency** of the activity: The number of times an exercise or group of exercises is performed within a certain time frame. Usually this is measured in sessions per week. How frequently you perform a certain exercise depends on the intensity of the exercise.
- **Intensity** of the activity: The amount of energy exerted while performing an exercise (e.g., usually guided by your heart rate in the case of cardiorespiratory exercise, and how much weight is lifted or force used for muscular strengthening).
- **Time** or duration of the activity: The measurement of how long an exercise or group of exercises takes to complete. For muscular strengthening this also includes how many repetitions or times a person lifts a weight.
- **Type** of activity: The classification of exercise. Daily activity, cardiorespiratory endurance, muscle strength, and flexibility are all different types of activities.

Table 4.2	**For Even *Greater* Health Benefits**

Adults should increase their activity to:

5 hours (300 minutes) each week of moderate-intensity aerobic activity **and**
muscle-strengthening activities on 2 or more days a week that work all major muscle groups (legs, hips, back, abdomen, chest, shoulders, and arms).

OR

2 hours and 30 minutes (150 minutes) each week of vigorous-intensity aerobic activity **and**
muscle-strengthening activities on 2 or more days a week that work all major muscle groups (legs, hips, back, abdomen, chest, shoulders, and arms).

OR

An equivalent mix of moderate- and vigorous-intensity aerobic activity **and**
muscle-strengthening activities on 2 or more days a week that work all major muscle groups (legs, hips, back, abdomen, chest, shoulders, and arms).

Source: Courtesy of the Centers for Disease Control and Prevention.

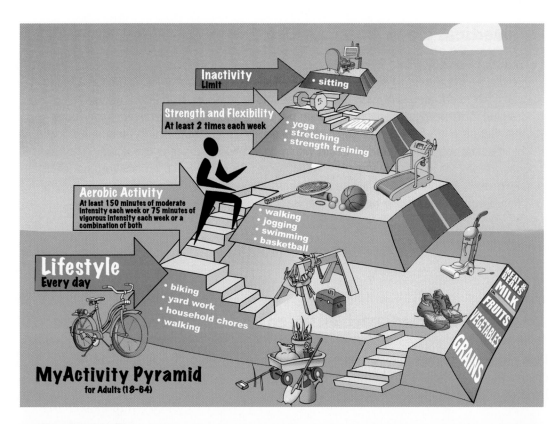

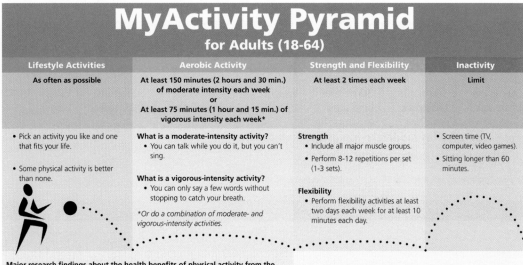

MyActivity Pyramid
for Adults (18-64)

Lifestyle Activities	Aerobic Activity	Strength and Flexibility	Inactivity
As often as possible	At least 150 minutes (2 hours and 30 min.) of moderate intensity each week **or** At least 75 minutes (1 hour and 15 min.) of vigorous intensity each week*	At least 2 times each week	Limit
• Pick an activity you like and one that fits your life. • Some physical activity is better than none.	**What is a moderate-intensity activity?** • You can talk while you do it, but you can't sing. **What is a vigorous-intensity activity?** • You can only say a few words without stopping to catch your breath. *Or do a combination of moderate- and vigorous-intensity activities.*	**Strength** • Include all major muscle groups. • Perform 8-12 repetitions per set (1-3 sets). **Flexibility** • Perform flexibility activities at least two days each week for at least 10 minutes each day.	• Screen time (TV, computer, video games). • Sitting longer than 60 minutes.

Major research findings about the health benefits of physical activity from the Physical Activity Guidelines for Americans:

• Regular physical activity reduces the risk of many adverse health outcomes like heart disease, type 2 diabetes and some cancers.

• Most health benefits occur with at least 150 minutes (2 hours and 30 min.) a week of moderate-intensity physical activity.

• For additional health benefits, adults should increase their aerobic physical activity to 300 minutes (5 hours) a week of moderate-intensity, 150 minutes a week of vigorous-intensity aerobic physical activity or a combination of both. Additional benefits include lower risk of colon and breast cancer, and prevention of unhealthy weight gain.

• People with disabilities can also benefit from physical activity.

Physical Activity Guidelines are also available for the following:

• Children and adolescents

• Older adults

• Women during pregnancy and the postpartum period

• Adults with disabilities

• People with chronic medical conditions

To learn more about these guidelines go online to *health.gov/paguidelines*

Figure 4.1

MyActivity Pyramid. (*Source:* Courtesy of Steve Ball, Ph.D., University of Missouri-Extension.)

4

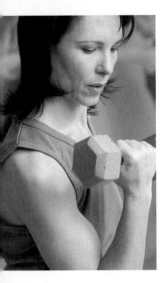

Medical News You Can Use

Bursts of Activity Can Trigger Heart Attacks

Researchers analyzed 14 studies of cardiac effects of episodic physical activity and found that it was associated with more than a three-fold increase in heart attack risk and a five-fold increase in sudden cardiac death risk in the short-term. Researchers concluded that there is a link between episodic physical activity (e.g., sexual activity) with the risk of heart attack and sudden cardiac death within one to two hours after the activity. The risk was greatest for those who are not engaged in regular exercise. To reduce your risk of heart attack and sudden cardiac death, researchers suggest to make your physical activity more frequent and regular rather than episodic.

Source: Data from Dahabreh I.J., Paulus J.K. Association of episodic physical and sexual activity with triggering of acute cardiac events. *Journal of the American Medical Association* 2011; 305(12):1225–1233.

Adding Exercise and Physical Activity to Your Life

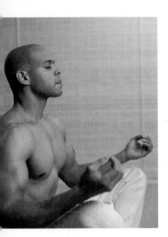

Pick physical activities that you enjoy and that match your abilities; this will help ensure that you stick with them (see **Lab 4-2**). If you are not sure where to start, here are some examples (see **Tables 4.3–4.8**):

Table 4.3	Example 1: Moderate-Intensity Activity and Muscle-Strengthening Activity						
Sunday	**Monday**	**Tuesday**	**Wednesday**	**Thursday**	**Friday**	**Saturday**
30-minute brisk walk	30-minute brisk walk	30-minute brisk walk	Weight training	30-minute brisk walk	30-minute brisk walk	Weight training

Total: 150 minutes moderate-intensity aerobic activity
+ 2 days muscle-strengthening activity

Source: Courtesy of the Centers for Disease Control and Prevention.

Table 4.4	Example 2: Vigorous-Intensity Activity and Muscle-Strengthening Activity						
Sunday	**Monday**	**Tuesday**	**Wednesday**	**Thursday**	**Friday**	**Saturday**
	25-minute jog		25-minute jog and weight training		Weight training	25-minute jog

Total: 75 minutes vigorous-intensity aerobic activity
+ 2 days muscle-strengthening activity

Source: Courtesy of the Centers for Disease Control and Prevention.

Table 4.5	Example 3: Mix of Moderate- and Vigorous-Intensity Activity and Muscle Strengthening Activity						
Sunday	**Monday**	**Tuesday**	**Wednesday**	**Thursday**	**Friday**	**Saturday**	
30-minute brisk walk	15-minute jog	Weight training	30-minute brisk walk	Weight training	15-minute jog	30-minute brisk walk	

Total: The equivalent of 150 minutes of moderate-intensity aerobic activity + 2 days muscle-strengthening activity

Source: Courtesy of the Centers for Disease Control and Prevention.

Here are six more examples.

Table 4.6	Moderate Aerobic Activity Routines							
	Monday	**Tuesday**	**Wednesday**	**Thursday**	**Friday**	**Saturday**	**Sunday**	**Physical Activity TOTAL**
Example 1	30 minutes of brisk walking	30 minutes of brisk walking	Resistance band exercises	30 minutes of brisk walking	30 minutes of brisk walking	Resistance band exercises	30 minutes of brisk walking	150 minutes moderate-intensity aerobic activity AND 2 days muscle strengthening
Example 2	30 minutes of brisk walking	60 minutes of playing softball	30 minutes of brisk walking	30 minutes of mowing the lawn		Heavy gardening	Heavy gardening	150 minutes moderate-intensity aerobic activity AND 2 days muscle strengthening

Source: Courtesy of the Centers for Disease Control and Prevention.

Table 4.7	Vigorous Aerobic Activity Routines							
	Monday	**Tuesday**	**Wednesday**	**Thursday**	**Friday**	**Saturday**	**Sunday**	**Physical Activity TOTAL**
Example 3	25 minutes of jogging	Weight lifting	25 minutes of jogging	Weight lifting	25 minutes of jogging			75 minutes vigorous-intensity aerobic activity AND 2 days muscle strengthening
Example 4	25 minutes of swimming laps		25 minutes of running	Weight training	25 minutes of singles tennis	Weight training		75 minutes vigorous-intensity aerobic activity AND 2 days muscle strengthening

Source: Courtesy of the Centers for Disease Control and Prevention.

4

| Table 4.8 | Mix of Moderate and Vigorous Aerobic Activity Routines |

	Monday	Tuesday	Wednesday	Thursday	Friday	Saturday	Sunday	Physical Activity TOTAL
Example 5	30 minutes of water aerobics	30 minutes of jogging	30 minutes of walking Yoga		30 minutes of brisk walking	Yoga		90 minutes moderate-intensity aerobic activity AND 30 minutes vigorous-intensity aerobic activity AND 2 days muscle strengthening
Example 6	45 minutes of doubles tennis Weight lifting	Rock climbing			30 minutes of vigorous hiking		45 minutes of doubles tennis	90 minutes moderate-intensity aerobic activity AND 30 minutes vigorous-intensity aerobic activity AND 2 days muscle strengthening

Source: Courtesy of the Centers for Disease Control and Prevention.

Overcoming the Excuses for Not Exercising or Being Physically Active

Given the health benefits of regular physical activity, we might have to ask why two out of three (60%) Americans are not active at recommended levels.

Many technological advances and conveniences that have made our lives easier and less active, and many personal variables, including physiological, behavioral, and psychological factors, may affect our plans to become more physically active. In fact, the 10 most common reasons adults cite for not adopting more physically active lifestyles are:

- do not have enough time to exercise;
- find it inconvenient to exercise;
- lack self-motivation;
- do not find exercise enjoyable;
- find exercise boring;
- lack confidence in their ability to be physically active (low self-efficacy);
- fear of being injured or have been injured recently;
- lack self-management skills, such as the ability to set personal goals, monitor progress, or reward progress toward such goals;
- lack encouragement, support, or companionship from family and friends; and
- do not have parks, sidewalks, bicycle trails, or safe and pleasant walking paths convenient to their homes or offices.

Understanding common barriers to physical activity and creating strategies to overcome them (Table 4.9) may help you make physical activity part of your daily life (see Lab 4-3).

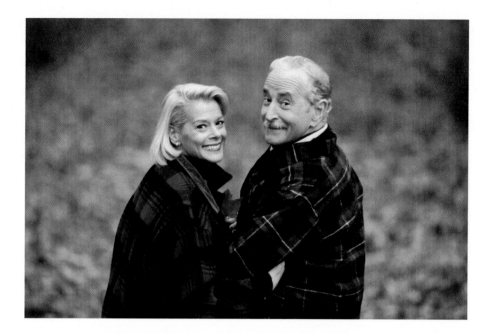

Table 4.9	Suggestions for Overcoming Physical Activity Barriers
Lack of time	Identify available time slots. Monitor your daily activities for one week. Identify at least three 30-minute time slots you could use for physical activity. Add physical activity to your daily routine. For example, walk or ride your bike to work or shopping, organize school activities around physical activity, walk the dog, exercise while you watch TV, park farther away from your destination, etc. Select activities requiring minimal time, such as walking, jogging, or stair climbing.
Social influence	Explain your interest in physical activity to friends and family. Ask them to support your efforts. Invite friends and family members to exercise with you. Plan social activities involving exercise. Develop new friendships with physically active people. Join a group, such as the YMCA or a hiking club.
Lack of energy	Schedule physical activity for times in the day or week when you feel energetic. Convince yourself that if you give it a chance, physical activity will increase your energy level; then, try it.
Lack of motivation	Plan ahead. Make physical activity a regular part of your daily or weekly schedule and write it on your calendar. Invite a friend to exercise with you on a regular basis and write it on both your calendars. Join an exercise group or class.
Fear of injury	Learn how to warm up and cool down to prevent injury. Learn how to exercise appropriately considering your age, fitness level, skill level, and health status. Choose activities involving minimum risk.
Lack of skill	Select activities requiring no new skills, such as walking, climbing stairs, or jogging. Take a class to develop new skills.

continues

Table 4.9	Suggestions for Overcoming Physical Activity Barriers, *continued*
Lack of resources	Select activities that require minimal facilities or equipment, such as walking, jogging, jumping rope, or calisthenics. Identify inexpensive, convenient resources available in your community (community education programs, park and recreation programs, worksite programs, etc.).
Weather conditions	Develop a set of regular activities that are always available regardless of weather (indoor cycling, aerobic dance, indoor swimming, calisthenics, stair climbing, rope skipping, mall walking, dancing, gymnasium games, etc.).
Travel	Put a jump rope in your suitcase and jump rope. Walk the halls and climb the stairs in hotels. Stay in places with swimming pools or exercise facilities. Join the YMCA or YWCA (ask about reciprocal membership agreement). Visit the local shopping mall and walk for half an hour or more. Bring your mp3 player with your favorite aerobic exercise music. Find an exercise DVD and use it in your room.
Family obligations	Trade babysitting time with a friend, neighbor, or family member who also has small children. Exercise with the kids—go for a walk together, play tag or other running games, get an aerobic dance or exercise tape for kids (there are several on the market) and exercise together. You can spend time together and still get your exercise. Jump rope, do calisthenics, ride a stationary bicycle, or use other home gymnasium equipment while the kids are busy playing or sleeping. Try to exercise when the kids are not around (e.g., during school hours or their nap time).
Retirement years	Look upon your retirement as an opportunity to become more active instead of less. Spend more time gardening, walking the dog, and playing with your grandchildren. Children with short legs and grandparents with slower gaits are often great walking partners. Learn a new skill you've always been interested in, such as ballroom dancing, square dancing, or swimming. Now that you have the time, make regular physical activity a part of every day. Go for a walk every morning or every evening before dinner. Treat yourself to an exercycle and ride every day while reading a favorite book or magazine.

Source: Courtesy of the Centers for Disease Control and Prevention.

Environmental Considerations

Exercising in the Heat

Exercising in hot weather puts extra stress on your body. If you do not take care when exercising in the heat, you risk serious illness. Both the exercise itself and the air temperature increase your core body temperature. To help cool itself, your body sends more blood to circulate through your skin. This leaves less blood for your muscles, which in turn increases your heart rate. If the humidity is high, your body faces added stress because sweat does not readily evaporate from your skin. That pushes your body temperature even higher.

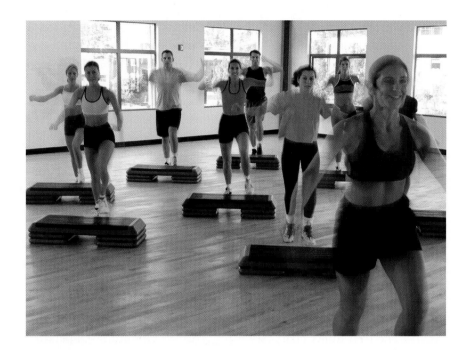

Heat-related problems can be avoided:

- Schedule outdoor exercise at the coolest time of day, either early morning or after sunset.

- Exercise in facilities with air conditioning.

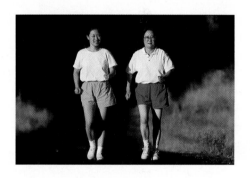

- Slow down. Lowering the intensity of your workout will reduce the strain on your body and improve its ability to regulate temperature.

- Drink water. A general recommendation is to drink 24 ounces of water 2 hours before exercise. Drinking an additional 8 ounces of water 30 minutes before exercise is also helpful. While you are exercising, break for a 6- to 8-oz. cup of water every 20 or 30 minutes. Replace your fluids, whether you feel thirsty or not.

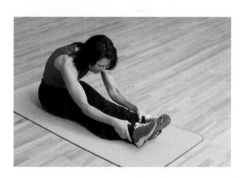

- Avoid too much water since it can dilute the electrolytes in the blood and cause a condition known as hyponatremia (also known as "water intoxication") which can result in unresponsiveness and death. If your workout exceeds an hour, you may substitute a sports drink to replace lost electrolytes (e.g., sodium) for water.

- Monitor the color of your urine. The darker your urine, the less hydrated you are and the greater your risk for heat injury. Drink enough fluids to keep your urine a very light color.

- Dress right. Do not wear waterproof cloths. These fabrics will prevent the evaporation of sweat from the skin and increase the risk of heat injury. Wear lightweight and light-colored clothing that is breathable.

- Protect against sun exposure with sunscreen (at least SPF 15 and sweat-resistant). Depending upon the type of activity, wear sunglasses and a hat.

- Get your body accustomed to the heat. It takes 7 to 10 days of combined heat exposure and exercise for your body to adapt to the heat. Once acclimatized, you will sweat sooner, sweat more, and lose fewer electrolytes through sweat, resulting in a lower body core temperature, a decreased heart rate response to exercise, and lower potential for dehydration and electrolyte depletion.

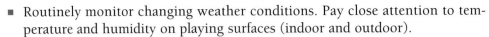

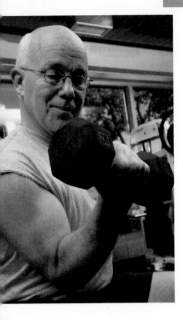

- Routinely monitor changing weather conditions. Pay close attention to temperature and humidity on playing surfaces (indoor and outdoor).
- When there are extreme heat and humidity conditions, consider postponing or canceling your activity.

Heat-related Illnesses. Under normal conditions, your skin, blood vessels, and perspiration level adjust to the heat. But these natural cooling systems may fail if you are exposed to high temperatures and humidity for too long, you sweat heavily, or you do not drink enough fluids. The result may be a heat-related illness. Heat-related illnesses occur along a continuum, starting out mild but worsening if left untreated. Heat illnesses include:

- heat syncope (fainting);
- heat cramps (muscle spasms);
- heat exhaustion (severe dehydration that, if untreated, progresses to heat-stroke); and
- exertional heatstroke (affects healthy, active people who are strenuously working or exercising in a warm environment; can cause death).

The heat index chart (see **Figure 4.2**) combines temperature and humidity to show the likelihood of heat disorders with prolonged exposure or strenuous activity. For more information about heat illnesses and first aid for them, go to Appendix A.

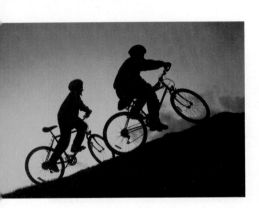

Sunburn. Sunburn is the skin's response to the ultraviolet (UV) radiation that results mainly from exposure to UVB radiation or, rarely, to UVA radiation. This is the most common burn, and the body's reactions begin 2 to 8 hours after exposure. Sunburns are first- and second-degree burns. For sunburn first aid, refer to Appendix A.

Exercising in the Cold

When you are out in the cold, your body's first priority is to maintain its core temperature. To do that, it shifts blood away from the extremities and toward the central organs—the heart and lungs. This increases the risk of frostbite to your

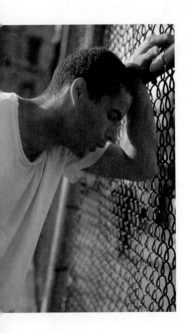

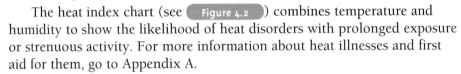

		Temperature (°F)														
		80	81	84	86	88	90	92	94	96	98	100	102	104	106	108	110
Relative Humidity (%)	40	80	81	83	85	88	91	94	97	101	105	109	114	119	124	130	136
	45	80	82	84	87	89	93	96	100	104	109	114	119	124	130	137	
	50	81	83	85	88	91	95	99	103	108	113	118	124	131	137		
	55	81	84	86	89	93	97	101	106	112	117	124	130	137			
	60	82	84	88	91	95	100	105	110	116	123	129	137				
	65	82	85	89	93	98	103	108	114	121	126	130					
	70	83	86	90	95	100	105	112	119	126	134						
	75	84	88	92	97	103	109	116	124	132							
	80	84	89	94	100	106	113	121	129								
	85	85	90	96	102	110	117	126	135								
	90	86	91	98	105	113	122	131									
	95	86	93	100	108	117	127										
	100	87	95	103	112	121	132										

Likelihood of Heat Disorders with Prolonged Exposure or Strenuous Activity

☐ Caution ☐ Extreme Caution ☐ Danger ☐ External Danger

Figure 4.2

NOAA's National Weather Service Heat Index. (*Source:* Courtesy of the National Weather Service/NOAA.)

toes, fingers, nose, and ears. When the body temperature drops, the body attempts to restore its normal temperature by shivering, which is a sign of mild hypothermia.

Generally, you will not be affected by the cold unless a lot of energy is expended on shivering. This is especially true during swimming, when heat is removed from the body more rapidly through conduction in the water (about 25 times faster than in air).

Moderate-intensity, land-based exercise usually generates enough heat to maintain the body's core temperature at as low as −22°F (−30°C) without the need for excessive heavy clothing.

When exercising in the cold, remember to stay hydrated by drinking water. Avoid alcohol and caffeinated beverages because they cause dehydration. Alcohol also dilates the skin's blood vessels, which results in more heat loss.

For a wind chill factor chart, see ⬭ Figure 4.3 ⬭. The wind chill factor combines temperature and wind speed. Notice the amount of time for frostbite to develop. For first aid information for frostnip, frostbite, and hypothermia, see Appendix A.

Clothing for Cold-Weather Physical Activity

Note the following pointers for clothing in cold weather to prevent heat loss.
- Wearing multiple layers of thin clothing is warmer than one heavy layer. Layers are also easier to add or remove to better regulate your core temperature. The body should be kept warm, but avoid sweating and prevent shivering (sign of mild hypothermia).
- Layers next to the skin should be made of wicking materials (e.g., polypropylene, silk, polyester).
- Wear a hat because up to 50% of your body heat can be lost through the head.
- Socks and glove liners should be synthetic material (e.g., polypropylene) or wool to ensure wicking of moisture from the extremities that are most susceptible to frostbite.
- Wearing a scarf or face mask over the nose and mouth during exercise will trap heat and water vapor that serves in warming and humidifying the inhaled air.

Exercising in Polluted Air

Exposure to air pollution can cause health problems even when you are not exercising. The combination of air pollution and exercise increases the potential health problems. For example, during aerobic activity you typically inhale more air, and you breathe it

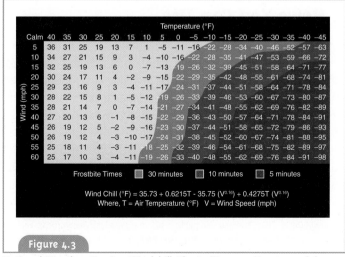

Figure 4.3

National Weather Service Windchill Chart. (*Source:* Courtesy of the National Weather Service/NOAA.)

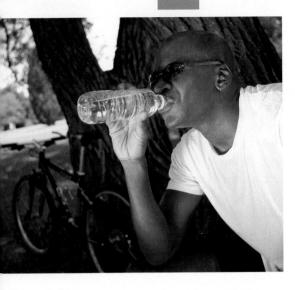

more deeply into your lungs. Since you are likely to breathe mostly through your mouth during exercise, the air you breathe in bypasses your nasal passages, which normally serve to filter airborne pollution particles.

Health problems associated with air pollution include:

- damage to the airways of the lungs;
- increased risk of asthma development;
- worsening of existing asthma;
- increased risk of heart attacks and strokes; and
- increased risk of death from lung cancer and cardiovascular disease.

What is not clear with air pollution and exercise is how much exposure is a danger, or how long you have to be exposed. Because exercise has definite health benefits, do not give up on exercise entirely, unless your healthcare provider has instructed you to do so. Instead, focus on ways to minimize the risks of the air pollution-and-exercise combination.

You can limit pollutions effects by:

- avoiding outdoor activity or reducing its intensity and duration when air quality alerts have been issued (completely avoid outdoor activity when high pollution levels exist);
- exercising indoors on poor air quality days; and
- avoiding high-pollution areas (e.g., near highways).

Exercising at High Altitudes

Decreased oxygen at high altitudes makes exercising and physical activities difficult. In unacclimatized persons, going above 8000 feet for several days can produce one of several types of altitude sickness (i.e., acute mountain sickness, high-altitude pulmonary edema, or high-altitude cerebral edema) because of lack of oxygen and decreased pressure in the blood and tissues. To reduce the likelihood of high-altitude illness, these measures are highly recommended:

- Make a gradual ascent to allow time for acclimatization. This usually requires several days. Some people will "climb high, but sleep low."

Medical News You Can Use

How Much Exercise Is Enough?

A low level of physical activity is one of the most important factors in the high rate of obesity in the United States. Those who exercise regularly at a moderate pace, doing activities such as gardening, yard work, walking, or dancing can burn an additional 150 calories per half-hour. Exercise guidelines released by the American Heart Association and the American College of Sports Medicine report that adults 65 and older should engage in at least 30 minutes of moderate-intensity aerobic exercise 5 days a week, or at least 20 minutes of vigorous-intensity exercise at least 3 days each week. These are the same recommendations for those of ages 18–65; however, the intensity of the exercise may need to be adjusted for younger individuals.

Source: Data from Nelson M.E., et al. Physical activity and public health in older adults: Recommendation from the American College of Sports Medicine and the American Heart Association *Circulation* 2007; 116(9):1094–1105.

- Eat high-carbohydrate foods. High altitudes may suppress your appetite and increase your energy needs.
- Keep hydrated. Adequate hydration is indicated by clear urine.
- If you have had past problems when at high altitudes, ask your physician for medication to lessen the symptoms of high-altitude illness.

Other environmental stresses at high altitudes include lower humidity, decreased temperatures, and increased ultraviolet radiation—all with medical consequences. Wear sunglasses and sunscreen (at least SPF 15) that is sweat resistant. Wear a hat.

Because of dry air at high altitudes, sore throat and coughing may develop. If they occur, drink fluids, apply an antibiotic ointment in the nostrils, and suck hard candy or throat lozenges.

Muscle Soreness

Expect to have muscle soreness after a strenuous physical activity workout or after starting a new type of exercise. Several remedies have been reported as helpful:

- *Rest:* Not using the affected muscles may take a week for the soreness to disappear, but if you desire, try some easy activities during the initial week.
- *Ice application:* An ice pack should be applied at the first sign of soreness.
- *Stretching:* The jury is still out and more research would be helpful in deciding if stretching helps to reduce muscle soreness. It may help—and cannot hurt.
- *Massage:* Some studies recommend gently massaging the muscle to stimulate blood flow to the area and diminish swelling.
- *Anti-inflammatory medicines:* These help relieve soreness and inflammation. Some people are sensitive to these medications.
- *Topical ointments/creams:* Whereas these give the sense of heat, they have no effect on the muscle.
- *Heat application:* This can help relax a stiff muscle and should be considered while recovering from muscle soreness.

Tipping Point

The American Orthopedic Foot and Ankle Society makes several recommendations for selecting a good fitting shoe (Figure 4.4 and Figure 4.5):

- Have both feet measured when they are at their largest: at the end of the day or after a run, walk, game, or practice.
- Wear your workout socks.
- Try on the shoes, because sizes vary by manufacturer.
- Make sure both shoes fit.
- Ensure that the shoe provides at least one thumb's width of space from the longest toe to the end of the toe box.

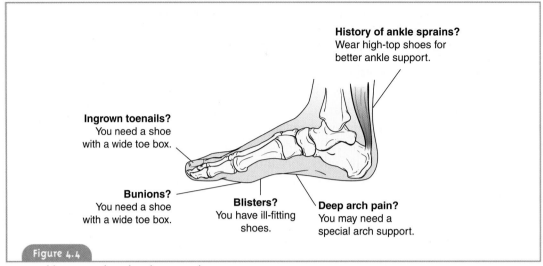

Figure 4.4

Foot problems may be related to your shoes.

Reflect ›››› Reinforce ›››› Reinvigorate

Knowledge Check

Answers in Appendix D

1. The component(s) of physical fitness include:

   A. Cardiorespiratory endurance

   B. Muscular endurance

   C. Flexibility

   D. All of the above

2. The fourth level of the Physical Activity Pyramid is reserved for:

   A. Muscular strength   B. Rest   C. Stretching   D. Cardiovascular endurance

3. Less than this percentage of adults achieve the recommended amount of regular physical activity.

   A. 16%   B. 27%   C. 39%   D. 50%

4. Mike has started going to the gym with his roommate. While lifting weights, Mike notices that his roommate can lift 30 pounds more than Mike can. Mike should not get discouraged because this disparity is due to:

   A. Individual differences

   B. Overload

   C. Consistency

5. Jim is on the track team. He used to stretch first thing when he went to practice, but recently his coach told the team that they should be stretching after their warm-ups.

   The coach changed the workout order because:

   A. The team was too impatient to stretch before their warm-up.

   B. Stretching is safer when the muscles are warmer.

   C. Stretching is not an important aspect of a workout.

6. Amelia needs to buy a new pair of shoes for exercising. She has a history of ankle sprains. She should find shoes that offer:

A variety of athletic shoes exist: running/jogging, walking, tennis, court, and cross-training. Properly sized socks help prevent blisters, ingrown toenails, and absorb perspiration.

Athletic shoes should have:

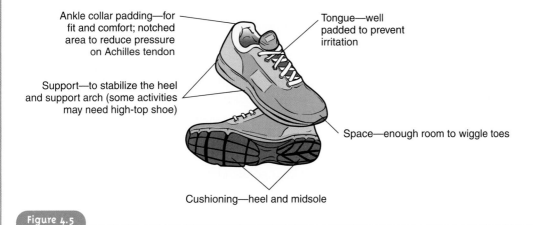

Ankle collar padding—for fit and comfort; notched area to reduce pressure on Achilles tendon

Tongue—well padded to prevent irritation

Support—to stabilize the heel and support arch (some activities may need high-top shoe)

Space—enough room to wiggle toes

Cushioning—heel and midsole

Figure 4.5

Select your athletic footwear carefully.

A. A wider toe box
B. Special arch support
C. A high-top style that offers more ankle support

7. Deciding to pursue leg extensions to work directly on the quad muscles in the legs is an example of:
   A. Progression
   B. Specificity
   C. Overload
   D. Consistency

8. Joanie used to work out all the time, and she was pleased with her body. Now she is rarely active; she has gained weight and feels sluggish. The change in Joanie reflects which principle of fitness?
   A. Reversibility
   B. Progression
   C. Overload
   D. Safety

9. What is the acronym used to remember the dimensions of designing a workout?
   A. SPLAT
   B. BUFF
   C. WORK
   D. FITT

10. Which of the following is not a general rule related to clothing for exercise?
    A. Wear cotton blends to absorb sweat effectively.
    B. Clothing should allow you to move freely.
    C. Wear protective gear when necessary.
    D. All are general rules for exercise.

Modern Modifications

Try these suggestions when you find yourself becoming sedentary:

- Take breaks from long periods of sitting. Get up and stretch every 15 minutes. Walk across the room a few times.
- While watching television, do a couple of simple exercises. Try sets of crunches, leg lifts, or modified push-ups during the commercials.
- While sitting in class or at a computer for an extended period of time, sit only on the front 6 inches of the seat, keeping your back straight. Correct posture will naturally engage your abs and other muscle groups as you sit.
- Do not use the remote. Get up to change the channels or turn the power on or off.

Critical Thinking

1. Leroy is a predominantly sedentary person but has decided to begin physical activity in 2 weeks. What stage is Leroy in? Based on the Physical Activity Pyramid, what activities should be in Leroy's plan for the first week?
2. Consider the activities you do around your house in the evening. Identify five moderate-level activities you could integrate into your evening routine.

Going Above and Beyond

Websites

American Alliance for Health, Physical Education, Recreation, and Dance

http://www.aahperd.org

American College of Sports Medicine

http://www.acsm.org

American Council on Exercise

http://www.acefitness.org

American Heart Association

http://www.heart.org/HEARTORG/

Canada's Physical Activity Guide

http://www.phac-aspc.ca/pau-uap/paguide

CDC Physical Activity Information

http://www.cdc.gov/physicalactivity/

Health A to Z

http://www.myoptumhealth.com/portal/

Medicine and Science in Sports and Exercise

http://journals.lww.com/acsm-msse/pages/default.aspx

Physician and Sports Medicine

http://www.physsportsmed.com

References and Suggested Readings

————. *Why Should I Be Active?* 2004. http://www.cdc.gov/physicalactivity/everyone /health/index.html [June 18, 2004].

American College of Sports Medicine. *ACSM's Guidelines for Exercise Testing and Prescription.* Baltimore, MD: Lippincott Williams & Wilkins, 2006.

Balady G. J. Survival of the fittest—More evidence. *New England Journal of Medicine* 2002; 346:852–854.

Blair S. N., Cheng Y., and Holder J. S. Is physical activity or physical fitness more important in defining health benefits? *Medicine and Science in Sports and Exercise* 2001; 33: S379–S399.

Edlin G. and Golanty E. *Health and Wellness,* 9th ed. Sudbury, MA: Jones and Bartlett, 2007.

Garber C. E., Blissmer B., Deschenes M. R., Franklin B. A., Lamonte M. J., Lee I. M., Nieman D. C., and Swain D. P. Quantity and quality of exercise for developing and maintaining cardiorespiratory, musculoskeletal, and neuromotor fitness in apparently healthy adults: Guidance for prescribing exercise. *Medicine and Science in Sports and Exercise* 2011; 7:1334–1359.

National Center for Chronic Disease Prevention and Health Promotion (NCCDPHP). *Components of Physical Fitness.* 2003. http://www.cdc.gov/physicalactivity/everyone /glossary/index.html

National Center for Health Statistics (NCHS) Vital Statistics System. *10 Leading Causes of Deaths, United States.* 2001. http://www.cdc.gov/injury/index.html [June 18, 2004].

Pescatello L. S. Exercising for health: The merits of lifestyle physical activity. *Western Journal of Medicine* 2001; 174:114–118.

Pfeiffer R., and Mangus B. *Concepts of Athletic Training,* 5th ed. Sudbury, MA: Jones and Bartlett, 2008.

U.S. Dept. of Health and Human Services (U.S. DHHS). *2008 Physical Activity Guidelines for Americans.* www.health.gov/paguidelines.

U.S. Dept. of Health and Human Services, Centers for Disease Control and Prevention, National Center for Chronic Disease Prevention and Health Promotion, and President's Council on Physical Fitness and Sports. *Physical Activity and Health: A Report of the Surgeon General.* Atlanta, GA: U.S. DHHS, 1996.

CHAPTER 5

Cardiorespiratory Endurance

Objectives

After reading this chapter, you should be able to:

- Differentiate between *aerobic* and *anaerobic* activities.
- Describe the benefits of cardiorespiratory exercises.
- Measure and assess your cardiorespiratory endurance.
- Design an appropriate cardiorespiratory exercise program.

The Doorway to Cardiorespiratory Activity

From a health standpoint, **cardiorespiratory endurance activity** is about as close as you can get to an elixir for physical health and well-being. It can help you lose weight, ease stress, boost your immune system, and reduce the risk of certain diseases.

There are a few *buzz words* that are basically synonymous with cardiorespiratory activity:

- Cardiovascular activity
- Cardiopulmonary activity
- **Aerobic exercise**

Merriam-Webster's Dictionary defines *aerobic* as "occurring only in the presence of oxygen." Linked with exercise, *aerobic* refers to any activity that increases oxygen intake and heart rate and keeps them elevated for at least 20 minutes.

When you exercise aerobically, you repeatedly contract large muscle groups, such as your legs and arms, and increase your breathing and your heart rate.

Examples of aerobic exercises include:

- walking (brisk pace);
- jogging/running;
- bicycling: road or mountain;
- in-line skating or rollerblading;
- swimming;
- cross-country skiing;
- treadmill;
- stationary bicycle;
- stair climber;
- rowing machine; and
- aerobic dancing.

To understand how you benefit from these kinds of activities, you must first have a basic understanding of how the cardiorespiratory system works.

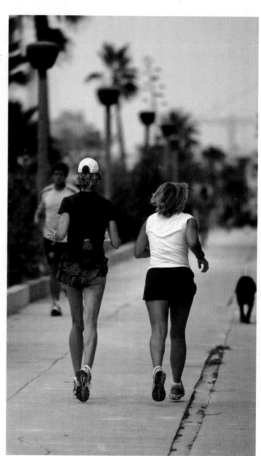

Basic Physiology

The cardiorespiratory system consists of the following components:

- **heart:** a muscle required to continuously deliver oxygen-rich blood to all the organs of the body;
- **lungs:** organs that provide the body with oxygen and rid the body of carbon dioxide through respiration; and
- **blood vessels:** a system of arteries, veins, and capillaries that transports blood to and from the heart.

Cardiovascular Processes

The processes of respiration and circulation (**pulmonary** and **systemic**) are connected within the cardiovascular system. Working together, the heart, lungs, and blood vessels deliver and transport oxygen to the body without stopping. **Figure 5.1** outlines this intricate process in eight basic stages.

> **What's the word...**
>
> **cardiorespiratory endurance activity**
> Exercise that contracts large muscle groups and increases breathing and heart rate.
>
> **aerobic exercise**
> Exercise that depends on oxygen for energy production.

> **What's the word...**
>
> **pulmonary circulation**
> Circulation between the heart and the lungs.
>
> **systemic circulation**
> Circulation between the heart and the rest of the body.

5

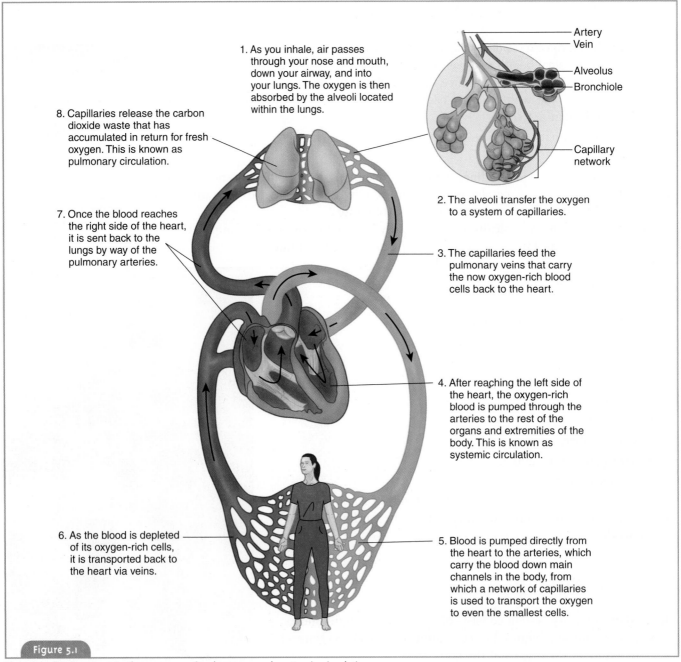

1. As you inhale, air passes through your nose and mouth, down your airway, and into your lungs. The oxygen is then absorbed by the alveoli located within the lungs.

Artery
Vein
Alveolus
Bronchiole
Capillary network

8. Capillaries release the carbon dioxide waste that has accumulated in return for fresh oxygen. This is known as pulmonary circulation.

7. Once the blood reaches the right side of the heart, it is sent back to the lungs by way of the pulmonary arteries.

2. The alveoli transfer the oxygen to a system of capillaries.

3. The capillaries feed the pulmonary veins that carry the now oxygen-rich blood cells back to the heart.

4. After reaching the left side of the heart, the oxygen-rich blood is pumped through the arteries to the rest of the organs and extremities of the body. This is known as systemic circulation.

6. As the blood is depleted of its oxygen-rich cells, it is transported back to the heart via veins.

5. Blood is pumped directly from the heart to the arteries, which carry the blood down main channels in the body, from which a network of capillaries is used to transport the oxygen to even the smallest cells.

Figure 5.1

The eight basic stages in the process of pulmonary and systemic circulation.

The ability of the body to deliver oxygen to and from the heart is critical. The more active you are, the more efficient your pulmonary and circulatory systems become. The less active you are, the weaker your heart muscle will be. Being sedentary and out of shape may have a more detrimental effect on your health than other well-known risk factors such as smoking, high blood pressure, and heart disease (Myers et al., 2002).

The basic idea underlying cardiorespiratory or aerobic training is to place greater demands on the heart than what is required during rest. By regularly overloading the heart in this fashion, it will become stronger. This results in the heart pumping more blood and delivering more oxygen to the body per heartbeat, creating a lower resting heart rate. See Lab 5-1 to determine your current resting heart rate.

Benefits of Cardiorespiratory Endurance Exercise

Regular endurance exercise can benefit the body in many healthy ways. Following are the short- and long-term benefits achieved by exercising regularly, using the cardiorespiratory system.

Short-Term Benefits

Many people start a physical activity program because of its long-term benefits; however, it is the short-term benefits that keep them motivated to continue the habit.

Relaxes and Revitalizes

Physical activity reduces mental and muscular tension and increases concentration and energy levels. Regular aerobic exercise releases endorphins.

Offers a Break from Daily Routine and Stress

Planned or unplanned physical activity can be enjoyable and provide a release from day-to-day stress and boredom.

Helps You Feel Good About Yourself

Physical activity can improve your self-esteem and self-confidence, and enhance your general sense of well-being.

Long-Term Benefits

Decreases Risk of Heart Disease

The leading health threat today is cardiovascular disease, which includes heart attack, stroke, hypertension, coronary artery disease (the buildup of fatty deposits on the inside of arteries), and congestive heart failure. Coronary artery disease (also called heart disease) and stroke are major causes of disability.

Prevents plaque buildup in arteries. Atherosclerosis is another key factor in cardiovascular disease. Fatty deposits called plaques build up as particles of low-density lipoprotein (LDL, or "bad" cholesterol) pass out of the bloodstream and lodge in weakened portions of artery walls, including the arteries supplying the heart and the brain. Over time, these plaques can narrow the vessels enough to deprive these organs of oxygen-rich blood. When this happens in the heart, it can lead to a heart attack. Blocked arteries in the brain can result in a stroke.

Moderate to vigorous aerobic exercise increases healthy high-density lipoprotein (HDL) cholesterol in our blood. HDL transports fats back to your liver for metabolism, preventing their accumulation along artery walls. Exercise also reduces the blood levels of unhealthy LDL cholesterol and triglycerides.

Protects arteries. Exercise can help keep arteries resilient. Regular expansion and contraction of arteries during exercise keeps the vessels "in shape."

Makes clots less likely. Exercise helps keep the inner lining of the arteries healthy and thereby less prone to injuries that set the stage for plaque formation. It also inhibits clot formation by making platelets less "sticky" and promotes the release of enzymes that break down clots. Higher activity levels lower inflammation in the arteries.

Promotes new coronary arteries. Aerobic exercise can lead to an increase in the size and number of coronary arteries feeding the heart. If an arterial blockage occurs, there is less risk of heart muscle damage because there are alternative channels to keep the blood supply flowing.

The Inside Track

Before menopause, women's risk for cardiovascular disease is lower than that of men. After menopause, women's risk becomes closer to that of men.

What's the word...

endorphins Proteins produced in your brain that serve as your body's natural pain-killer. Endorphins also reduce stress, depression, and anxiety.

The Inside Track

Women's bone density is typically greatest in their mid-20s to mid-30s, but then declines slowly until menopause, which is a time of rapid bone loss. Physical activity in younger years will help women maintain good bone mass at menopause. Even physical activity begun later in life or during menopause will help slow the loss of bone.

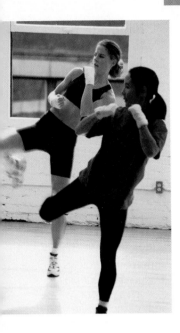

Decreases Risk of Cancer

Exercise increases circulation and respiration, accelerates the movement of food through the bowels, improves energy metabolism and immune function, and affects hormone levels. All of these may help protect against most types of cancer.

Lowers Blood Pressure

Exercise helps protect you from cardiovascular disease in numerous ways. The less active you are, the more likely you are to develop hypertension. Chronic hypertension doubles or triples the risk for developing congestive heart failure and can lead to heart disease, brain hemorrhage, aortic aneurysms, kidney disease and failure, and damage to other organs.

Increases Stamina

Exercise may cause fatigue immediately after the activity. Over the long term, though, it will increase stamina and reduce fatigue.

Lowers Body Fat

Exercise can counter creeping weight gain. Approximately 70% of the energy burned every day is taken up by bodily functions; the remaining 30% depends on our level of activity, so exercise choices certainly make a difference.

For people who are already overweight, exercise is an integral part of any weight-loss program. The most effective way to lose weight is to increase your level of activity and to reduce the calories you consume.

Cutting back on calories leads to faster weight loss than from exercising. Because you need to burn 3500 calories to lose a single pound, it may take a few weeks of regular, moderate exercise to successfully do so. However, consuming 500 less calories a day will result in the loss of a pound a week.

If you only cut back on calories, however, you are more likely to regain the weight lost. That is because your body reacts to weight loss as if it were starving and, in response, slows its metabolism. When your metabolism slows, you burn less calories. Increasing your physical activity will counteract the metabolic slowdown caused by reducing calories.

Exercise raises your energy expenditure while you are exercising and also while you are resting when the workout is done. Pounds lost by increasing your activity level consist almost entirely of fat.

Improves Muscular Health

Aerobic exercise stimulates the growth of blood vessels and capillaries in the muscles, providing for more efficient oxygen delivery to the muscles and helping to remove irritating metabolic waste products such as lactic acid. This can reduce pain in those who have fibromyalgia and chronic low-back pain.

Reduces the Number of Sick Days

Many studies report that people who exercise regularly are less susceptible to minor viral illnesses, such as colds or flu, because of an improved immune system.

Decreases the Chance of Premature Death

In 1986, results from the Harvard Alumni Health Study published in the *New England Journal of Medicine* for the first time linked exercise with increased life spans. Since then, additional research has supported this finding.

Decreases Cholesterol and Triglyceride Levels

High blood cholesterol and triglyceride levels increase the risk of heart disease. Regular exercise raises the level of good cholesterol (HDL), which may help to clear blood vessels and to lower the level of bad cholesterol (LDL). HDLs and LDLs are discussed further in the text.

Decreases the Risk of Diabetes

Untreated or poorly treated diabetes can lead to blindness, kidney disease, and the loss of limbs. It is also a major factor in heart disease and stroke.

All cells need sugar as a source of energy. Insulin, a hormone produced by the pancreas, helps cells extract sugar from the blood. When you have diabetes, your body is unable to make or use insulin efficiently, so you have excess sugar (glucose) in your blood. About 5% to 10% of people with diabetes cannot make insulin at all; this condition is called type 1 diabetes. Those who have type 1 diabetes must take daily insulin shots.

Type 2 diabetes accounts for 90% to 95% of cases of diabetes. In type 2 diabetes, the pancreas can pump out more insulin for a time, but eventually it cannot keep up with the greater demand, and blood glucose levels rise. Type 2 diabetes often can be controlled by diet and exercise, although medications or insulin may eventually be needed.

Exercise lowers modest amounts of blood glucose and boosts the body's sensitivity to insulin. This can help control existing diabetes and, most important, stave off the onset of type 2 diabetes.

Decreases the Risk of Osteoporosis

Weight-bearing exercise is necessary to stimulate the growth of new bone tissue. When demands are put on a bone, it responds by becoming stronger and denser.

Any activity that works against gravity can potentially build bone. Examples of such activities include running, walking, weight lifting, and stair climbing. However, activities such as swimming or biking, which are not weight-bearing, do not build bone. Higher-impact activities or resistance exercises (e.g., strength training) have a greater effect on bone than lower-impact exercises (e.g., walking) do. Only the bone that actually bears the load of the exercise will benefit, however. For example, walking or running protects bones in the lower extremities. A well-rounded strength training plan can help all of your bones.

Decreases Arthritis Symptoms

Overuse of certain joints can set the stage for arthritis, but regular moderate activity does not raise the risk for this disease developing in normal joints. Instead, moderate exercise—whether aerobic or resistance—actually helps to reduce swelling in joints and relieve pain. When joints are not used, the cartilage thins and softens, making the joint more vulnerable to arthritis. Exercise can also control weight. Overweight and obesity put people at a much higher risk for developing arthritis.

> **What's the word...**
>
> **type 2 diabetes** A disease that involves the inability to produce an adequate amount of insulin.
>
> **obesity** Excessive amounts of body fat.

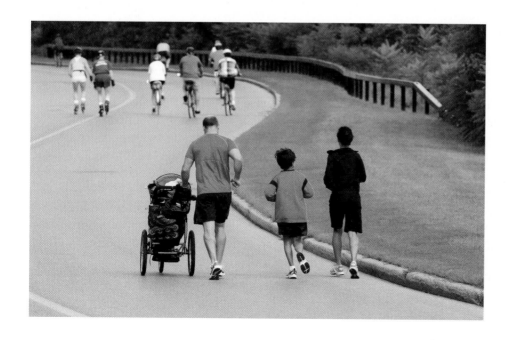

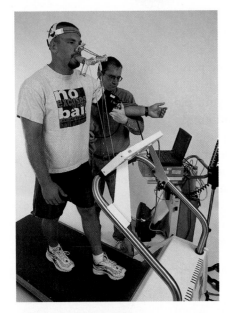

Assessing Cardiorespiratory Fitness/Endurance

Cardiorespiratory fitness or endurance is largely determined by physical activity. As defined earlier in the chapter, aerobic, or cardiorespiratory, exercise involves oxygen. When you assess your cardiorespiratory endurance, you are actually measuring how efficiently your system is using oxygen.

Maximal Oxygen Uptake

Determining maximal oxygen uptake (VO_{2max}):
- is the best measure of cardiorespiratory fitness;
- reveals how much oxygen is delivered to body tissues; and
- requires an exercise physiology laboratory with trained personnel to analyze a person's oxygen intake.

Maximal tests can be substituted with field tests, which are a comparable way to score the VO_{2max}. They are less expensive, require little to no equipment, and are, therefore, more practical.

What's the word...

maximal oxygen uptake (VO_{2max}) How efficiently the cardiorespiratory system uses oxygen.

Field Tests

Field tests can give a fairly good estimate of VO_{2max}. The following are among the field tests features:
- Monitoring your heart rate is necessary for these tests.
- Large numbers of people can be tested at one time.
- The tests require little equipment.
- Test results can be affected by a person's motivation and pacing ability.

The following tests are commonly used to judge cardiorespiratory endurance. The instructions for each are provided in the corresponding lab:
- Rockport Fitness Walking Test™ (**Lab 5-2** , Activity 1)
- YMCA Step Test (**Lab 5-2** , Activity 4)
- Cooper's 1.5-Mile Run/Walk Test (**Lab 5-2** , Activity 3)

Complete the PAR-Q, **Lab 4-1** , before taking any of these tests.

Designing a Cardiorespiratory Endurance Exercise Program

The Inside Track

A common mistake is to do stretching exercises before the muscles are warmed up; not only is it difficult to stretch cold muscles, but there are also risks to exercising heavily on muscles that are not warm, especially as you get older.

Cardiorespiratory exercise, also called aerobic exercise, consists of physical activities in which people move their large muscles in a rhythmic manner for a sustained period. Running, brisk walking, bicycling, playing basketball, dancing, and swimming are all examples of aerobic activities. Aerobic activity makes a person's heart beat more rapidly to meet the demands of the body's movement. Over time, regular aerobic activity makes the heart and the cardiovascular system stronger and fitter.

The purpose of the aerobic activity does not affect whether it counts toward meeting the recommended exercise amounts. For example, physically active occupations can count toward meeting the recommendations, as can active transportation choices (walking or bicycling). All types of aerobic activities can count as long as they are of sufficient intensity and duration. Time spent in muscle strengthening activities does not count toward the aerobic activity guidelines.

Table 5.1	2008 Physical Activity Guidelines for Adults

- All adults should avoid inactivity. Some physical activity is better than none, and adults who participate in any amount of physical activity gain some health benefits.
- For substantial health benefits, adults should do at least 150 minutes (2 hours and 30 minutes) a week of moderate-intensity, or 75 minutes (1 hour and 15 minutes) a week of vigorous-intensity aerobic physical activity, or an equivalent combination of moderate- and vigorous-intensity aerobic activity. Aerobic activity should be performed in episodes of at least 10 minutes, and preferably, it should be spread throughout the week.
- For additional and more extensive health benefits, adults should increase their aerobic physical activity to 300 minutes (5 hours) a week of moderate-intensity, or 150 minutes a week of vigorous-intensity aerobic physical activity, or an equivalent combination of moderate- and vigorous-intensity activity. Additional health benefits are gained by engaging in physical activity beyond this amount.
- Adults should also do muscle-strengthening activities that are moderate or high intensity and involve all major muscle groups on 2 or more days a week, as these activities provide additional health benefits.

Source: Reproduced from the 2008 Physical Activity Guidelines for Americans. Courtesy of the U.S. Department of Health & Human Services.

It is important to consider the total amount of activity, as well as how often to be active, for how long, and at what intensity (see **Table 5.1**). Every person has individual needs. Your exercise program should consist of physical activities that are right for your body and your endurance level and that make you feel good, both mentally and physically. As you proceed with your program, make sure that you:

- warm up and cool down;
- follow the FITT (Frequency, Intensity, Time, Type) guidelines; and
- progress safely.

Warm-up

Begin each exercise session with a warm-up.

- Usually, the warm-up involves the same activity as the workout, but at a low intensity.
- You can also simply swing your arms from side-to-side for a couple of minutes or walk around at a steady pace.
- After 5 to 10 minutes, stretch the primary muscles used in the warm-up before proceeding to the cardiorespiratory endurance exercise.

Cool-down

End each exercise session with a cool-down.

- The cool-down should last 5 to 10 minutes and be done at a low intensity.
- Allow your heart rate, breathing, and circulation to return to normal.
- Stretch the primary muscles used.

The Inside Track

Those who are considered obese should avoid vigorous-intensity workouts and should consult a doctor before beginning an exercise regimen.

FITT Guidelines

After the warm-up, the FITT formula is an easy way to design an effective aerobic exercise program.

F = Frequency

Aerobic physical activity should preferably be spread throughout the week. Studies consistently show that activity performed on at least 3 days a week produces health benefits.

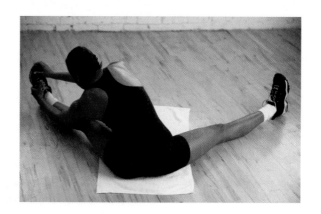

5

Spreading physical activity across at least 3 days a week may help to reduce the risk of injury and avoid excessive fatigue.

Both moderate- and vigorous-intensity aerobic activity should be performed in episodes of at least 10 minutes. Episodes of this duration are known to improve cardiovascular fitness and some risk factors for heart disease and type 2 diabetes.

I = Intensity

Adults should focus on two levels of intensity: moderate-intensity activity and vigorous-intensity activity. Adults can do either moderate-intensity or vigorous-intensity aerobic activities, or a combination of both. It takes less time to get the same benefit from vigorous-intensity activities than from moderate-intensity activities. A general rule of thumb is that 2 minutes of moderate-intensity activity counts the same as 1 minute of vigorous-intensity activity. For example, 30 minutes of moderate-intensity activity a week is roughly the same as 15 minutes of vigorous-intensity activity.

Table 5.2 lists some examples of activities classified as moderate-intensity or vigorous-intensity based on absolute intensity. Either absolute or relative intensity can be used to monitor progress in meeting the guidelines.

There are several ways to monitor exercise intensity:

- heart rate reserve (HRR);
- perceived exertion;
- calories; and
- talk-test.

The Inside Track

Resting between high-intensity workouts is essential to preventing injury and promoting recovery.

Calculating Intensity Training Range Using the Heart Rate Reserve Method

Your heart rate is the most precise way to monitor the intensity of your exercise. Heart rate is the number of heartbeats per minute (bpm). Heart rate can vary as the body's need to absorb oxygen and excrete carbon dioxide changes as during exercise or sleep.

Table 5.2	Examples of Different Aerobic Physical Activities and Intensities

Moderate Intensity

- Walking briskly (3 miles per hour or faster, but not race-walking)
- Water aerobics
- Bicycling slower than 10 miles per hour
- Tennis (doubles)
- Ballroom dancing
- General gardening

Vigorous Intensity

- Racewalking, jogging, or running
- Swimming laps
- Tennis (singles)
- Aerobic dancing
- Bicycling 10 miles per hour or faster
- Jumping rope
- Heavy gardening (continuous digging or hoeing, with heart rate increases)
- Hiking uphill or with a heavy backpack

Note: This table provides several examples of activities classified as moderate-intensity or vigorous-intensity. This list is not all-inclusive. Instead, the examples are meant to help people make choices.

Source: Data from the *2008 Physical Activities for Americans.* Courtesy of the U.S. Dept. of Health and Human Services.

The Heart Rate Reserve (HRR) is preferred for individuals determining their heart rate intensity training range. Other methods are either not as accurate or difficult to understand, and few people are familiar with them. Follow these steps to determine your heart rate intensity training range:

Step 1: Determine Your Maximum Heart Rate

Your maximum heart rate (HRmax) is the highest heart rate you can safely achieve through exercise. It depends on age. You can use a formula to estimate HRmax.

For exercisers, the typical way we once calculated HRmax was with the formula: HRmax = 220 − age. While it is easy to remember and calculate, it is not considered to be accurate by reputable health and fitness professionals. The formula is a bit controversial because it does not reflect the differences in heart rate according to age.

A more accurate formula involves a bit more math than the original equation. The better formula is: HRmax = 208 − (0.7 × age). Here is an example for a 25-year-old: 208 (0.7 × 25) = 190.5.

Step 2: Determine Your Resting Heart Rate

The resting heart rate (HRrest) refers to the number of times your heart beats in 1 minute while at rest. To take your resting heart rate, feel your pulse the first thing in the morning. For tips on taking your pulse, see ⬤ Box 5.1 . You can also take your pulse after resting for 20–30 minutes if you are not able to do it in the morning. You should try for at least three different readings on separate days and calculate the average heart rate reading. Locate your pulse by placing your index finger and middle finger together on either your radial artery on your wrist or your carotid artery on your neck. After you find the pulse beat, count the number of beats in 60 seconds.

As your cardiorespiratory system gets better, your resting heart rate decreases because your stronger heart is now capable of pumping more blood with each beat.

Step 3: Calculate Your Heart Rate Reserve

To determine your heart rate reserve (HRR), subtract your resting heart rate (HRrest) from your maximum heart rate (HRmax). For example, a 25-year-old with a HRmax of 190.5 and HRrest of 70 has a HRR = 190.5 − 70 = 120.5.

Step 4: Calculate the Low End of Your Heart Rate Training Zone

To calculate the low end of your heart rate training zone, select either the moderate intensity or vigorous intensity unless you are unfit (see ⬤ Table 5.3 for the classifications and heart rate training zones). The formula is: HRR × intensity % + HRrest for the low end of a moderate heart rate training zone.

Example: For a 25-year-old with a resting pulse of 70, selecting a vigorous intensity training range:
190.5 × 0.6 + 70 = 142 bpm for the low end of a heart rate vigorous training range.

Step 5: Calculate the High End of Your Heart Rate Training Range

In the previous step, you used the formula (known as the Karvonen formula) to calculate the lower end of your moderate exercise heart rate training zone. You use the same formula to calculate the higher end.

Example: For a 25-year-old with a resting pulse of 70, selecting a vigorous intensity exercise program:
190.5 × 0.8 + 70 = 166 beats per minute for the high end of a vigorous heart rate training range.

5

Box 5.1	Pulse-Taking Tips

Pulse Palpation Sites

Baroreceptors in the carotid sinus can be sensitive to pressure, causing a reduced heart rate in some individuals. A thicker fat layer over the radial pulse site may make it more difficult to obtain a pulse in some individuals. Other palpation-accessible sites include the brachial artery and temporal (skull).

Bradycardia

Generally, a lower pulse rate is good. It is possible, however, that one's heart rate can be too low. A heart rate of less than 60 bpm is known as bradycardia, a condition that can be dangerous, especially when blood pressure is also low. Symptoms seldom occur until the rate drops below 50 bpm. These symptoms include weakness, fatigue, and fainting. Medical attention should be sought immediately if these symptoms are present.

Trained athletes can have pulse rates as low as 40 to 60 BPM. Resting bradycardia in athletes should not be considered abnormal if the individual has no symptoms associated with it.

Monitoring Time

A 15-second pulse is recommended for taking heart rate during rest and exercise. If an accurate pulse cannot be obtained during exercise, it is acceptable to stop exercising and immediately take a pulse. Since post-exercise heart rate decreases rapidly, a 6- or 10-second pulse should be taken.

- An error of 1 bpm during a 6-second count results in an error of 10 bpm.
- An error of 1 bpm during a 10-second count results in an error of 6 bpm.
- An error of 1 bpm during a 15-second count results in an error of 4 bpm.

Heart Rate Monitoring

- At submax work intensity, it may take about 3 minutes before the heart rate stabilizes after an increase in exercise intensity.
- Manual monitoring:
  - If time is started at the first beat, the first beat is counted as "0."
  - If heart rate is monitored immediately after the start of time (as in a group setting), the first beat is counted as "1."
- The maximum heart rate in the horizontal position is 10 to 15 beats lower than that in the vertical position, because the heart does not have to work as much against gravity in the horizontal position as in the vertical position.

Warnings

- Do not press too hard on your neck, as pressing too hard can stimulate a reflex mechanism that can slow down the heart.
- Do not palpate both carotid arteries on your neck simultaneously, as it will decrease the blood circulation to the brain.
- If you notice skipped beats while doing this procedure, seek medical attention.
- If you notice that your heartbeat is really fast—above 135—and is not normal for you, seek medical advice.
- If you can obviously tell that your heartbeat is irregular as well as really fast, follow up with medical attention.

Table 5.3	Classification of Cardiorespiratory Endurance Exercise Intensity
Intensity	**Heart Rate Reserve (HRR) Percentage**
Very light	<20%
Light	20–39%
Moderate	40–59%
Hard	60–84%
Very hard	>85%

Source: Adapted from Howley E. T. Type of activity: Resistance, aerobic and leisure versus occupational physical activity. *Medicine and Science in Sports and Exercise* 2001; 33(6 Suppl):S364–S369.

In the example of a 25-year–old, he or she has a heart rate training zone between 142 to 166 beats per minute for a vigorous exercise program. If you have fractions in the calculations, you can round numbers off. Lab 5.2 provides an opportunity to calculate your heart rate training range.

Your next step is to figure out how to use these numbers in your workout to make sure you are working at the right intensity. For the example of the 25-year-old, when this person exercises, he or she should try to reach the heart rate training zone (142 to 166 bpm) and maintain it for the duration of the cardiorespiratory activity. Several times or halfway through the aerobic activity, he or she should take a 6-second pulse check and add a 0 to get the 1-minute figure (you could also do a 10-second count and multiply by 6 or a 15-second count and multiply by 4). The longer pulse counts are more accurate. However, the heart rate will slow within a minute of stopping an activity; so, to be accurate, you must be quick to count the pulse beats.

Exercise classified as moderate-intensity or vigorous-intensity in Table 5.2 meets the recommended programs for adults. In this table, exercise intensity of near-maximal to maximal should be performed only by those in excellent aerobic condition. Exercise in this range cannot be sustained for long time periods and is primarily performed to develop the anaerobic capabilities and improve performance in activities such as sprinting and bursts of speed.

Now that you know how to calculate your training zone, determining the intensity level at which you should exercise is quite simple. Exercising within the training range enables most individuals to achieve good health, fitness, and weight management goals.

When starting an exercise program, aim at the lowest value of your training range during the first few weeks. Gradually build up to the higher values of your training range—this may take at least 1 month or up to 6 months or more. Progressing gradually in a cardiorespiratory exercise program helps to avoid muscle aches, pain, and discouragement.

You should always be able to catch your breath and speak comfortably while moderately exercising. Feeling effort or maybe even slight discomfort is normal during some exercises. Always warm up slowly and cool down gradually.

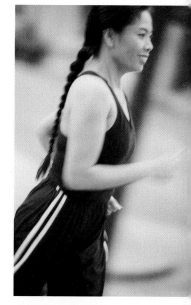

Perceived Exertion

Exercise intensity can be monitored by your subjective feelings of exertion and fatigue. Very simply, when your exercise feels "somewhat hard" to "hard," you may be within your recommended **target heart rate range**. Use your perceived exertion by measuring your heart rate while in the target heart rate zone and then associate it with how you feel when you are exercising in the zone. For future workouts, exercise hard enough to experience what you felt when you were within your target heart rate zone. Some believe this method is easier than stopping for a 10-second **pulse** count.

What's the word. . .

target heart rate range A range of heart rates used to maintain optimal effects during aerobic exercise.

pulse The surge of blood that can be felt on certain points on the body each time the heart pumps blood into the arteries.

5

What's the word...

rate of perceived exertion (RPE) A person's own perception of the intensity of his or her exercise.

However, use caution when you depend on your perceived exertion to judge exercise intensity because individuals vary as to what is "somewhat hard" or "hard." This may be especially true for those with an aversion to strenuous physical activity. Additionally, feelings of exertion and fatigue may be influenced by the type of exercise, psychological factors, and environmental conditions. Studies related to the **ratings of perceived exertion (RPE)** scales revealed inconsistencies about the strength of the relationship between ratings of perceived exertion and various physiological criterion measures (e.g., heart rate, VO_{2max}, etc.).

Talk-Test Method

The talk-test method of measuring intensity is simple. A person who is active at a light-intensity level should be able to talk while doing the activity. One who is active at a moderate-intensity level should be able to carry on a conversation comfortably while engaging in the activity. If a person becomes winded or too out-of-breath to carry on a conversation, the activity can be considered vigorous.

Calories: Not Just for Dieting

Calories per hour is the amount of energy that an exerciser expends when maintaining the same exercise intensity for an hour. This value can be roughly calculated by most exercise machines and pedometers. Please see **Box 5.2** for instructions on how to use a pedometer.

It is possible, of course, to calculate the number of calories you would burn by participating in a variety of activities. The basic formula is to multiply your weight (in pounds) by the number of minutes in the activity and by a caloric expenditure figure. Caloric expenditures for several common activities are found in **Table 5.4**.

For example, if you weighed 120 pounds and you bicycled at a moderate pace for 30 minutes, you would take $120 \times 30 \times 0.05$. The result indicates that you burned 180 calories during that activity.

T = Time

When adults do the equivalent of 150 minutes of moderate-intensity aerobic activity each week, the benefits are *substantial*. These benefits include lower risk of premature death, coronary heart disease, stroke, hypertension, type 2 diabetes, and depression.

Medical News You Can Use

Walking Tops Weight Training for Metabolic Syndrome

Eight months of resistance training had little impact on metabolic syndrome (increased risk of cardiovascular disease and diabetes) in overweight adults with poor lipid profiles. But the same duration of aerobic exercise resulted in greater benefits for weight, waist circumference, triglycerides, and overall metabolic syndrome score. The combination of weights and aerobic exercise had significant benefits. However, doing both types of exercises was not significantly more effective than aerobics alone. For practical reasons, when weighing the time commitment versus the health benefit, to improve cardiovascular health, aerobic training alone was the most efficient method of exercise. These conclusions agree with guidelines from the American Heart Association supporting aerobic exercise over resistance training to improve cardiovascular health.

Source: Data from Bateman L.A., Comparison of aerobic versus resistance exercise training effects on metabolic syndrome (from the Studies of a Targeted Risk Reduction Intervention through Defined Exercise—STRRIDE-AT/RT). *American Journal of Cardiology* 2011. 108(6):838–844.

| Box 5.2 | Using a Pedometer To Track Walking |

For adults who prefer walking as a form of aerobic activity, pedometers or step counters are useful in tracking progress toward personal goals. Popular advice, such as walking 10,000 steps a day, is not a Guideline per se, but a way people may choose to meet the Guidelines. The key to using a pedometer to meet the Guidelines is to first set a time goal (minutes of walking a day) and then calculate how many steps are needed each day to reach that goal.

Episodes of brisk walking that last at least 10 minutes count toward meeting the Guidelines. However, just counting steps using a pedometer doesn't ensure that a person will achieve those 10-minute episodes. People generally need to plan episodes of walking if they are to use a pedometer and step goals appropriately.

As a basis for setting step goals, it's preferable that people know how many steps they take per minute of a brisk walk. A person with a low fitness level, who takes fewer steps per minute than a fit adult, will need fewer steps to achieve the same amount of walking time.

One way to set a step goal is the following:

- To determine usual daily steps from baseline activity, a person wears a pedometer to observe the number of steps taken on several ordinary days with no episodes of walking for exercise. Suppose the average is about 5,000 steps a day.
- While wearing the pedometer, the person measures the number of steps taken during 10 minutes of an exercise walk. Suppose this is 1,000 steps. Then, for a goal of 40 minutes of walking for exercise, the total number of steps would be 4,000 (1,000 × 4).
- To calculate a daily step goal, add the usual daily steps (5,000) to the steps required for a 40-minute walk (4,000), to get the total steps per day (5,000 + 4,000 = 9,000).

Each week the person gradually increases the time walking for exercise until the step goal is reached. Rate of progression should be individualized. Some people who start out at 5,000 steps a day can add 500 steps per day each week. Others, who are less fit and starting out at a lower number of steps, should add a smaller number of steps each week.

Source: Reprinted from the *2008 Physical Activity Guidelines for Americans.* Courtesy of the U.S. Department of Health and Human Services.

Not all health benefits of physical activity occur at 150 minutes a week. As a person moves from 150 minutes a week toward 300 minutes (5 hours) a week, he or she gains *additional* health benefits. Additional benefits include lower risk of colon and breast cancer and prevention of unhealthy weight gain.

Also, as a person moves from 150 minutes a week toward 300 minutes a week, the benefits that occur at 150 minutes a week become *more extensive.* For example, a person who does 300 minutes a week has an even lower risk of heart disease or diabetes than a person who does 150 minutes a week.

The benefits continue to increase when a person does more than the equivalent of 300 minutes a week of moderate-intensity aerobic activity. For example, a person who does 420 minutes (7 hours) a week has an even lower risk of premature death than a person who does 150 to 300 minutes a week. Current science does not allow identifying an upper limit of total activity above which there are no additional health benefits.

Table 5.4	Caloric Expenditures					
Activity	**Calories per Minute per Pound**	**Calories per Hour per 150 Pounds**		**Activity**	**Calories per Minute per Pound**	**Calories per Hour per 150 Pounds**

Archery	0.034	305		Rowing
				  Light (2.5 mph)
				  Vigorous
					0.036
					0.118
						325
						1062

Badminton
  Moderate
  Vigorous
	0.039
	0.065
		350
		585
				Running
				  6 mph (10-min mile)
				  10 mph (6-min mile)
				  12 mph (5-min mile)
					0.079
					0.1
					0.13
						710
						900
						1170

Basketball Moderate	0.047	423		Soccer	0.06	540

Baseball	0.031	279		Swimming
				  25 yd/min
				  50 yd/min
					0.058
					0.071
						520
						640

Bicycling
  Slow (5 mph)
  Moderate (10 mph)
  Fast (15 mph)
	0.025
	0.05
	0.072
		225
		450
		550
				Table tennis	0.025	225

Dancing
  Moderate
  Fast
	0.045
	0.064
		405
		575
				Tennis
				  Moderate
				  Vigorous
					0.046
					0.06
						415
						540

Fishing	0.018	165		Volleyball
				  Moderate
				  Vigorous
					0.036
					0.065
						325
						585

Gardening	0.024	220		Walking
				  2 mph
				  3 mph
				  4 mph
				  5 mph
					0.022
					0.03
					0.039
					0.064
						200
						270
						350
						576

Golf	0.029	260				
Hill climbing	0.06	540				
Jogging (4.5 mph)	0.063	565				
Karate	0.087	785		Wrestling	0.091	820

A cardiorespiratory endurance session should vary from 20 or more minutes—even a multiple of 10-minute sessions—to gain significant aerobic and fat-burning benefits. This does not include the warm-up and cool-down phases of your program. All beginners, especially those who are out of shape, should take a very conservative approach and train at low intensities for 10 to 25 minutes. As you get into better shape, you can gradually increase the length of time you exercise.

Gradually increase the duration of exercise before you increase the intensity. For example, when beginning a brisk walking program, be more concerned with increasing the number of minutes of the exercise session before you increase how fast you walk or add a hilly terrain.

T = Type of Aerobic Exercises

To choose the best exercises for you, consider the following:

- Choose an exercise that involves major muscle groups and that is continuous, rhythmic in nature, and weight-bearing. This will require the greatest amount of energy and oxygen to perform.

- Choose the exercises that you enjoy the most.
- Alleviate boredom and decrease your risk for injuries by cross-training or alternating the types of exercise you perform.

Table 5.5 provides a few choices of indoor and outdoor aerobic activities, and the pros and cons of why you may or may not choose one of these activities for your exercise.

Walking Technique

Most people of all ages and fitness levels can walk. You burn almost the same number of calories in briskly walking 1 mile as you do in jogging the same distance. Moreover, brisk walking usually involves less jarring of the joints. Practice these good walking techniques:

- Land on your heel and roll forward onto the ball of your foot, pushing off from your toes.
- Point your toes straight ahead.
- Take long, easy strides. To go faster, take quicker steps instead of longer ones.
- Hold your head up; keep your back straight.
- Let your arms swing loosely at your sides. To go faster, bend your elbows at a 90° angle and swing the arms more.

Here is a way to measure your walking speed. If on level ground, you can count your steps per minute to determine your speed:

- Slow = 80 steps per minute
- Moderate to brisk = 100 steps per minute
- Fast = 120 steps per minute
- Race walking = more than 120 steps per minute

Cross-Training

Cross-training involves different types of exercises, making your fitness routine more fun and beneficial. The American Academy of Orthopaedic Surgeons says that the benefits of cross-training program may include:

- toning the entire body because of the variety of activities;
- better likelihood of sticking with your exercise routine;
- better preparation of muscles for new exercises and working more muscle groups;
- reduced risk of overuse injury; and
- in case of injury, you are still able to perform some of your unusual exercises, with some modifications.

Interval Training

Interval training is a type of physical training that involves bursts of high-intensity exercise. This high-intensity workout is alternated with periods of recovery (which may involve complete rest and/or lower-intensity activity). The training can be used in any

5

Table 5.5	Types of Indoor and Outdoor Aerobic Activity	
Activity	**Pros**	**Cons**
Walking 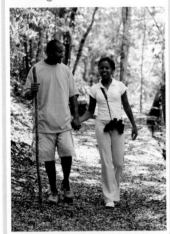	• Most popular of all activities • No age limit—a lifetime activity • Convenient • Easily incorporated into lifestyle • Little skill involved • No cost • Fewer injuries than jogging or running • You can take in seasonal changes or walk through city streets and people watch • This is a weight-bearing exercise • Uses most major lower-body muscle groups	• Not active enough for some • Takes three times longer to get the same aerobic benefit as from running • Injuries can occur, such as shin splints and blisters

Jogging/running
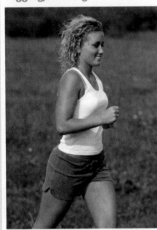
	• Convenient
	• High levels of cardiorespiratory fitness benefits in short time periods
	• Few skills needed
	• Impact on hard surface builds stronger bones and offers protection against osteoporosis
	• Euphoric feeling or "runner's high"
	• In bad weather, you can run on an indoor track, if one is available
	• Low cost—just need a good pair of running shoes
	• Because it is often done outdoors, you get to view nature and a change of scenery
		• Frequent, chronic injuries from impact to muscles, tendons, ligaments, and bones
		• Injuries such as shin splints and stress fractures due to:
		  • Improper warm-up
		  • Excessive distances
		  • Impact of feet and legs on ground
		  • Wearing inadequate shoes
		• Dangerous when done on roads with traffic
		• Poor outdoor conditions (i.e., snow, pollution) may prohibit

Bicycling: road or mountain 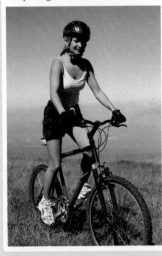	• No age limit—a lifetime activity • Fewer injuries than running because there is less impact on legs and feet • Because it is done outdoors, you get to view nature and a change of scenery	• May be difficult to locate a safe place to ride • Injuries include painful knees, feet, back, and saddle soreness • Cost for the bike and other gear such as helmet, gloves, water bottle, sunscreen, and glasses

Table 5.5	Types of Indoor and Outdoor Aerobic Activity, *continued*	
Activity	**Pros**	**Cons**
In-line skating or rollerblading 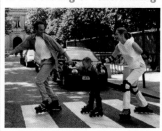	• Lots of fun—curving, turning, gliding, sprinting, and spinning • Change of scenery • Works thighs, hips, and buttocks muscles	• There is a learning curve, which could make the beginning stages a bit dangerous • May be difficult to locate a safe place to skate • Some people have difficulty stopping • Injuries may result from collisions, falling, and blisters • Requires skill and balance • Coasting loses the aerobic effects • Costs for skates, helmet, wrist guards, knee guards, elbow guards, and gloves
Swimming 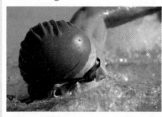	• Fewer injuries because there is no impact on legs and feet • Good for people who are: • Injured and want to keep exercising • Pregnant • Overweight • Works every part of the body, with an emphasis on the upper body • Refreshing • No age limit—lifetime activity	• You must locate a swimming pool and an available lane for swimming laps • Requires skill • Repetitive arm motions can result in pain and inflammation, leading to tendonitis and bursitis • Swimming laps can be repetitive and seem boring • Not a social activity • Since this exercise doesn't involve impact, it does not help build bone density • Risk of infections in the ears, eyes, and sinuses
Cross-country skiing 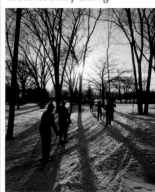	• Involves both lower and upper body, including most major muscle groups when poles are used • Rigorous workout obtained when at higher altitudes, in cold weather, and from added weight of clothing • Scenery changes • Low impact	• Exposure to cold conditions can lead to frostnip, frostbite, or hypothermia • Requires accessibility to snow • Skiing downhill decreases the aerobic effect
Treadmill 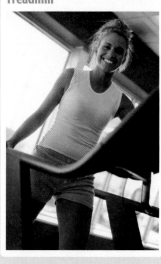	• Easily accessible no matter what the weather conditions • Good for beginners, many levels • Easy to use • Easier on joints than walking or jogging on asphalt and concrete surfaces • Can watch TV while exercising • Some machines have various personal high-tech computer programs that monitor heart rate	• Can get monotonous • Can stumble and slide off • Expensive to own; may require health club membership

continues

Table 5.5 | Types of Indoor and Outdoor Aerobic Activity, *continued*

Activity	Pros	Cons
Stationary bicycle 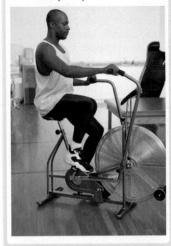	• Great thigh workout • Gives knees a rest • Can read or watch TV while exercising • Easy to use	• With stationary bikes you have added convenience, but lose the ability to ride outdoors • Expensive to own; may require health club membership
Rowing machine 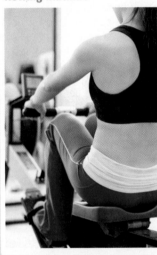	• Total body workout using most major muscle groups • Can watch TV while exercising • Will prepare you for outdoor rowing or paddling on a canoe or kayak	• Can strain back if not performed correctly • Repetitive motion can become boring • Requires coordination

Aerobic dancing 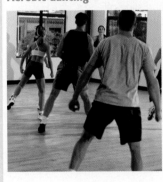	• Enjoyable
	• Can be done with a class or individually at home with a video or a televised class
	• Camaraderie can develop within a group of people working out together
	• Low injury rates
	• Different styles and variations of classes may be classified as below:
	  - High impact—more jumping and faster movement
	  - Low impact—less jumping and slower movement
	  - Aquatic—done in the water
	  - Step aerobics using a 6- to 12-inch step—increase impact and weight-bearing movement
	  - Kick boxing—uses movements of kick boxing for added variety and strength
	  - Circuit—uses weights and aerobics to work out upper body as well as to increase aerobic endurance
		• Possible injuries could occur, such as shin splints, tendonitis, muscle strain, back strain, and stress fracture
		• Cost of class or travel time to a gym

Medical News You Can Use

Drinking Chocolate Milk May Help Your Workout

Drinking low-fat chocolate milk after a workout helps endurance, builds muscle, and seems to improve performance. The drink seems to have the right combination of carbohydrates and protein. When recovering from exercise, two things you want to do is replenish sugar stores in the muscle and turn on protein synthesis and stop protein breakdown. The low-fat chocolate milk beat out two other drinks tested—a no-calorie beverage and a carbohydrate drink with no protein.

Source: Data from Ferguson-Stegall L., et al. Aerobic exercise training adaptations are increased by postexercise carbohydrate-protein supplementation. *Journal of Nutrition and Metabolism* Epub 2011 Jun 9; Article ID 623182.

cardiovascular workout (e.g., cycling, running, jogging). Interval training has been shown to better improve cardiorespiratory fitness, blood lipoproteins, and glucose levels than does single-intensity exercise. This type of training adds variety and helps you avoid boredom.

No single formula for the ratio between hard work and rest or moderate work exists. However, the high-intensity phase should be long and strenuous enough that you are out of breath—usually 1 to 4 minutes of exercise at 80% to 85% of your HRmax. Recovery periods should not be too long to reach the resting rate.

Stair Workouts

One form of interval training is walking or running stairs. Many athletes run stairs at a stadium, but you can also look for a local outdoor stairway or a stairwell in a building with about a hundred steps. If you have not done stair workouts before, you should plan to start slowly and gradually build up your time and intensity. Stair workouts use muscles you may not have used before and overdoing your first workout will result in unnecessary muscle soreness. Start out by walking or climbing the stairs. Later and depending upon your fitness level, you could try running up the stairs. Whether you walk or run *up* the stairs, you should walk *down* the stairs. Use caution especially when going down the stairs because falling by a misstep or inattentiveness can cause severe injuries.

Medical News You Can Use

Less Weight Gain with Biking, Fast Walking

Study participants who reported walking briskly or bicycling gained less weight over a 16-year period than those who did not participate in those activities. Researchers said that you should walk as if you were late for the bus. If you walk at 120 steps or fewer per minute, you are walking too slow. Bicycling is another option for those not comfortable with walking briskly. In the study, 39% of study participants reported walking briskly at baseline and 48% reported bicycling. However, by the end of the study, only 1.2% of participants were biking more than 30 minutes per day. Brisk walking appears to be the activity of choice to lose weight among study participants.

Source: Data from Lusk A., et al. Bicycle riding, walking, and weight gain in premenopausal women. *Archives of Internal Medicine* 2010; 170(12):1050–1056.

Progression

There is a tendency, when first beginning a fitness regimen, for people to do too much too quickly. Keep in mind that not meeting your goal the first day does not mean that you will not get there eventually. Slow and consistent improvement is the safe way to train. If you have been sedentary, begin by taking a brisk walk or by bouncing on an exercise ball for 5 to 10 minutes. Gradually increase the duration of the activity by 10% per week until you can perform 20 to 60 minutes continuously. Your training intensity during these exercise sessions should be between 70% and 85% of your HRmax.

Rules for Progression

1. Increase only one FITT component at a time. It is best to increase duration first.
2. Increase your exercise workout by no more than 10% per week. Increasing too fast can lead to injury.
3. Stop exercising and seek immediate health care if you experience any of the following:
   - tightness in your chest;
   - severe shortness of breath;
   - chest pain or pain in your arms or jaw, often on the left side;
   - heart palpitations; and
   - dizziness, faintness, or feeling sick in the stomach.

Overtraining

Overtraining occurs when an individual does not give the body sufficient time to recover between workouts. Some signs that you may be suffering from excessive training are:

- general aches and pains that do not seem to subside;
- leg, muscle, and joint soreness or injury;
- insomnia;
- inability to relax or irritability;
- feeling drained of energy;
- decreased workout performance;
- dehydration; and
- more likelihood for sickness (e.g., colds, sore throat, other minor ills).

Medical News You Can Use

Intense Exercise May Protect Aging Brain

Older people who regularly exercise at moderate to intense levels may have a 40% lower risk of developing brain damage linked to strokes, certain kinds of dementia, and mobility problems. Those who exercise at higher levels were significantly less likely to show brain damage caused by blocked arteries that interrupt blood flow—markers for strokes—than people who exercised lightly. There is no difference between those who engaged in light exercise and those who did not exercise at all.

Source: Data from Willey J., et al. Lower prevalence of silent brain infarcts in the physically active: The Northern Manhattan Study. *Neurology* 2011; 76(24):2112–2118.

If you begin to recognize these symptoms, the best option is to stop your routine and allow your system to recover. The body can heal only during rest, and it is important to listen to your body when it tells you to slow down! You may want to visit a physician to rule out any significant ailment. Once you have given yourself time to recover, you should be able to return to a reasonable level of activity (use the Physical Activity Pyramid as your guide).

Conclusion

Aerobic activity can increase your overall wellness by boosting your immune system, easing stress, improving your self-image, and reducing the risk of certain diseases. When you exercise, you strengthen your heart, making it pump oxygen-rich blood to the rest of the body more efficiently. Field tests assess how efficiently the cardiorespiratory system uses oxygen.

When designing your fitness program, make sure to follow the FITT guidelines.

Always warm up and cool down, and progress slowly. Choose activities that are appropriate for your fitness level, patience, interests, and schedule. Most important, have fun!

5

Reflect >>>> Reinforce >>>> Reinvigorate

Knowledge Check

Answers in Appendix D

1. Circulation between the heart and lungs is called:
   A. Pulmonary circulation
   B. Systemic circulation
   C. Cardiovascular circulation

2. What does aerobic mean?
   A. Exercising with a pain in your chest
   B. Exercising using oxygen
   C. Exercising for more than 60 minutes

3. The body's natural painkiller that is produced in the brain is:
   A. Histamine
   B. Endorphins
   C. Oxygen

4. Gary is 18 years old and would like to improve his cardiorespiratory health. What should be his first step toward putting together an effective exercise program?
   A. Take a submaximal test to find his current cardiorespiratory fitness level
   B. Begin running 2 miles per week
   C. Bike for 40 minutes per day and gradually add other activities

5. Marcia is 23 years old and has been told that stretching is an important component of cardiorespiratory training. When is the best time for Marcia to stretch?
   A. First thing when she gets to the gym
   B. Fifty minutes after exercising, when her muscles have cooled down
   C. After she warms up for 5 to 10 minutes but before she starts her routine

6. Sylvia is 20 years old, walks 15 minutes per day, and would like to increase her level of activity. What is the safest way for Sylvia to progress with her cardiorespiratory training?
   A. Jog for the 15 minutes instead of walking
   B. Increase the duration of her walks by 10% each week until she feels comfortable walking for 60 minutes continuously
   C. Try running a mile once a week in addition to her daily walks

7. What is the recommended frequency for aerobic endurance workouts?
   A. Once each week
   B. 3–5 times each week
   C. Daily

8. How many calories will a 180-pound person burn by hill-climbing for 45 minutes?
   A. About 400
   B. About 500
   C. About 700

9. James is in the middle of his aerobic routine. He can still speak with his partner, but occasionally he must stop talking to catch his breath. At what intensity level is James most likely working?
   A. Light
   B. Moderate
   C. Hard

10. Aerobic workouts should last for how long each session?
   A. 10 to 20 minutes
   B. 20 to 60 minutes
   C. 60 to 90 minutes

Modern Modifications

Try a few of these suggestions to add a little more heart-friendly activity to your daily routine:

- Park at the farthest spot in the parking lot and walk briskly or jog to the door.
- Take the stairs—avoid the escalator and elevator as much as possible.
- Turn up the stereo and dance. Cut loose for a couple of minutes when your favorite song comes on the radio.
- When shopping, walk the length of the mall between entering stores.
- Put away the leaf-blower and snow-blower—pick up a rake or shovel instead.
- After you take the dog for a walk, stay outside and play with the dog for an extra 30 minutes.
- Join an intramural team. It is great exercise, you meet new people, and it is a fun way to spend a few hours!

Critical Thinking

Now that you have a basic understanding of cardiorespiratory endurance, consider the role that it plays in your life. At what stage of change are you regarding cardiorespiratory endurance? What would an appropriate target zone be for you to begin a new routine? After reviewing the variety of activities in Table 5.4, which three are most appropriate for you? Why? What strategies can you employ to counter the "cons" of the activities you have chosen?

Going Above and Beyond

Websites

American Academy of Orthopaedic Surgeons
http://aaos.org

American Heart Association
http://www.heart.org/HEARTORG/

Cooper Institute for Aerobics Research
http://www.cooperinstitute.org/

MedlinePlus: Exercise and Physical Fitness
http://www.nlm.nih.gov/medlineplus/exercisephysicalfitness.html

Physician and Sports Medicine
http://www.physsportmed.com

Runner's World Online
http://www.runnersworld.com

Shape Up America! Fitness Center
http://shapeup.org/fitness

Walking
http://walking.about.com/

References and Suggested Readings

American College of Sports Medicine (ACSM). *ACSM's Guidelines for Exercise Testing and Prescription*. Philadelphia: Lippincott Williams & Wilkins, 2006.

American College of Sports Medicine (ACSM). ACSM position stand: The recommended quantity and quality of exercise for developing and maintaining cardiorespiratory, muscular fitness and flexibility in healthy adults. *Medicine and Science in Sports and Exercise* 1998; 30:975–991.

ACSM. Quantity and Quality of Exercise for Developing and Maintaining Cardiorespitory, Musculoskeletal, and Neuromotor Fitness in Apparently Healthy Adults: Guidance for Prescribing Exercise. *Medicine and Science in Sports and Exercise*. DOI: 10.1249/MSS.0b0138213fefb

American Heart Association. Cholesterol. http://www.heart.org/HEARTORG/Conditions/Cholesterol/Cholesterol_UCM_001089_SubHomePage.jsp. Accessed September 25, 2011.

American Heart Association. Diabetes mellitus. http://www.heart.org/HEARTORG/Conditions/Diabetes/Diabetes_UCM_001091_SubHomePage.jsp. Accessed September 25, 2011.

———. Resting heart rate. 2004c. http://www.heart.org/HEARTORG/ [June 14, 2004].

———. Target heart rate. 2004d. http://www.heart.org/HEARTORG/ [June 14, 2004].

American Heart Association (AHA). A statement on exercise: Benefits and recommendations for physical activity programs for all Americans. *Circulation* 1995; 91:580.

Blair S. N. and Jackson A. S. Physical fitness and activity as separate heart disease risk factors: A meta-analysis. *Medicine and Science in Sports and Exercise* 2001; 33:762–764.

Borg G. A. Psychophysical basis of perceived exertion. *Medicine and Science in Sports and Exercise* 1982; 14:377.

Carroll J. F. and Kyser C. K. Exercise training in obesity lowers blood pressure independent of weight change. *Medicine and Science in Sports and Exercise* 2002; 34:596–601.

Cooper K. H. *The Aerobics Program for Well-Being*. Toronto: Bantam Books, 1982.

Erikssen G. Physical fitness and changes in mortality: The survival of the fittest. *Sports Medicine* 2001; 31:571–576.

Fletcher G., et al. American Heart Association: Statement on exercise. *Circulation* 1992; 86:726.

Garber C. E., Blissmer B., Deschenes M. R., Franklin B. A., Lamonte M. J., Lee I-M., Nieman D. C., and Swain D. P. Quantity and Quality of Exercise for Developing and Maintaining Cardiorespiratory, Musculoskeletal, and Neuromotor Fitness in Apparently Healthy Adults: Guidance for Prescribing Exercise. *Medicine in Science and Sports and Exercise* 2011; 43(7): 1334–1359,

Myers J., Prakash M., Froelicher V., Do D., Partington S., and Atwood J. E. Exercise capacity and mortality among men referred for exercise testing. *New England Journal of Medicine* 2002; 346:793–801.

Haskell W. L., Lee I. M., Pate R. R., Powell K. E., Blair S. N., Franklin B. A., Macera C. A., Heath G. W., Thompson P. D., and Bauman A. American College of Sports Medicine, American Heart Association. Physical activity and public health: Updated recommendation for adults from the American College of Sports Medicine and the American Heart Association. *Circulation* 2007; 116(9):1081–1093. http://circ.ahajournals.org /content/116/9/1081.full.pdf

Public Health Service. *Surgeon General's Report on Physical Activity and Health*. Washington, DC: U.S. Government Printing Office, 1996.

UC Davis Health System. The well-connected report: Exercise. March 2000. http://www .ucdmc.ucdavis.edu/healthconsumers/health/wellconnected/exercise29.html [June 14, 2004].

U.S. DHHS. *2008 Physical Activity Guidelines for Americans*. www.health.gov/paguidelines.

CHAPTER 6

Flexibility

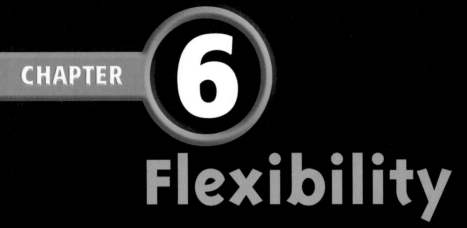

Objectives

After reading this chapter, you should be able to:

- Define flexibility and describe the benefits of increased flexibility.
- Explain the factors influencing flexibility.
- Assess flexibility.
- Explain the difference between ballistic, static, dynamic, and proprioceptive neuromuscular facilitation (PNF) stretching.
- Describe various types of stretching exercises.
- Implement stretching into an exercise program.
- Explain how low-back pain can be prevented.
- Describe which exercises can help prevent back pain.
- List ways to improve your posture.

What Determines Flexibility?

Flexibility is the ability of a joint and its surrounding muscle to move through their full range of motion.

- Flexibility is an important part of physical fitness, but it is often overlooked during workouts.
- Flexibility is achieved by stretching. Stress causes muscles to contract and tighten. Stretching helps muscles relax, relieving pain from muscular stress.
- There are two recommended kinds of stretching: static and dynamic.

Factors That Influence Flexibility

- *Muscle temperature.* Warm muscles stretch more easily than cold muscles.
- *Physical activity.* Sedentary individuals are less flexible; active individuals tend to maintain or even increase flexibility.
- *Injury.* Injury can limit range of motion, but a good rehabilitation program can help regain all or part of a joint's flexibility.
- *Body composition.* Most muscular individuals have good flexibility because they have trained their muscles through a full range of motion. Overly bulky muscles may limit movement. Fat can also limit movement and flexibility.
- *Age.* As a person ages, flexibility declines due more to inactivity than to the aging process itself. Flexibility can be maintained by doing stretching activities regularly.
- *Disease.* Diseases such as arthritis can make it uncomfortable or even painful to move joints. Arthritic individuals can improve their joint mobility through exercise.
- *Gender.* Females tend to have a slightly greater range of motion in most joints than males.

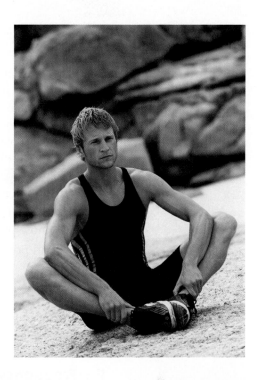

What's the word. . .

flexibility Ability to move a joint smoothly through a full range of motion.

stretching Primary method of improving flexibility.

static or passive stretching Muscle is stretched naturally without force being applied.

dynamic or active stretching Muscle is taken beyond its normal range of motion with help from a partner.

Ask Yourself ❓

• Am I doing some light activity before I attempt to stretch out?

What Are the Benefits of Flexibility?

Flexibility offers the following benefits:

- Increases joint movement (mobility)
- Improves circulation, bringing nutrients to keep tissues healthy and transporting wastes out of the tissues
- Improves performance in some activities (e.g. golfing, dancing)
- Improves posture and personal appearance
- Assists in the cool-down phase of a workout
- Reduces the risk of low-back problems
- Improves coordination and balance, which helps maintain an independent and active lifestyle in the elderly
- Helps reduce excess stress by lowering anxiety and boosting feelings of self-confidence

6

Creating a Flexibility Program

The adage "use it or lose it" applies especially to flexibility. Joint flexibility decreases with aging; however, it can be improved through exercises.

Each muscle–tendon group joint is different; we need to do exercises specific for each joint to maintain or improve its range of motion. There is no test of overall flexibility, so you should plan a program of stretching exercises that involves most of your joints (e.g., shoulder, chest, neck, trunk, lower back, hips, and posterior and anterior legs) (see **Table 6.1**).

Precautions involving stretching include:

- Do not stretch swollen or painful joints without a healthcare professional's advice.
- Do not stretch a surgically repaired joint without a healthcare professional's advice.
- Avoid potentially harmful stretching exercises (see **Table 6.2**).

Using the FITT Formula

The goal of a flexibility program is to develop the range of motion in the major joints.

F = Frequency

Performing flexibility exercises 2 to 3 days per week is effective, but greater gains in joint range of motion can be obtained with daily flexibility exercise.

I = Intensity

Stretch to the point of mild discomfort or tightness.

T = Time

Holding a stretch for 10–30 seconds at the point of tightness or slight discomfort enhances joint range of motion. Holding it longer offers no additional benefit except in older persons who may gain greater improvements in range of motion with a 30- to 60-second stretch. For PNF stretching, a 20% to 75% maximum contraction held for 3–6 seconds followed by a 10- to 30-second assisted stretch is recommended.

Repeating each flexibility exercise two to four times is effective. The goal is to gain 60 seconds of total stretching time per flexibility exercise (e.g., 60 seconds of stretch time can be met by two 30-second stretches or four 15-second stretches).

Completing a daily set of flexibility exercises can be completed within 10 minutes.

When to stretch? Do not stretch to warm up. Flexibility exercise is most effective when the muscles are warmed through light-to-moderate cardiorespiratory or muscular endurance exercise or through external-moist heat packs or hot baths. You will gain the most flexibility by stretching after your cardiorespiratory or resistance exercise is completed. Flexibility exercise can be done alone—not involving other types of exercise.

T = Types of Stretching

Stretching techniques include static stretches, dynamic stretches, ballistic stretches, and PNF (proprioceptive neuromuscular facilitation).

Static Stretching

Static stretching is the most common and practical type of stretching. It is effective, causes less pain, and usually is easier to do. Perform a static stretch by slowly and gently stretching the muscle to the point of tightness and holding that position for 10–30 seconds.

See Table 6.1 for proper stretching exercises and Table 6.2 for potentially harmful exercises that should be avoided.

Dynamic Stretching

Dynamic or slow-movement stretching involves a gradual transition from one body position to another and a progressive increase in reach and range of motion as the movement is repeated several times. This involves moving a joint through its full range of motion with little resistance. The movement can be through the range of motion used in a specific exercise or sport.

Ballistic Stretching

Ballistic stretching uses bouncing, repetitive movements to force a stretch past the normal range of motion. When properly performed, it is as effective as static stretching and may be considered for those engaged in ballistic movements (e.g., basketball).

Proprioceptive Neuromuscular Facilitation

Proprioceptive neuromuscular facilitation (PNF) involves tightening a muscle (isometric contraction) as hard as you can, followed by a static stretching of the same muscle. The theory behind PNF is that the act of tightening or squeezing results in the muscle becoming relaxed and more receptive to the stretch.

PNF usually requires a partner, takes more time, and can cause more muscle soreness. It is largely impractical for most exercisers. There are several PNF techniques. Here is an example of one method of performing a PNF stretch:

- Do a 20% to 75% 3- to 6-second isometric contraction of the muscle you wish to stretch.
- Immediately relax the muscle for 2 seconds, then have a partner push the muscle into a static stretch for 10 to 30 seconds.

Informal Stretching

Stretching can be done virtually anywhere. When you need a quick break, want a short stress reliever (during a test, for instance), or sense discomfort in a muscle group during the day, use stretching as a means to relieve the pain. In addition, these activities can be fun if you choose to do them with a friend, while listening to music or watching television, or during your own time. Here is an example of a routine you can do anywhere, anytime:

- Clasp your hands together and stretch out in front of you.
- In the same position, stretch your hands over your head.
- While standing or sitting, lean right.
- While standing or sitting, lean left.
- Clasp your hands behind your back and open up your chest area.
- Stretch your wrists by bending your wrists back, then down, then in a circle.
- Lift your shoulders up to your ears, then down and back. Do that five times.
- Take your right hand and put it on your left shoulder. With your left hand, gently push your right elbow, pushing your right hand past your shoulder and stretching the back of your right arm.
- Stretch your left arm in the same manner.
- Put your hands flat on your desk, palms down, and push your chair out, stretching your back.
- Feel free to add more stretches for variety and to avoid boredom!

The Inside Track

Physiology of Stretching

Areas within your muscles and tendons protect them from overstretching or tearing during a quick stretch by creating a stretch reflex. For example, someone tapping your leg just below the kneecap quickly stretches the quadriceps muscle. This makes your thigh contract and kick out your lower leg. The quicker the stretch, the stronger the reflex. The protective action of tendons causes a stretched muscle attached to the tendon to relax and signals its opposing muscle to contract. This protects the stretched muscle and tendon from tearing. By stretching slowly during exercise, you avoid contracting the muscle you are trying to stretch. As a stretch is held, your muscles and tendons adapt to the new length.

The Inside Track

Time and Place

A stretch workout can be done at any time and at any place (e.g., first thing in the morning or last thing at night, while watching television, while waiting for someone, or while in a line), and during or after long periods of sitting, standing, or sleeping.

Table 6.1	Proper Form for Stretching Exercises

Neck

Ear to shoulder | Chin to chest | Look right and left

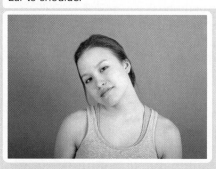 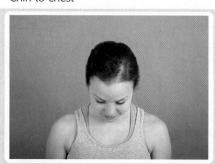 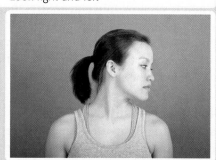

Shoulders, chest, upper back, and abdominals

Shoulder roll | Back scratch | Handcuff stretch | Rack stretch

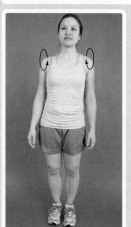 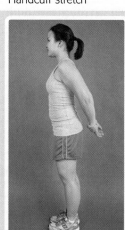 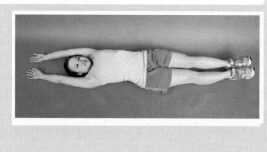

Reach up | Slow arm circles | Wall press

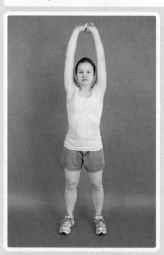 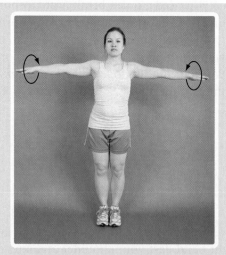 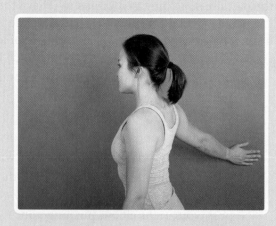

Hamstrings, groin, and lower back

Supine hamstring stretch

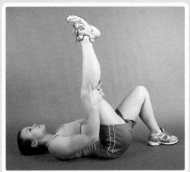

Modified hurdler

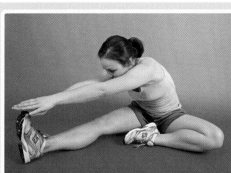

Single knee-to-chest

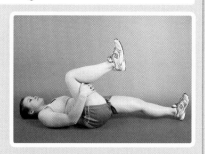

Double knee-to-chest

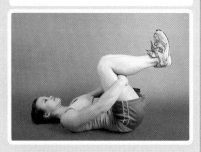

Calf

Calf stretch

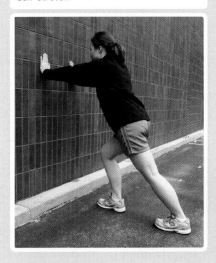

Quads, inner thigh, and hips

Standing heel-to-buttock (do not perform without your health-care provider's advice if you have knee pain or knee surgery)

Butterfly stretch

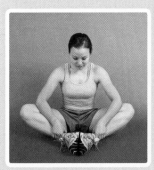

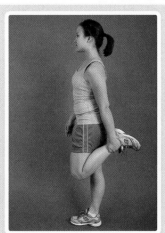

Standing lunge

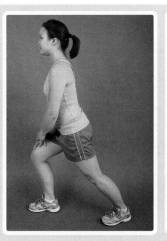

Side (skater) lunge

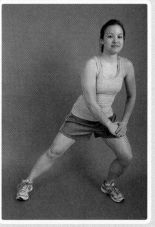

6

Table 6.2   Potentially Harmful Exercises to Avoid

Don't	Do

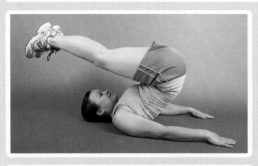

Yoga plough

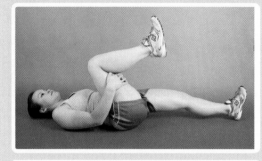

Single knee-to-chest
Hug the thigh, not the knee

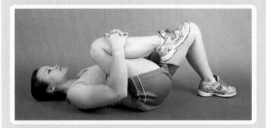

Single knee-to-chest

Don't	Do

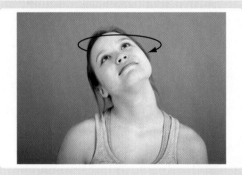

Full head circles

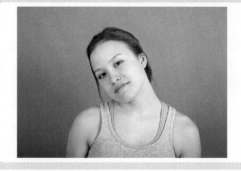

Ear to shoulder

Don't	Do

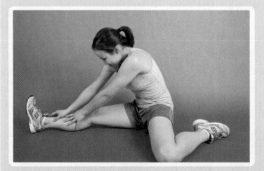

Hurdler stretch

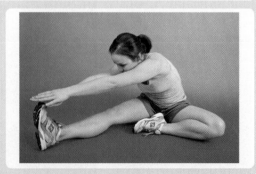

Modified hurdler stretch

Don't

Do

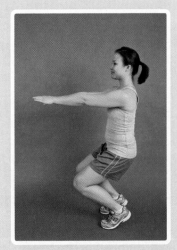

Full squat

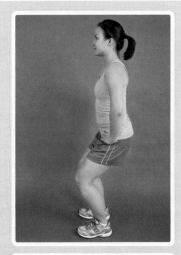

Half-knee bend

Don't

Do

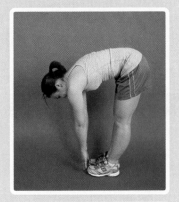

Standing toe touch

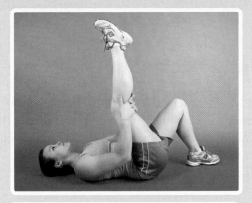

Lying hamstring stretch

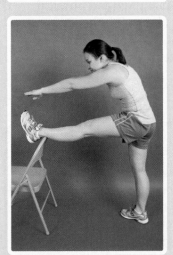

Ballet bar leg stretch

continued

Table 6.2	Potentially Harmful Exercises to Avoid, *continued*

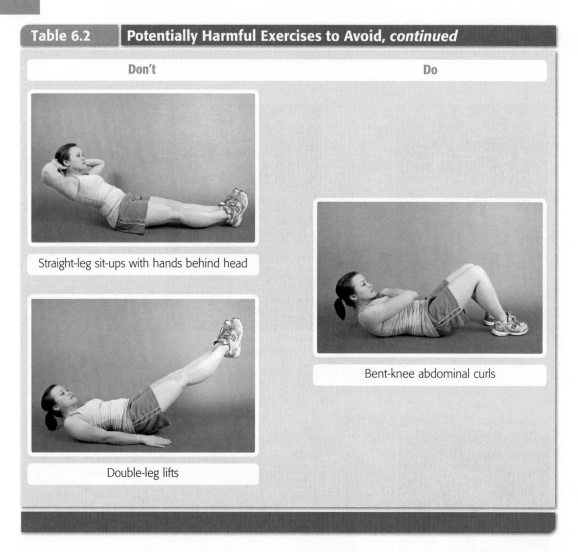

Don't	Do

Straight-leg sit-ups with hands behind head

Bent-knee abdominal curls

Double-leg lifts

Flexibility and Back Pain

More than 80% of North Americans suffer back pain in their lifetime. Low-back pain, both acute and chronic, centers on the muscles supporting the spine. Age and physical condition are the major factors associated with low-back pain, along with the trauma of lifting something in the wrong way or injuring yourself in an activity or sport. Being overweight, poor posture, stress, and occupation (e.g., computer programmers and

Tipping Point

Caution

• Avoid ballistic stretching—for example, bending forcefully to touch your toes with your knees straight and bouncing while you reach. Ballistic stretching may do more harm than good, because the muscles may shorten reflexively. This type of stretching is not recommended for most people. However, some athletes believe that controlled ballistic stretching can better prepare a muscle for sustained activity, especially one requiring a burst of speed.

truck drivers) may contribute to the pain. There is also recent research indicating a link between smoking and lower-back pain.

Preventing Low-Back Pain

To prevent low-back pain:

- Exercise regularly to improve the strength of your back and abdominal muscles.
- Maintain correct posture in sitting and standing, especially while studying and working on a computer.
- Warm up before engaging in physical activity.
- Keep the spine straight up and down when lifting an object. Do not bend over. Use the muscles of your legs and hips to lift.

Exercises for the Lower Back

The following exercises will help to stretch and strengthen your lower back:

- Curl up

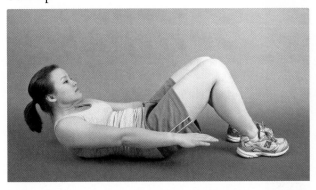

- Knee-to-chest

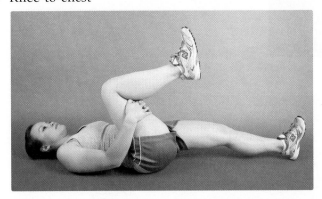

- Elbow-to-knee stretch

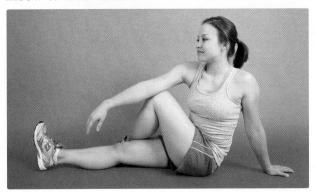

- Cat and camel

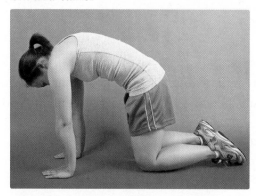 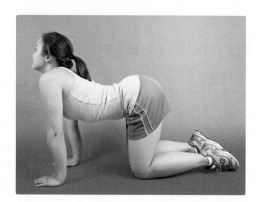

- Lunge stretch

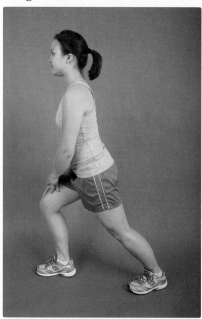

- Modified chest lift

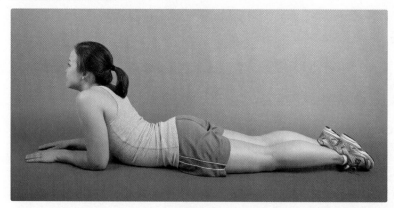

Body Posture

You can evaluate your posture by standing in front of a three-panel mirror of the kind often found in fitting rooms. See **Figure 6.1** for guidance on good and poor posture.

Why Have Good Posture?

- Good posture makes your bones align properly.
- Correct bone alignment allows for muscles, joints, and ligaments to work properly.
- With good posture, internal organs are in the right position and can work more effectively (allows for deep breathing and proper digestion).
- Good posture lessens the risk of lower-back pain.
- Good posture can project the body image that you are strong and proud.

Signs of Poor Posture

- Head aligned in front of center of gravity (can cause headaches; dizziness; and neck, shoulder, and arm pain)
- Too much outward curve in upper back (can shorten breath by squeezing the lung area; can cause neck, shoulder, and arm pain)
- Too much inward curve in lower back (can cause low-back pain, painful menstruation)
- Abdomen sticks out too far (can cause lordosis, low-back pain, painful menstruation)
- Knees extend backward too much (can cause knee injury and lordosis) (see Figure 6.2)

Ways to Improve Your Posture

- **Sit correctly:** Distribute your weight evenly on both hips, bend knees at a right angle, legs should not be crossed and feet should be flat on the floor, keep back straight and shoulders back.
- **Stand correctly:** Hold head up with chin in, ears should be in line with shoulders, shoulders should be back, chest forward, knees straight, stomach tucked in.
- **Lift correctly:** Keep back straight and bend at knees and hips, keep feet in wide stance, lift object using leg muscles, moving in a steady motion.
- **Lie in bed correctly:** Lie on your side with your hips and knees slightly bent; put a flat pillow between your knees (see Figure 6.3).

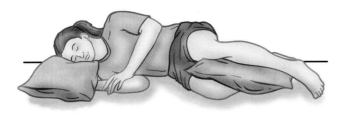

Figure 6.3

To improve your posture, sleep on your side with your hips and knees slightly bent.

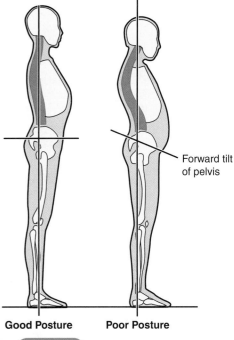

Forward tilt of pelvis

Good Posture　**Poor Posture**

Figure 6.1

Good posture depends on the pelvic tilt and abdominal muscles. Only when the pelvis is level is it at its strongest.

What's the word. . .

lordosis Excessive pelvic tilt.

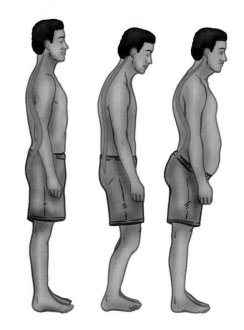

Figure 6.2

Left to right: good posture (pelvic tilt); poor posture (lordotic back, pelvis tilted too far forward; pelvis tilted too far back).

6

Reflect >>>> Reinforce >>>> Reinvigorate

Knowledge Check

Answers in Appendix D

1. In assessing your flexibility, you should:

   A. Warm up before you do a stretch test

   B. Do fast moves to get your muscles warm

   C. Bounce at the end of each movement

2. What are three basic types of stretching?

   A. Fast, slow, ballistic

   B. Static, ballistic, PNF

   C. Active, passive, quick

3. You can help prevent low-back pain by:

   A. Lying flat on your back while sleeping

   B. Always standing with your legs at least 2 feet apart

   C. Exercising your back and abdominal muscles regularly

Scenario One: After standing around waiting for a delayed gun, you bolt from the starting line of a 5K, feeling fit and ready to have a great race. As you sizzle through the first half-mile, you marvel at how fast you are running and how easy the pace feels to you. Suddenly, agonizing pain stabs you, and you are forced to hobble to a complete stop. You realize that you have torn your hamstrings so badly that you probably will not run at anything faster than a very slow jogging pace for at least 6 to 8 weeks.

4. Can stretching before exercising help prevent muscle injuries?

   A. Yes

   B. No

5. Which is the safest type of stretching for most people?

   A. Ballistic

   B. Static

   C. Proprioceptive neuromuscular facilitation (PNF)

Scenario Two: Craig, as a dentist, bends over patients daily for long hours. When he was younger, he experienced no back problems. However, in middle age, he has experienced severe back pain.

6. Does flexibility decrease as a person ages?

   A. Yes

   B. No

7. Could having a "pot belly" affect Craig's flexibility?

   A. Yes

   B. No

8. The best sleeping position for your posture is:

   A. On your back, with your face and toes pointed toward the ceiling

   B. On your stomach, facing downward

   C. On your side, with your knees slightly bent

9. How long should you hold each stretch during your exercise routine?

   A. 5–10 seconds

   B. 10–30 seconds

   C. 30–45 seconds

10. When first starting your exercise routine, how often should you perform stretching exercises?

    A. Rarely, because injury may occur

    B. Only on days where aerobic activity is performed

    C. Daily, to improve flexibility

Modern Modifications

Think about the activities you do and the postures you assume each day. Are there ways you can improve your flexibility and posture just by changing the way you do these activities? When you are sitting or standing, are you:

- Arching your back?
- Rounding your shoulders?
- Letting your head slump forward?

When you are lying down, are you:

- Tilting your pelvis down?
- Arching your back?

While lying on your back, you should have just enough room between the small of your back and the floor to slide a computer mouse under there. You know your posture is bad if your back is touching the floor (squishing the mouse) or arching (the mouse could do jumping jacks).

Consciously change what you do during each activity or posture. For instance:

- While sitting, keep your back straight, lean slightly forward, and use a footrest to keep your knees higher than your hips.
- While standing, use a footrest to raise one leg to help you keep your back straight.
- When lifting, bend at the knees, not at the waist, lift slowly, and push with your legs. Do not twist.
- Do one different stretching exercise each morning, at noon, and each evening before going to bed.

Critical Thinking

1. Consider your current level of activity. What role do flexibility and stretching play in your workouts? Identify three to five ways you can improve your flexibility based on the suggestions in the text.

2. What rationalizations do you believe you might hear from someone who does not practice stretching as a portion of his or her routine? What are the risks the individual may be taking by avoiding this piece of the routine?

Going Above and Beyond

Websites

American Academy of Orthopaedic Surgeons

http://aaos.org

MedlinePlus

http://www.nlm.nih.gov/medlineplus

National Institute on Aging

http://www.nia.nih.gov

Physician and Sports Medicine

http://www.physsportsmed.org

References and Suggested Readings

————. Stretching during warm-up: Do we have enough evidence? *Journal of Physical Education, Recreation and Dance* 2000; 70:271–277.

American College of Sports Medicine. Quantity and Quality of Exercise for Developing and Maintaining Cardiorespiratory, Musculoskeletal, and Neuromotor Fitness in Apparently Healthy Adults: Guidance for Prescribing Exercise. *Medicine and Science in Sports and Exercise.* DOI: 10.1249/MSS.0b0138213fefb

Canham-Chervak M., et al. Does stretching before exercise prevent lower-limb injury? *Clinical Journal of Sport Medicine* 2000; 10:216.

Garber, C.E., et al. Quantity and quality of exercise for developing and maintaining cardiorespiratory, musculoskeletal, and neuromotor fitness in apparently healthy adults: Guidance for prescribing exercise. *Medicine and Science in Sports and Exercise* 2011; 43(7): 1334–1359.

Gleim G. W. and McHugh M. P. Flexibility and its effect on sports injury and performance. *Sports Medicine* 1997; 24:289–299.

Hodges P. and Jull G. Does strengthening the abdominal muscles prevent low-back pain? *Journal of Rheumatology* 2000; 27:2286–2288.

Knudson D. Stretching: From science to practice. *Journal of Physical Education, Recreation and Dance* 1998; 69:38–42.

Patel A. T. and Ogle A. A. Diagnosis and management of acute low back pain. *American Family Physician* 2000; 61:1779–1786.

Shrier I. and Gossal K. Myths and truths of stretching. *Physician and Sports Medicine* 2000; 28:57–63.

Shrier I. Stretching before exercise: An evidence-based approach. *British Journal of Sports Medicine* 2000; 34:324–325.

U.S. DHHS. *2008 Physical Activity Guidelines for Americans*. www.health.gov/paguidelines

CHAPTER 7

Muscular Strength and Endurance

Objectives

After reading this chapter, you should be able to:

- Explain the difference between muscular strength and muscular endurance and identify how training differs for each.
- Describe the changes that occur in your body as a result of muscle training.
- Explain the differences in muscle fibers and their functions.
- Assess muscular strength and endurance.
- Describe effective individual muscle-training exercises.
- Design an effective muscle-training program.

Weight training is one of the key elements of an overall fitness program. The training described here emphasizes a general physical fitness rather than bodybuilding. Everyone can become stronger. Everyone can see a marked difference after 6 to 10 weeks of conscientious strength training.

Unused muscles ultimately atrophy, and even underused muscles quickly lose strength. The adage "use it or lose it" readily applies to muscles.

It is one thing to understand the importance of weight training. It is another thing to put that knowledge to work for you. For muscles to become stronger, you need to demand more of them than their usual workload.

Muscular Endurance

Muscular endurance describes how long or how many times (number of repetitions) you can lift and lower a given weight (often referred to as resistance). It can be assessed by determining the time or the number of repetitions of a particular exercise that can be performed.

For most people, developing muscular endurance is more important than muscular strength. Muscular endurance is usually more important in carrying out everyday activities.

> **What's the word. . .**
>
> **muscular endurance** The ability of muscles to apply force repeatedly.
>
> **muscular strength** The force muscles can exert against resistance.

Muscular Strength

As you lift and lower a weight, your muscle must generate enough force to move that weight. Muscular strength can be assessed by determining the amount of weight that can be lifted in one repetition of an exercise. Strength can be developed by increasing the amount of weight that can be lifted in an exercise.

Fundamentals of Weight Training

- To get stronger, use a few repetitions (6–8) with maximum weight. The number of repetitions performed without stopping to rest is called a set.
- To gain endurance, use many repetitions (12–15) with minimum weight to complete the set of repetitions.

> **What's the word. . .**
>
> **repetition (rep)** A single lifting and lowering of the weight.
>
> **set** Number of reps performed without stopping to rest.

Developing Different Types of Muscle Fiber

Muscles consist of many muscle fibers. Larger muscle fibers mean a larger and stronger muscle (hypertrophy). When muscle fiber size diminishes, the muscle fiber is said to atrophy.

Two types of muscle fibers exist according to their contraction speed and energy source:

- Type I slow-twitch fibers do not contract as rapidly or strongly as fast-twitch fibers. They are fatigue-resistant and rely on aerobic energy metabolism.
- Type II fast-twitch fibers contract quickly and forcefully but fatigue more rapidly than slow-twitch fibers. They rely on anaerobic energy metabolism.

Endurance activities (i.e., jogging) use slow-twitch fibers; power and strength activities (i.e., sprinting) use fast-twitch fibers. Weight training can increase the size and strength of both fiber types.

> **What's the word. . .**
>
> **hypertrophy** Increase in bulk or size by thickening of muscle fibers.
>
> **atrophy** Progressive loss (wasting) of muscle mass.

Everyone has both types of muscle fiber. Your genetics determine the proportion of each type of fiber in your body.

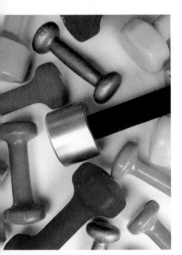

How Does Weight Training Change Body Composition and Metabolism?

Exercising the muscles changes the ratio of fat to muscle fiber and speeds up weight loss. The more muscle, the higher the metabolic rate and the more calories your body will burn on its own. It will be easier to keep your weight where you want it by eating right and exercising.

Exercising also slows degeneration of muscle and nerves with age. It keeps the bones strong, helping you to avoid osteoporosis. Being stronger when you are older keeps you from falling down as easily. Falls are the number one cause of injury for seniors.

Weight training keeps more of your motor nerves connected to the muscles they control. And you are better able to make quick and powerful moves.

Benefits of Muscular Strength and Endurance

Muscular strength and endurance are important components of physical fitness. The benefits of strength and endurance training:

- Improve the capabilities of performing physical work, sports, recreation, and activities of daily living (e.g., walking).
- Raise confidence by the way you look and help fight mild to moderate depression.
- Help prevent osteoporosis (porous and less-dense bones), which makes the bones fragile and more vulnerable to fractures. Strength training can slow bone loss and even help build bone.
- Prevent falls and fractures by improving balance and preserving power to correct missteps. By age 65, one in three people suffers a fall. Because bones also weaken over time, one out of every 20 of these falls causes a fracture, usually of the hip, wrist, or leg (National Safety Council 2007).
- Relieve some of the load carried by the heart. Strong muscles pluck oxygen and nutrients from the blood much more efficiently than weak ones do. That means any activity requires less cardiac effort and puts less strain on your heart.

The Inside Track

Will Weight Training Give Women Bulky Muscles?

Women do not develop large muscle mass as a result of weight training because they lack the male hormones in the quantity necessary for significant hypertrophy to occur.

The principal advantages of weight training for women are (1) greater strength as they age, (2) better bone density, and (3) easier maintenance of desired weight without fat.

Medical News You Can Use

More Muscle May Reduce the Odds of Developing Diabetes

Researchers from the University of California, Los Angeles (UCLA), found that for each 10% increase in the skeletal muscle index (the ratio of muscle mass to total body weight), there was a corresponding 11% decline in insulin resistance and a 12% reduction in pre-diabetes (a condition characterized by higher-than-normal blood sugar levels). The findings represent a departure from the usual focus on just losing weight to improve metabolic health. Instead, this research suggests a role for maintaining fitness and building muscle. This is good news for many overweight people who experience difficulty in achieving weight loss, as any effort to get moving and keep fit should be seen as being beneficial.

Source: Data from Srikanthan P., Karlamangla A. S. Relative muscle mass is inversely associated with insulin resistance and prediabetes. Findings from the third National Health and Nutrition Examination Survey. *Journal of Clinical Endocrinology and Metabolism* 2001; 96(9):2898-2903.

- Help control blood glucose—strong muscles are better at absorbing sugar in the blood and helping the body stay sensitive to insulin, which helps cells remove sugar from the blood. In this way, strong muscles can help keep blood glucose levels in check, which in turn helps prevent or control type 2 diabetes.

- Increase metabolism even while resting, resulting in more calories burned and, thus, helping keep weight within a healthy range.

- Better manage stress and anxiety.

- Improve posture.

- Relieve arthritic pain and expand a limited range of motion.

- Ease back and neck pain.

Assessing Your Muscular Strength and Endurance

Muscular fitness is determined by assessing muscular strength and endurance.

- Muscular strength: Because muscular strength is specific to a muscle group, testing one group of muscles does not provide accurate information about the strength of other muscle groups. For a comprehensive assessment, strength testing must involve several major muscle groups. Standard tests use free weights. The heaviest weight you can lift only one time through the full range of motion for a specific muscle group is considered your maximum strength for that muscle group.

- Muscular endurance: Muscular endurance is also specific to each muscle group. Few tests of muscular endurance have been developed. The YMCA developed a bench-press test for muscular endurance using a standard weight. (Using the bench press to test strength is preferred by some experts. It is not a fair test for smaller, lighter individuals, however.) See Lab 7-1, Activity 1 for complete instructions on how to perform this assessment.

Also see Labs 7-2 and 7-3 for assessing muscular strength and endurance.

Gender Differences for Weight Training

Men are, on average, larger and stronger than women, because they have more muscle mass. But women have about the same strength in the lower body and only a small percentage less in the upper body. Why? Men have more androgens (hormones that cause facial hair, deep voice, and other sex-linked characteristics). Also, male muscles tend to activate faster, adding to muscle power.

Designing a Muscular Fitness Program Using the FITT Formula

F = Frequency

Completing a strength training routine two to three times per week can result in gains of muscle function and size. The fastest gains are made in the first 4 to 8 weeks; after that, gains are slower. Once you reach your goal, you can keep working out two to three times a week if you would like to make further gains. Or you can reduce your training to twice or even once a week to maintain the gains you have made.

Training can be done with "whole body" training sessions, exercising all muscle groups in the same session during the two to three times a week, or by using a "split-body" (upper body/lower body) routine, where a few muscle groups are trained during one session and the remaining muscle groups in the next. Both methods are effective as long as each muscle group is trained 2 to 3 days per week. Whichever routine is used, always allow at least 48 hours for muscles to recover between training workouts.

I = Intensity

Intensity is the most critical part of resistance training. The basis of such training is progressive overloading. Progressive overloading strengthens individual muscle fibers and engages a larger proportion of available fibers in an activity. This makes you stronger.

Once you understand exactly how to do each exercise, choose a weight that allows you to do 12 repetitions. The last one or two repetitions should be difficult. If you cannot lift the weight at least eight times, use a lighter weight.

After a while, your muscles will gradually adapt to the weight you are using so you can do more repetitions. When you can comfortably perform 12 repetitions without completely tiring the muscle, it is time to increase the amount of weight.

Strength training focuses on tiring the muscles being worked. Once you have attained the desired level of strength and/or size, you can maintain that level of training—it is not necessary to increase the resistance, sets, or training sessions per week. Strength may be maintained by training just 1 day per week if the resistance and intensity keeps constant.

Resting for 2 to 3 minutes between sets produces the best strength gains in a general fitness program.

T = Time

Warm-up

Begin with a 5- to 10-minute warm-up. This will:
- Prepare the heart muscle and circulatory system for exercise
- Warm the muscles, making them more flexible

To warm-up, use low-intensity exercises (i.e., biking, stair-climbing, treadmill/jogging, or even low resistance with a high number of repetitions). When you begin to sweat, you are warmed up.

During the Workout

Strength training should:
- Enhance muscular fitness gradually over time to realize gains. You can do this several ways: (1) increase the number of repetitions, (2) increase the number of sets for a muscle group, or (3) increase the resistance by adding weight. Use only one of these options at a time to avoid injury.
- Have rhythmic movement, which means moving the weights smoothly without jerking.
- Involve moving the weights at a moderate to slow speed.
- Involve a full range of motion.
- Involve all of the major muscle groups (i.e., arms, shoulders, chest, back, legs).
- Not cause labored breathing (see the next section, T = Types of Resistance, for exercises, **Table 7.1**, Training with Weights, and **Table 7.2**, Training Without Weights).
- Change the exercises you perform for each muscle group every 4 to 8 weeks, even if you keep the same set and repetition routine. Changing exercises will overload the muscles differently, increase your strength gains, and alleviate boredom. (See Lab 7-3 for tracking your muscular training workouts.)

What's the word...

progressive overloading Increasing, from one session to another, the amount of weight you lift during a set.

Table 7.1	Advantages and Disadvantages of Weight Machines
Advantages	**Disadvantages**
<ul><li>Recommended for beginners</li><li>Convenient</li><li>Safe: weight cannot fall on you</li><li>Less clutter: no weights scattered around</li><li>No spotters needed</li><li>No lifter needed to balance bar</li><li>Offer variable resistance</li><li>Ensure correct lifting movements, which prevents cheating when tired</li><li>Easy to use: require less skill than **free weights**</li><li>Easy to move from one exercise to the next</li><li>Easier to adjust</li><li>Easier to isolate specific muscle groups</li><li>Back support (on most machines)</li><li>Some offer high-tech options like varying resistance during lifting motion</li></ul>	<ul><li>Limited availability: may need to go to a club</li><li>Expensive</li><li>Require a lot of space</li><li>Do not allow natural movements</li><li>Most machines have only one exercise</li><li>Less motivation: only working against resistance on a machine</li></ul>

What's the word...

free weights Use barbells or hand weights.

exercise machines Have a stack of weights that is lifted through an assortment of pulleys.

Table 7.2	Advantages and Disadvantages of Free Weights
Advantages	**Disadvantages**
<ul><li>Allow dynamic movements</li><li>Allow a greater variety of exercises</li><li>Widely available</li><li>Require minimal space</li><li>Strength transfers to daily activities</li><li>Inexpensive</li><li>Offer greater sense of accomplishment</li><li>Most serious bodybuilders and lifters use free weights</li></ul>	<ul><li>Not as safe as **exercise machines**: weights can fall off the end of the bar or can pin or smash you when muscles tire</li><li>Balancing is required, which can be difficult and dangerous (e.g., weights overhead or while doing squats)</li><li>Require spotters for some exercises</li><li>Allow cheating by swinging for momentum when muscles tire</li><li>Require more time to change weights</li><li>Can cause blisters and calluses</li><li>Clutter creates hazard when weights are scattered</li></ul>

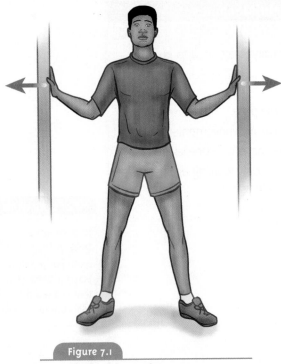

Figure 7.1

Isometric (static) exercise.

Exercise Order

The sequence of exercises during a workout can vary:

- Do large muscle group exercises before doing small muscle group exercises.
- Do multiple-joint exercises (e.g., squats) before doing single-joint exercises (e.g., arms curl). Why? Because single-joint exercises fatigue the smaller muscle groups needed to perform multiple-joint exercises. An example of a multiple-joint exercise is the bench press, because your upper and lower arms move at the shoulder and elbow joints. An example of a single-joint exercise is a biceps curl, because only your lower arm moves at the elbow. To determine which exercises are multiple-joint exercises, watch and feel how many joints move while you perform the exercise.
- Lower-back and abdominal exercises should be done at the end of your workout because these muscles are used during other exercises for balance and posture. If they are fatigued before doing the other exercises, you may not be able to do those exercises properly.
- Use Lab 5-3 to help you design your workout and to record your progress.

Cool-Down

Cool down for 2 to 5 minutes with a mild activity (e.g., walking, jogging, or cycling). Stretch after exercising—warm muscles stretch farther and are less likely to tear.

T = Types of Resistance Exercises

Resistance training can involve different types of equipment, such as free weights, machines with stacked weights or pneumatic resistance, and rubber bands. Each major muscle group (e.g., chest, shoulders, abdomen, back, legs, and arms) should be involved.

Types of Exercise for Developing Muscular Strength and Endurance

Isometric (Static) Exercises

Isometric (static) exercise contracts muscle without changing muscle length (does not involve joint or muscle movement) (see **Figure 7.1**).

- Do these exercises against an immovable object (e.g., stand between door frames and push) to provide resistance.
- You can use isometric exercises to strengthen muscles after an injury or surgery.

Advantages:

- Require little or no equipment or expense
- Low risk of muscle soreness
- Can be done in a small space
- Rapid strength improvement

Disadvantages:

- Difficult to devise a full-body workout
- Not very motivating

Isotonic Exercises

Isotonic (dynamic) exercise contracts muscle in a way that changes muscle length (involves muscle and joint movement). Isotonic is the most popular type of exercise for increasing muscle strength. It can be performed with weight machines (see **Figure 7.2**, free weights,

---

What's the word...

multiple-joint exercise An exercise in which two or more joints move together.

What's the word...

isometric Muscle contraction without movement at the joint

isotonic Muscle contraction where tension is constant while length increases.

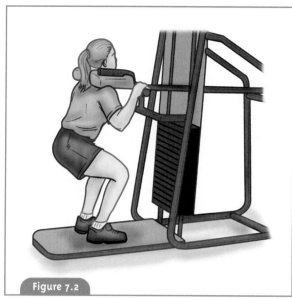

Figure 7.2

Isotonic (dynamic) exercise using a weight machine.

or your own body (i.e., push-ups). There are two kinds of muscle contractions (see **Figure 7.3**):

- Concentric contractions occur when the muscle applies force as it shortens and the joints move.
- Eccentric contractions occur when the muscle applies force as it lengthens and the joints move.

For example, during an arm curl, the biceps muscle works concentrically as the weight is raised toward the shoulder and eccentrically as the weight is lowered.

Advantages:

- Improve strength across the entire range of motion
- Help improve joint flexibility
- More motivating

Disadvantages:

- Require more exercise equipment
- Higher risk of muscle soreness

Isokinetic Exercises

Isokinetic exercise combines the advantages of both isometric and isotonic exercises. It uses special apparatus to provide a maximum resistance to the muscles, as in isometric exercise, but throughout the full range of motion, as in isotonic exercise. This equipment is often used by individuals who are in rehabilitation (see **Figure 7.4**).

What's the word...

isokinetic Muscle contraction where the maximum tension is generated in the muscle as it contracts at a constant speed over the full range of motion of the joint.

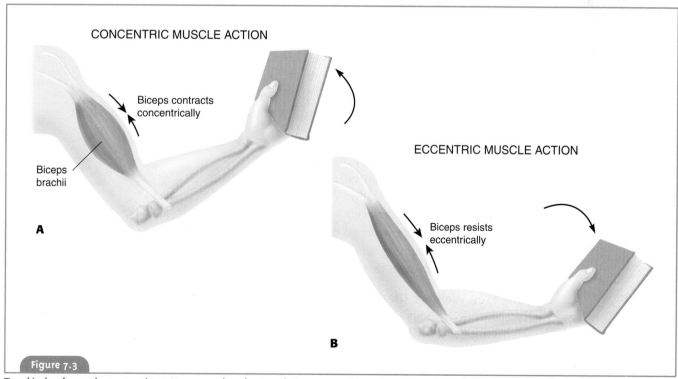

CONCENTRIC MUSCLE ACTION

Biceps contracts concentrically

Biceps brachii

A

ECCENTRIC MUSCLE ACTION

Biceps resists eccentrically

B

Figure 7.3

Two kinds of muscle contractions. Your muscles shorten during concentric action (A) and lengthen during eccentric action (B).

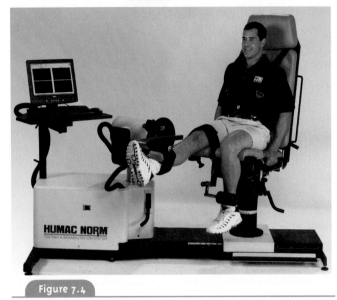

Figure 7.4
Isokinetic exercise apparatus.

Plyometric Exercises

Plyometrics involves doing abrupt, explosive movements, such as bounding on and off a box or jumping off a platform and immediately leaping upward. It develops quick-twitch muscle fibers but risks incurring injury. Do plyometric exercises only after you have developed well-conditioned muscles. These exercises may especially benefit some athletes.

Where Should You Exercise?

At a Health Club/Gym: Advantages

- Availability of professional supervision and trainers
- Many exercise options, including aerobic options
- Social climate: meet new friends
- Influence of motivated exercisers

At Home: Advantages

- Convenient: no concerns about appearance, travel time, parking, gym hours
- Private: avoids strangers, not intimidating if you feel weak and awkward
- No waiting in line; no noise from loud music and talking
- Cleaner: the germs on the bench and bars are yours
- Less expensive: no monthly payments for health club membership

Fundamentals of Weight Training

Use **Figure 7.5** to identify muscles in **Tables 7.3 and 7.4**.

Weight-Machine Training Safety

- Keep away from moving weight stacks.
- Stay away from moving parts of the machine that could pinch your skin.
- Do not lift in an awkward position.
- Beware of broken bolts, frayed cables, broken chains, or loose cushions.
- Be alert to what is happening around you.
- Be aware of the advantages and disadvantages of using weight machines (see Table 7.1).

Weight Machines: Circuit Training

Circuit training combines aerobic and strength exercises.
- Each exercise station takes 30 to 45 seconds to do.
- Stations alternate between upper and lower body exercises.
- The circuit is repeated two or more times per session.
- Do a circuit-training workout three times each week for aerobic conditioning and moderate increases in strength.

Using Free Weights (Barbells, Dumbbells)

Olympic-style barbells with a narrow center bar for gripping and wider ends for loading weights are the most common in gyms.
- The bar is 5 to 7 feet long and weighs 30 to 45 pounds.
- The bell plates used to load the bars come in pounds and kilograms. They range from 2.5 to 45 lb (1.25 to 20 kg).

What's the word...

plyometrics A form of training where muscles are subjected to rapid alternation of lengthening and shortening while resistance is continuously applied.

The Inside Track

What Kinds of Equipment Do You Need?

- Standard workout clothing
- Supportive shoes
- Fitted lifting gloves (optional)
- Exercise machine or free weights

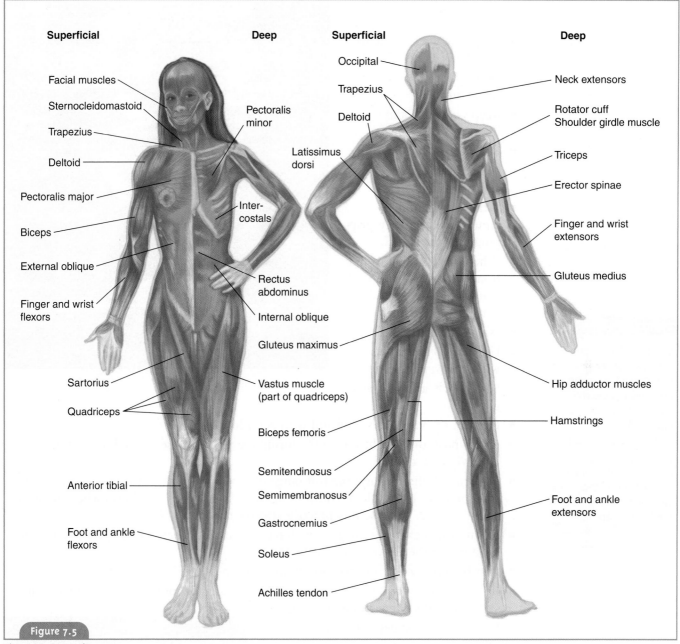

Superficial   **Deep**   **Superficial**   **Deep**

Facial muscles
Sternocleidomastoid
Trapezius
Deltoid
Pectoralis major
Biceps
External oblique
Finger and wrist flexors
Sartorius
Quadriceps
Anterior tibial
Foot and ankle flexors

Pectoralis minor
Inter-costals
Rectus abdominus
Internal oblique
Gluteus maximus
Vastus muscle (part of quadriceps)
Biceps femoris
Semitendinosus
Semimembranosus
Gastrocnemius
Soleus
Achilles tendon

Occipital
Trapezius
Deltoid
Latissimus dorsi

Neck extensors
Rotator cuff
Shoulder girdle muscle
Triceps
Erector spinae
Finger and wrist extensors
Gluteus medius
Hip adductor muscles
Hamstrings
Foot and ankle extensors

Figure 7.5

The major muscle groups.

- Know if your gym uses plates in pounds or kilograms: 1 kg is 2.2 lbs. Use adjustable collars to keep plates on the bar.
- Depending on the style of collar, a pair of bells can add 1 to 5 lb to your bar.
- Be aware of the advantages and disadvantages of using free weights (see Table 7.2).

Tipping Point

Determining Your Repetition Maximum
- Adjust the exercise intensity by knowing your **repetition maximums (RM)**. Use free weights to determine your RM for each muscle group.

What's the word...

repetition maximums (RM) The maximum weight you can lift successfully once while using proper form.

7

Proper Free-Weight Lifting Techniques

- Keep weights as close to your body as possible.
- Do most of the lifting with your legs.
- Keep your hips and buttocks tucked in.
- Keep your hands dry.
- Wear gloves to prevent calluses and blisters.
- Wrap your thumbs around the bar when gripping it.
- When picking up a weight from the ground, keep your back straight and your head level or up.
- Warm up before lifting.
- Use spotters and collars with free weights.
- Start slowly and progress gradually.
- Perform exercises smoothly and with good form.
- Lift or push the weight forcefully during the active phase of the lift and then lower it slowly with control.
- Perform all lifts through the full range of motion to reduce the chance of injury and soreness. Do not lock (fully straighten) your knees or elbows when involved in an exercise, because this practice stresses the joint.
- Exhale when exerting the greatest force, and inhale when moving the weight into position for the active phase of the lift.
- Rest between sets if you perform more than one set of each exercise.
- If you feel pain during an exercise, stop immediately. Continue only if the pain subsides, but reduce the amount of weight.
- Soreness the next day is normal when first starting to exercise or when increasing the amount of weight you lift.
- Cool down after a workout.

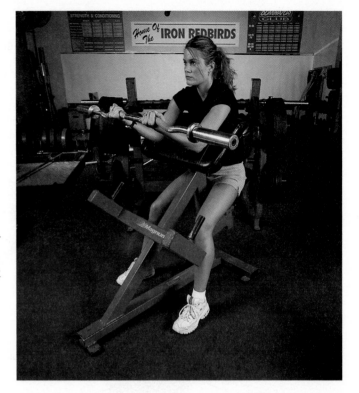

What's the word...

spotter Another person who can help if the weight tilts or can help move a weight into position before or after a lift.

collars Devices used to secure weights to a barbell or dumbbell. Without collars the weights on one side of the bar will slip off.

The Inside Track

Holding your breath can make you dizzy and faint and could bring on a condition known as the *Valsalva maneuver*. Your windpipe is blocked, and as pressure builds up in your lungs, your blood pressure will shoot up. This increases the risk of a heart attack, stroke, or hemorrhage.

Improper Free-Weight Lifting Techniques

Do not do the following:

- Bend at the waist with legs straight;
- Twist your body while lifting;
- Jerk weights; lift smoothly and slowly;
- Bounce weights against your body during an exercise;
- Arch your back when lifting a weight;
- Lift beyond the limits of your strength; or
- Hold your breath when lifting.

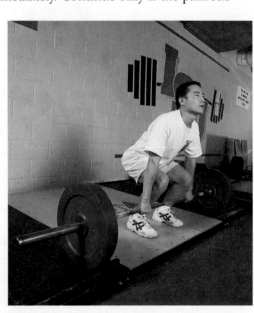

Table 7.3	Training with Weights

These exercises may be done with free weights or with circuit-training machines.

Exercise

Muscles Developed and Technique/Procedure

Bench Press

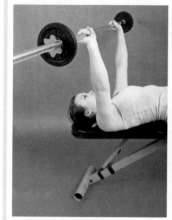 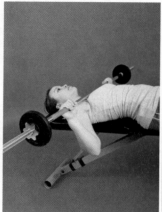

Muscles developed: pectoralis major, triceps, deltoids
- Lie facing up on a bench, your feet flat on the floor, with your head, shoulders, and buttocks pressed down firmly.
- Grip the bar with your hands about shoulder width apart or slightly wider. Push the bar from a low point on your chest to a high point over your chin.
- Extend your arms, pause momentarily, and then lower them slowly. Repeat.
- **Do not** arch your back or raise your buttocks during lifting.
- **Do not** bounce the bar off of your chest.

Shoulder (military press)

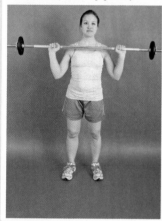 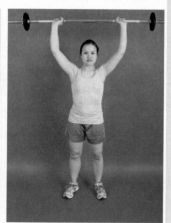

Muscles developed: deltoids, triceps, trapezius
Stand or sit with your feet shoulder-width apart. Keep your eyes straight ahead and your back straight. Place your hands shoulder-width apart. Push the bar overhead to arm's length, pause, and then slowly lower it. Repeat.

Biceps Curl

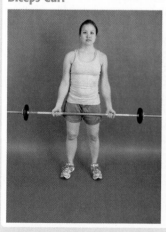 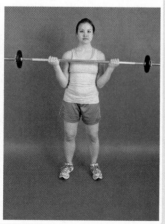

Muscles developed: biceps, brachialis
Stand with your feet spread shoulder-width apart, palms facing out. In the starting position, the bar should rest against your thighs. Keep your elbows by your sides, bend your arms slowly to raise the weight up to your chest, pause, and then slowly lower it. Repeat.

continues

7

Table 7.3	Training with Weights, *continued*

These exercises may be done with free weights or with circuit-training machines.

Exercise	**Muscles Developed and Technique/Procedure**
Triceps Curl 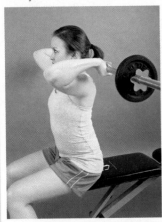 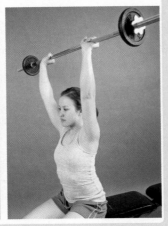	Muscles developed: triceps Sit erect with your elbows and palms facing up, the bar resting behind your neck on your shoulders. Your hands should be shoulder-width apart. Slowly curl the weight overhead, pause, and slowly lower it. Repeat.
Half Squat 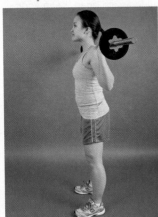 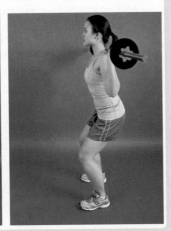	Muscles developed: quadriceps, gluteus maximus, hamstrings, gastrocnemius • Stand erect with the bar resting on your trapezius muscles (shoulder muscles), not your neck. • Use an overhand grip, with your hands and feet spread shoulder-width part. • Lower your weight by bending at the knees to a 90° angle, pause, and slowly return to an upright position. Repeat. • Keep your back straight; do not bend forward at the waist. • **Do not** squat beyond halfway or bounce at the bottom. • Place a bench behind you so that you can sit down if you lose your balance. Use spotters.
Heel Raise 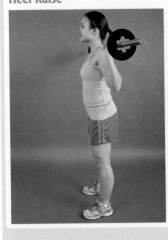 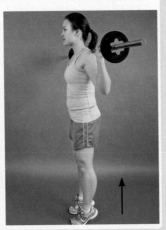	Muscles developed: gastrocnemius, soleus • Stand erect with your hands and feet spread shoulder-width apart. • Hold the bar resting on your shoulders (see half squat) or hold a dumbbell in each hand. Use an overhand grip. • With your feet flat on the floor, slowly push down on your toes while lifting your heels as high as possible, pause momentarily, and then lower slowly. Repeat. • You can also do this exercise by placing the front one-third of each foot on the edge of a bottom stair or wood block, with the backs of your feet hanging off.

| Table 7.3 | Training with Weights, *continued* |

These exercises may be done with free weights or with circuit-training machines.

Exercise | **Muscles Developed and Technique/Procedure**

Upright Rowing

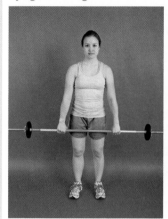 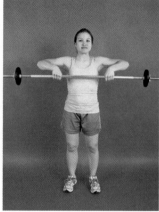

Muscles developed: trapezius, deltoids, biceps
- In a standing position, grip the bar with palms down and 4 to 8 inches apart.
- Keep your eyes straight ahead and chest high.
- Raise the bar until it reaches chin height, pause momentarily, and then lower slowly. Repeat.
- Keep your weight close to the front of your body, and make sure that your elbows stay higher than your hands.

Lunge

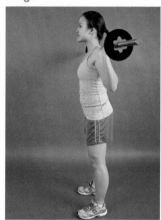 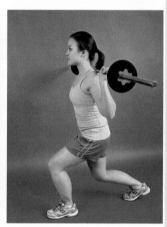

Muscles developed: thigh, gluteal
- Place the barbell behind your head or use a dumbbell in each hand.
- Keep the weight of the bar mainly on your trapezius muscles, not your neck.
- Your hands should be shoulder-width apart.
- Keep your head up and look forward, with your back straight.
- Slowly take a step forward and allow your leading leg to drop so that it is nearly parallel with the floor. The lower part of your leg should be nearly vertical and your back should be kept upright.
- Pause momentarily, and then take a stride with your other leg to return to a standing position.
- Repeat with your other leg.

Lateral Raise

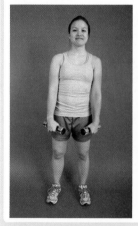 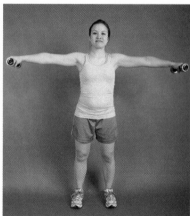

Muscles developed: deltoids
- Start with a dumbbell in each hand and feet apart.
- Slowly lift weights with elbows slightly bent.
- Lift weights until level with shoulders.
- Slowly lower the weights to starting position.

Table 7.4 — Training Without Weights

Exercise	Muscles Developed and Technique/Procedure

Push-ups

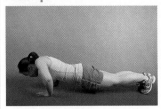 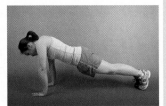

Muscles developed: triceps, deltoids, pectoralis major, abdominals, and erector spinae
- Keep your back as straight as possible. Flex your elbows. Lower your body until it almost touches the floor; pause momentarily, and then raise yourself back up to the starting position and repeat.
- You can use a bench, chair, or stairway to support your hands, rather than the floor. Increase resistance by having someone push down on your way up.
- If you are unable to do push-ups as described, do modified push-ups by placing your lower body on your knees rather than on your feet.

Modified Push-up

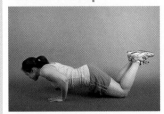 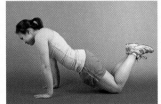

Modified Dip

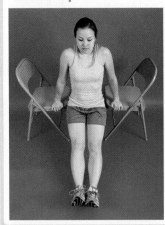 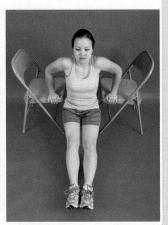

Muscles developed: triceps, deltoids, and pectoralis major
- Place your hands on opposite chairs or use parallel bars.
- With your knees slightly bent, dip down to at least a 90° angle at the elbow joint, pause momentarily, and then raise yourself back up to the starting position. Repeat. Increase resistance by having someone push down on your way up.

Pull-up or Chin-up

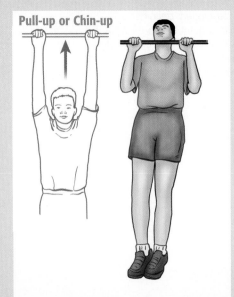

Muscles developed: biceps, triceps, trapezius, and latissimus dorsi
- Suspend yourself by your hands and arms from a bar.
- Pull-ups: Use an overhand grip, palms away, to develop the triceps.
- Chin-ups: Use an underhand grip, palms facing you, to develop the biceps. Pull your body up until your chin is above the bar, pause momentarily, and then lower yourself to the starting position. Repeat.
- If you are unable to do a pull-up or chin-up in this way, use a lower bar with your feet on the floor, or have a spotter help by pushing upward at the waist, hips, or legs during the exercise.

Table 7.4	Training Without Weights, *continued*
Exercise	**Muscles Developed and Technique/Procedure**
Arm Curl 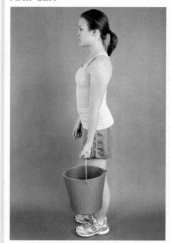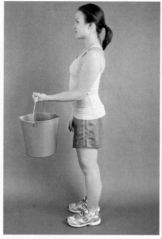	Muscles developed: biceps • Use a palms-up grip to raise a bucket filled with rocks, sand, or dirt. • Start with one arm completely extended. Curl up your arm as far as possible, pause momentarily, and then extend your arm back to the starting position and repeat. • Repeat the exercise with your other arm.
Curl-ups or Crunches 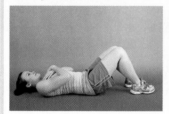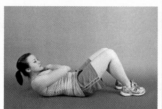	Muscles developed: abdominals and hip flexors • Lie face up on the floor or an exercise pad with your knees bent at an angle and both feet flat on the floor. • Fold your arms across your chest or place hands over your ears—do not lock your fingers behind your head. • Slowly raise your upper torso in a curling motion until your shoulders have totally cleared the floor. • Pause momentarily, and then slowly return to the starting position. Repeat. *Twisting Curl-up* • Perform the crunch (preceding section), but as you raise your shoulders off the floor, twist your upper torso to bring your left shoulder toward your right knee. • Slowly lower yourself back to the starting position. • Repeat by doing each twist to an alternate side, or alternate sides from one rep to another.
Lunges 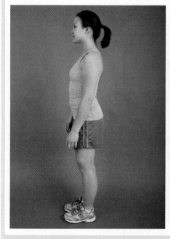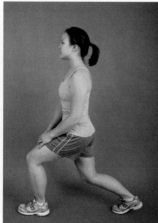	Muscles developed: thigh, gluteal • These exercises are completed in the same fashion as lunges with weights. • Look straight ahead. • From the "standing upright" position, step out and allow your leading leg to come almost parallel to the floor. • Your back leg should come to a nearly vertical position. • Pause, and return to the standing position. • Repeat with your other leg.

continues

Table 7.4	Training Without Weights, *continued*
Exercise	**Muscles Developed and Technique/Procedure**
Step-up 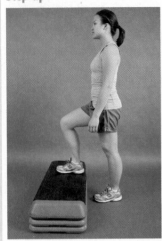 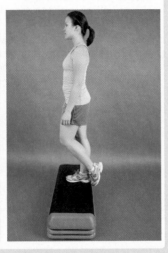	Muscles developed: gluteus maximus, quadriceps This exercise requires a firm box, aerobic step, or step of a stairwell to complete. • Position yourself facing the step. • Step in an "up, up, down, down" cadence. • Alternate the initial "step-up" leg. • As your strength develops, you can increase the height of the step or quicken the pace of the cadence.

Cautions About Supplements and Drugs

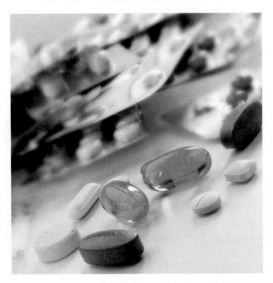

Many people take drugs and supplements to enhance the results of their weight training. This practice can be expensive and dangerous. The most common of these substances are anabolic steroids, synthetic derivatives of testosterone. Using this kind of drug helps bodybuilders develop abnormally large muscle mass—along with some undesirable secondary sexual characteristics.

Steroids increase protein synthesis, which promotes muscle growth and improves the ability of muscle to respond to training and recovery.

Drugs with Undesirable Side Effects

- Testosterone has the same benefits and similar side effects as steroids (see the following description of steroids).
- Human growth hormone promotes muscle growth but can cause gigantism: abnormal enlargement of the joints, jaw, and skull.
- Amphetamines increase motor activity and delay fatigue but can cause chest pains, extreme confusion, aggressiveness, irritability, and hallucinations.
- Creatine is said to increase performance in brief, high-intensity exercises such as sprinting. Side effects include diarrhea, dehydration, and muscle cramping and tearing.
- Caffeine also increases motor activity and delays fatigue, but can cause insomnia and abnormal heart rhythm.
- Androstenedione dehydroepiandrosterone (andro-DHEA) promotes muscle growth. It has similar side effects as steroids.
- Erythropoietin increases red blood cells and the ability to transport oxygen to the muscles. A bad side effect is thickened blood, which can lead to strokes or heart problems.

Even though steroids have been used in the sports and athletic arenas for some time, their long-term effects are not completely understood. Well-known athletes from many sports such as track, football, and professional baseball have admitted to using such performance enhancers to improve the quality of their play. But the problem goes well beyond these individuals. Participants in cycling, bodybuilding, and even "scripted" sports, such as professional wrestling, use performance-enhancing drugs.

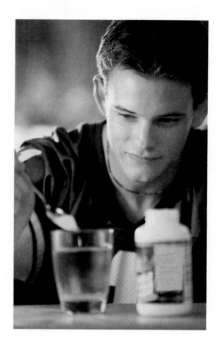

The challenge in denouncing steroids is that deaths can only be circumstantially attributed to use. The steroid itself does not kill the user; rather death results from long-term, high-level use. Lyle Alzado, a former professional football player, died from brain cancer he said was caused by more than 20 years of steroid use. As many as 10 professional wrestlers with a known history of heavy and consistent steroid use have died from complications directly related to the use of the drug in the last 5 years—either heart, liver, or emotional problems. It is estimated that more than 80 professional cyclists have died from drug use in the last 10 years. Countless reports of aggression, including some high-profile cases of suspected murder, are found in police blotters related to individuals known to have used performance-enhancing drugs. The numbers are not staggering, but the relationship between steroid use and these problems becomes clearer all the time.

According to the professionals at Exercise Prescription (ExRx.com), this is what we know about performance-enhancing drugs:

- Because each person is unique, each responds differently to the use of steroids. However, people choose steroids based on what has worked for others—a dangerous proposition at best.
- The extent of the side effects experienced is affected by the type of enhancer used, dose, length of time and frequency of use, age at first use, and use of other drugs while on steroids.
- Most physical effects are reversible after the drug is discontinued for several months, with the notable exception of damage to the myocardium—the inner muscle of the heart.

Possible side effects in men include:

- Multiple changes in the risk factors for heart disease, including the previously noted changes in the myocardium, increased triglyceride levels, increased cholesterol levels, and hypertension
- Damage to the liver's ability to function properly
- Damage and/or changes to the reproductive system, including reduced sperm count and mobility, reduced testicle size, and gynecomastia (breast development)
- Reduced ability to fight disease
- For injected forms of steroids, increased risks for HIV/AIDS, hepatitis, and other blood-borne diseases

Possible side effects in women include:

- Menstrual abnormalities and changes in clitoris size
- Masculinization, including voice changes, breast shrinkage, baldness, body hair development, and increased levels of testosterone
- Some are irreversible effects

Both men and women have reported a fairly consistent pattern of emotional effects related to steroid use, although the relationship seems to reflect the type of steroid, not the amount taken. Most commonly reported are bouts of anger and violence, significant mood swings, depression, and changes in the perception of one's body.

7

Reflect >>>> Reinforce >>>> Reinvigorate

Knowledge Check

Answers in Appendix D

1. What is the measure of muscle strength?

    A. Number of repetitions in a set
    B. Length of muscle stretch
    C. Force against resistance
    D. Time taken to complete a workout

2. Which mode of exercise is most popular for increasing strength?

    A. Isometric
    B. Isotonic
    C. Plyometric
    D. Isokinetic

3. Which of the following is an effect of muscle training on a person's body?

    A. Higher muscle-to-fat ratio
    B. Stronger bones
    C. Higher rate of metabolism
    D. All of the above

4. When the number of desired repetitions is accomplished during an exercise, it is the completion of one:

    A. Block
    B. Form
    C. Set
    D. Activity

5. Gradually increasing the weight one uses during a workout is called:

    A. Repetition maximum
    B. Progressive overload
    C. Specificity
    D. Muscular gain

6. Which of the following exercises is designed to help build muscles in the arm?
   A. Curls
   B. Squats
   C. Deadlift
   D. Extensions

7. Which of the following is an advantage of using machine weights?
   A. They are available everywhere.
   B. They are inexpensive.
   C. They are easier for beginners to use.
   D. They take up little space.

8. Which of the following would be a reason someone might choose not to use free weights?
   A. Lack of variety in exercises
   B. Limited availability
   C. No spotters available
   D. Too costly to purchase

9. A person who can help complete your lift if you cannot complete the exercise on your own is called a(n):
   A. Spotter
   B. Assistant
   C. Grabber
   D. Collar

10. Once an individual can lift a weight _____ times, it is recommended to increase the weight being used.
    A. 6
    B. 9
    C. 12
    D. 20

Modern Modifications

Take a moment to look at your lifestyle in terms of strength training. Would you like to be stronger and more fit? Try these simple suggestions to get started:

- Do a set of push-ups (modified or regular, whichever you are comfortable with) first thing each morning. Only do 1 set of however many push-ups you can perform at the moment: 5, 10, 15, or whatever that number may be. Every week try adding 1 to 2 more push-ups to your routine.
- Do a wall squat while you are waiting for class or a meeting to start.
- Take a stress ball to work or class—improve your grip strength and your mood at the same time.
- Grab a can of soup and do some bicep curls while watching television.

Critical Thinking

1. As Susan has gotten older, her upper arms have become flabby. She is very self-conscious when she raises an arm while wearing short sleeves. Describe the type of activities Susan can do to address her problem. Discuss specific types and forms of exercise as well as FITT principle descriptors. What may be the reason for her lack of firmness in the upper arms?

2. Phil wants to start a strength-training program. He has been told that exercise machines are better for beginners than free weights. Discuss the pros and cons of weight machines versus free weights. What would you suggest to Phil?

Going Above and Beyond

Websites

American College of Sports Medicine
http://www.acsm.org

Exercise Prescription
http://www.exrx.net

National Strength and Conditioning Association
http://www.nsca-cc.org

National Council of Strength and Fitness
http://www.ncsf.org

Physician and Sports Medicine
http://www.physsportsmed.com

References and Suggested Readings

————. Prescription of resistance training for health and disease. *Medicine and Science in Sports and Exercise* 1999; 31:38–45.

American College of Sports Medicine (ACSM). The recommended quantity and quality of exercise for developing and maintaining cardiorespiratory and muscular fitness and flexibility in healthy adults. *Medicine and Science in Sports and Exercise* 1998; 30:975–991.

American College of Sports Medicine. Quantity and Quality of Exercise for Developing and Maintaining Cardiorespiratory, Musculoskeletal, and Neuromotor Fitness in Apparently Healthy Adults: Guidance for Prescribing Exercise. *Medicine and Science in Sports and Exercise.* DOI: 10.1249/MSS.0b0138213fefb

Braill P. A., et al. Muscular strength and physical function. *Medicine and Science in Sports and Exercise* 2000; 32:412–416.

Ebben W. P. and Jensen R. L. Strength training for women. *Physician and Sports Medicine* 1998; 26:86.

Feigenbaum M. S. and Pollock M. L. Strength training: Rationale for current guidelines for adult fitness programs. *Physician and Sports Medicine* 1997; 25:44.

Garber, C. E., et al. Quantity and quality of exercise for developing and maintaining cardiorespiratory, musculoskeletal, and neuromotor fitness in apparently healthy adults: Guidance for prescribing exercise. *Medicine in Science and Sports and Exercise* 2011; 43(7):1334–1359.

National Safety Council. *Inquiry Facts.* Itasca, IL: National Safety Council, 2007.

Stamford B. Weight training basics. Part 1: Choosing the best options. *Physician and Sports Medicine* 1998; 26:115–116.

U.S. DHHS. *2008 Physical Activity Guidelines for Americans.* www.health.gov/paguidelines.

CHAPTER 8

Nutrition

Objectives

After reading this chapter, you should be able to:

- Identify the main nutrients and their functions in the body.
- Describe how the body converts nutrients to energy.
- Describe how the body uses energy during exercise.
- List the recommendations of nutrition guidelines and assessments useful in selecting a proper diet.
- Evaluate foods and supplements using their labels.
- Recognize the problems you might encounter in changing your diet and describe the ways to deal with them.

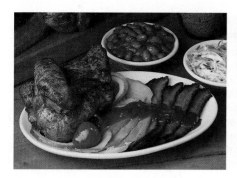 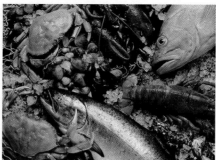 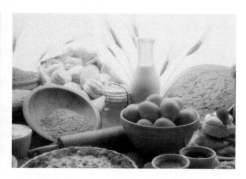

What Is a Healthy Diet?

Eating is one of life's greatest pleasures. Since there are many foods and many ways to build a healthy diet and lifestyle, there is plenty of room for choice.

Eating is also a necessity. Nutrients must come from what you eat because some nutrients cannot be made in the body at all and others are not in sufficient quantities.

Poor diet and physical inactivity are associated with major causes of death and disability. These include cardiovascular disease, hypertension, type 2 diabetes, osteoporosis, and some types of cancer (see [Table 8.1]). These diet and health associations make a strong and urgent case for improved nutrition and physical activity choices.

The six classes of nutrients are proteins, fats, carbohydrates, vitamins, minerals, and water.

- Proteins, fats, carbohydrates, and water are macronutrients.
- Vitamins and minerals are micronutrients.

What's the word. . .

nutrients Substances in food that the body needs for normal function and good health.

protein Nutrient made up of amino acids that is needed for growth, to build, repair, and maintain body tissues.

macronutrients Nutrients needed by your body in relatively large amounts.

micronutrients Nutrients needed by your body in relatively small amounts.

Medical News You Can Use

Study Finds Americans are Eating More

Researchers from the University of North Carolina at Chapel Hill examined surveys of the daily eating habits of U.S. adults over a 30-year period. In the top decile, the number of daily meals rose from five to seven. Americans were also consuming 570 more calories per day than they did in the late 1970s. Americans now consume 220 more calories per day just from drinking sugar-sweetened soft drinks than they did in the 1960s. Dr. Kiyah Duffey of the UNC Interdisciplinary Obesity Center suggests that the number of eating occasions is the driving change. Food is available everywhere and the decline in regular mealtimes may be driving the increase in caloric intake. "People aren't sitting down to three meals anymore," she said. "We sort of think about eating all through day." Some sources say eating frequent, small meals throughout the day increases metabolism and controls hunger and may be healthier than eating three big meals. The study concludes that what and how much you eat over the course of a day are more important than how often you eat. If you find yourself eating seven times a day, reach for healthy snacks like an apple rather than finishing off yesterday's pizza or eating salty snacks.

Source: Data from Duffey K.J., Popkin B.M. Energy Density, Portion Size, and Eating Occasions: Contributions to Increased Energy Intake in the United States, 1977–2006. *PLoS Medicine* 2011; 8(6): e1001050.

| Table 8.1 | Heavy Toll of Diet-Related Chronic Diseases |

Cardiovascular Disease
- 81.1 million Americans—37 percent of the population—have cardiovascular disease. Major risk factors include high levels of blood cholesterol and other lipids, type 2 diabetes, hypertension (high blood pressure), metabolic syndrome, overweight and obesity, physical inactivity, and tobacco use.
- 16 percent of the U.S. adult population has high total blood cholesterol.

Hypertension
- 74.5 million Americans—34 percent of U.S. adults—have hypertension.
- Hypertension is a major risk factor for heart disease, stroke, congestive heart failure, and kidney disease.
- Dietary factors that increase blood pressure include excessive sodium and insufficient potassium intake, overweight and obesity, and excess alcohol consumption.
- 36 percent of American adults have prehypertension—blood pressure numbers that are higher than normal, but not yet in the hypertension range.

Diabetes
- Nearly 24 million people—almost 11 percent of the population—ages 20 years and older have diabetes. The vast majority of cases are type 2 diabetes, which is heavily influenced by diet and physical activity.
- About 78 million Americans—35 percent of the U.S. adult population ages 20 years or older—have pre-diabetes. Pre-diabetes (also called impaired glucose tolerance or impaired fasting glucose) means that blood glucose levels are higher than normal, but not high enough to be called diabetes.

Cancer
- Almost one in two men and women—approximately 41 percent of the population—will be diagnosed with cancer during their lifetime.
- Dietary factors are associated with risk of some types of cancer, including breast (post- menopausal), endometrial, colon, kidney, mouth, pharynx, larynx, and esophagus.

Osteoporosis
- One out of every two women and one in four men ages 50 years and older will have an osteoporosis-related fracture in their lifetime.
- About 85 to 90 percent of adult bone mass is acquired by the age of 18 in girls and the age of 20 in boys. Adequate nutrition and regular participation in physical activity are important factors in achieving and maintaining optimal bone mass.

Source: Reproduced from the *Dietary Guidelines for Americans*, 2010. Courtesy of the U.S. Department of Health & Human Services.

Proteins

Protein is found throughout the body (i.e., skin, hair, muscle, bone). Twenty or so basic building blocks, called amino acids, provide the raw material for all proteins. Nine are called **essential amino acids** because the body cannot make them; they must be obtained from the diet. That is why you must eat protein—to take in the essential amino acids. Because the body does not store amino acids as it does fats and carbohydrates, it needs a daily supply of amino acids to make new protein.

Complete and Incomplete Proteins

Eating protein made up of amino acids is necessary for good health. There are two types of proteins: complete and incomplete.

Complete proteins are found in animal products (e.g., meats, milk, fish, and eggs). They contain all the amino acids needed to build new protein.

Incomplete proteins generally have one amino acid in insufficient quantity. Grains, legumes, and nuts are sources of incomplete proteins.

If you choose not to consume animal products, you must be sure to consume a variety of incomplete protein sources to acquire the necessary amino acids. Vegetable sources of protein, such as beans, nuts, and whole grains are good choices, and they offer fiber, vitamins, and minerals. Nuts also offer healthy fat.

What's the word...

essential amino acids The nine protein amino acids that the body cannot make and, therefore, must come from the foods you eat.

complete protein A protein that contains all the essential amino acids.

incomplete protein A protein lacking one or more of the essential amino acids.

Fish and poultry offer the best animal protein choices. If you like red meat (e.g., beef, pork, or lamb), choose the leanest cuts, use moderate portions, and eat them only occasionally.

How Much Protein Do You Need?

Many people eat high-protein foods because they think that proteins make them grow bigger and stronger. Also, high-protein diets (i.e., Atkins) for weight loss have brought increased attention to protein.

- Each day adults need about 4 grams of protein for every 10 pounds of body weight (your ideal weight, that is) to keep from slowly breaking down their own body tissues. Athletes may need a bit more. Beyond this, there is little solid information on the ideal amount of protein in the diet.

- You can estimate your protein needs and intake by using food labels, MyPlate, and other guidelines to get an ample amount of protein.

Protein and Health

Cardiovascular disease: Some believe that eating diets high in protein and fat and low in carbohydrates can harm the heart. Research provides evidence that eating a lot of protein does not harm the heart. Actually, eating more protein, especially vegetable protein, while cutting back on carbohydrates may benefit the heart.

Diabetes: Protein in the diet does not appear to be a factor in the development of type 2 diabetes (formerly called adult-onset diabetes); however, more research is needed. A recent study of women reported that eating a low-carbohydrate diet high in vegetable sources of fat and protein may modestly reduce the risk for type 2 diabetes.

Cancer: A greater risk for colon cancer exists among those who eat much red meat and processed meat (i.e., hotdogs, bacon, ham).

Weight control: One of the best studies was reported in the *Journal of the American Medical Association* in 2007 and compared four diets: (1) Atkins (eat as much protein and fat as desired with some carbohydrates), (2) Zone (30% percent of calories from protein, 40% from carbohydrates, and 30% from fat), (3) Ornish (low-fat), and (4) LEARN (low-fat, moderately high in carbohydrates). The women in all four groups steadily lost weight for the first 6 months, with the most rapid weight loss occurring among the Atkins dieters. Those eating mostly fat and protein (i.e., Atkins diet) not only lost more weight but their blood lipids (i.e., HDL cholesterol, triglycerides) and blood pressure also improved.

Why do high-protein, low-carb diets seem to work more quickly than low-fat, high-carbohydrate diets at least for a short time? A couple of possible reasons include: (1) high-protein foods slowly moves from the stomach to the intestine—this means that you feel full longer and hunger is delayed, and (2) protein avoids the quick rise in blood sugar that happens after eating an easily digested carbohydrate (i.e., white bread or baked potato). It has yet to be determined what the long-term effects of eating high-protein and high-fat diets with little or no carbohydrates might be.

Lack of protein: Protein deficiency can cause growth failure, loss of muscle mass, decreased immunity, weakening of the heart and the respiratory system, and death. Protein deficiency is a common form of malnutrition in the developing world. It can manifest in two forms: kwashiorkor and marasmus. Kwashiorkor occurs mostly in children. Affected children tend to have swollen body tissues, particularly hands and feet, and bloated bellies. Marasmus results from lack of food. The chronic protein deficiency results in severe wasting of body fat and muscles. Those with marasmus have skeletal bodies.

Excessive amounts of protein: Eating a lot of protein increases your fluid needs and thus may dehydrate you if you do not drink enough fluids. Also, eating excessive amounts of protein for a long time increases calcium excretion, which could then contribute to bone mineral loss.

What's the word. . .

lipids Fats or fat-like substances characterized by their insolubility in water or solubility in fat.

cholesterol Wax-like substance made by the body's liver and found in animal foods.

wasting Occurs when the diet lacks protein; the body breaks down body tissue (e.g., muscle) and uses it as a protein source.

8

Medical News You Can Use

Eggs May Help Prevent Heart Disease and Cancer

Eggs are well-known to be an excellent source of proteins, lipids, vitamins, and minerals. Researchers have recently found eggs to contain antioxidant properties, which helps prevent cardiovascular disease and cancer. Results of the study show that two egg yolks in their raw state have almost twice as many antioxidants as an apple and about the same as half a serving (25 grams) of cranberries. When fried or boiled, the antioxidant properties were reduced by about half and a little more than half when microwaved. This still leaves the antioxidant properties about equal to that of an apple.

Source: Data from Nimalaratne C., et al., Free aromatic amino acids in egg yolk show antioxidant properties. *Food Chemistry,* 2011. 129(1):155.

Fats and Cholesterol

Fats may have a bad reputation, but not all fats are the same (see Table 8.2).

Benefits of Fat Intake

Fats provide a major form of stored energy; they provide energy during exercise, in cold environments, and if starvation occurs. They:

- insulate your body;
- cushion internal organs;
- help carry other nutrients throughout your body;
- serve a structural role in making and repairing cells; and
- satisfy hunger and add taste to many foods.

For decades the advice has been to eat a low-fat, low-cholesterol diet. This advice was given as a way to lose weight and prevent or control heart disease and other chronic conditions. Thousands of foods are labeled as low fat or fat free. While some may have benefited from the low-fat approach to eating, in the United States it has not helped to control weight or become healthier. In the 1960s, about 45% of our calories came from fats and oils; about 13% of us were obese, and fewer than 1% had type 2 diabetes. Today, we get about 33% of our calories from fats and oils. However, 34% of us are obese and 8% have diabetes (mostly type 2, which is weight-related).

Table 8.2	Dietary Fats	
Type of Fat	**Main Sources**	**Effect on Blood Cholesterol Levels**
Monounsaturated	Olives; olive oil, canola oil, peanut oil; cashews, almonds, peanuts, and most other nuts	Lowers LDL; raises HDL
Polyunsaturated	Corn, soybean, safflower oil; fish	Lowers LDL; raises HDL
Saturated	Whole milk, butter, cheese, ice cream; red meat; chocolate; coconuts	Raises both LDL and HDL
Trans fatty acids	Most margarines; vegetable shortening; partially hydrogenated vegetable oil; deep-fried chips; many fast foods; most commercial baked goods	Raises LDL and lowers HDL

Reducing fat from the diet has not worked. The *total* amount of fat in the diet is not linked with weight or disease. The culprit is the *type of fat* in the diet. Trans and saturated fats (both bad fats) increase the risk for certain diseases. Monounsaturated and polyunsaturated fats (both good fats), do just the opposite. The heart and most other parts of the body benefit from them.

Lipoproteins

Almost all foods (even fat-free foods such as carrots and lettuce) have some fat. Fat provides a source of energy and also serves as a place for storing it. Cholesterol is involved in making estrogen, testosterone, vitamin D, and other vital compounds (see **Table 8.3**).

Fat and cholesterol do not dissolve in water or blood; the body solves this problem by putting fat and cholesterol into tiny particles called lipoproteins. Lipoproteins that carry fat can mix easily with blood and flow with it. Some of the lipoproteins in the bloodstream are large and buoyant; others are small and dense. When you have your cholesterol checked, the results will show your total blood cholesterol level. If you fasted overnight before giving a blood sample, the test should also show separate counts for your high-density lipoprotein (HDL) and low-density lipoprotein (LDL).

- **Low-density lipoproteins (LDL)** carry cholesterol from the liver to the rest of the body. When there is excessive LDL cholesterol in the blood, they form deposits in the walls of the coronary arteries and other arteries throughout the body. These deposits, known as plaque, narrow the arteries and limit blood flow. A heart attack or stroke can result when plaque breaks apart. Because of this, LDL cholesterol is often referred to as bad cholesterol.

- **High-density lipoproteins (HDL)** collect cholesterol from the bloodstream and from artery walls and transport it back to the liver for disposal. Because of this action, HDL cholesterol is often called good cholesterol.

- **Triglycerides** compose most of the fat that you eat and that travels through the bloodstream. As the body's main vehicle for transporting fats to cells, triglycerides are important for good health. However, excessive amounts can be unhealthy.

The higher your LDL and the lower your HDL, the greater is your risk for heart disease and other chronic conditions. The National Cholesterol Education Program suggests specific targets for lipoprotein levels (after 9- to 12-hour fasting).

What's the word...

saturated fat Fat from meat, poultry, dairy products, and hardened vegetable fat.

lipoprotein Allows cholesterol to dissolve in the blood and carries it through the bloodstream to all parts of the body; the two main types are high-density lipoprotein (HDL) and low-density lipoprotein (LDL).

low-density lipoprotein (LDL) Carries cholesterol from the liver to the rest of the body. When there is too much LDL cholesterol in the blood, it can be deposited on the walls of the coronary arteries. LDL is often referred to as *bad* cholesterol.

high-density lipoprotein (HDL) Carries cholesterol from the blood back to the liver, which processes the cholesterol for elimination from the body. HDL is often referred to as *good* cholesterol.

Table 8.3	What Your Cholesterol Levels Mean
LDL Cholesterol	
<100	Optimal
100–129	Near optimal/above optimal
130–159	Borderline high
160–189	High
>190	Very high
Total Cholesterol	
<200	Desirable—lower risk for heart disease
200–239	Borderline high
>240	High—increased risk for heart disease
HDL Cholesterol	
<40	Low—a major risk factor for heart disease
>60	High—considered protection against heart disease

Source: Courtesy of the National Heart, Lung and Blood Institute.

Medical News You Can Use

Diet Soda Tied to Vascular Risk

Researchers found that drinking diet soda, but not regular soda, was associated with a greater risk of stroke, heart attack, or vascular death in an older, multiethnic cohort. Results showed that those who drink diet soda every day were 48% more likely to have a vascular event after more than 9 years of follow-up. The American Heart Association (AHA) recommends consuming less than 1500 mg a day of dietary sodium. Only 12% of participants in an additional study met that recommendation. The average daily intake for participants was 3031 mg, with one fifth of the study participants consuming more than 4000 mg a day. Those who consumed more than 4000 mg/day had a 2.67-fold increased risk of stroke when compared to those who met the AHA target. Focusing on dietary behavior will help promote ideal cardiovascular and brain health.

Source: Data from Gardener H., et al. Soda consumption and risk of vascular events in the Northern Manhattan Study. *American Stroke Association* 2011; Abstract P55 and from Gardener H., et al. Dietary sodium intake is a risk factor for incident ischemic stroke: the Northern Manhattan Study (NOMAS). *American Stroke Association* 2011; Abstract 25.

Unsaturated Fats

Unsaturated fats are also known as good fats because they can improve blood cholesterol levels, ease inflammation, stabilize heart rhythms, as well as doing other beneficial roles. Unsaturated fats are mainly found in foods from plants, such as vegetable oils, nuts, and seeds. They are liquid at room temperature.

There are two types of unsaturated fats:

- Monounsaturated fats are found in high concentrations in canola, peanut, and olive oils; avocados; nuts such as almonds, hazelnuts, and pecans; and seeds such as pumpkin and sesame seeds.
- Polyunsaturated fats are found in high concentrations in sunflower, corn, soybean, and flaxseed oils and also in foods such as walnuts, flax seeds, and fish. Omega-3 fats are an important type of polyunsaturated fat. They must come from food since the body does not make them. Eating fish at least two times a week provides a good way to get omega-3. Flax seeds, walnuts, and oils, such as flaxseed, canola, and soybean, also represent good plant sources of omega-3 fats.

When polyunsaturated and monounsaturated fats are eaten in place of carbohydrates, these good fats decrease levels of harmful LDL and increase good HDL. When a diet rich in unsaturated fat (i.e., monounsaturated fat) replaces a carbohydrate-rich diet, lower blood pressure, improved lipid levels, and reduced cardiovascular risk result.

Most people are deficient of these healthful unsaturated fats each day. Exact guide-lines have not been established regarding how much to consume. Nevertheless, choose unsaturated fats over saturated whenever possible.

Saturated Fats

Saturated fat is bad because it contributes to producing cardiovascular disease. We don't need to eat any of it because our bodies make all the saturated fat we need. Sources of saturated fats include meat, seafood, poultry with skin, and whole-milk dairy products (i.e., cheese, milk, and ice cream). Some plant foods also contain high amounts of satu-rated fats, such as coconut and coconut oil, palm oil, and palm kernel oil. Saturated fats boost total cholesterol by elevating harmful LDLs. Unsaturated fat lowers the bad choles-terol and raises the good (see **Table 8.4**).

Medical News You Can Use

Reduced-Calorie Diets Result in Weight Loss

A study randomly assigned 811 overweight adults to one of four diets. The diets consisted of similar foods and met guidelines for cardiovascular health. At the end of the two-year study, weight loss remained similar in those who were assigned to a diet with 15% protein and those assigned to a diet with 25% protein; in those assigned to a diet with 20% fat and those assigned to a diet of 40% fat; and in those assigned to a diet with 65% carbohydrates and those to a 35% carbohydrate diet. The study concludes that reduced-calorie diets result in meaningful weight loss regardless of which macronutrients the diet emphasizes.

Source: Data from Sacks F.M., et al., Comparison of weight-loss diets with different compositions of fat, protein, and carbohydrates. *New England Journal of Medicine*, 2009. 360(9):859–873.

Table 8.4	**Differences in Saturated Fat and Calorie Content of Commonly Consumed Foods**

This table shows a few practical examples of the differences in the saturated fat content of different forms of commonly consumed foods. Comparisons are made between foods in the same food group (e.g., regular cheddar cheese and low-fat cheddar cheese), illustrating that lower saturated fat choices can be made within the same food group.

Food Category	Portion	Saturated Fat Content (grams)	Calories
Cheese			
• Regular cheddar cheese	1 oz	6.0	114
• Low-fat cheddar cheese	1 oz	1.2	49
Ground beef			
• Regular ground beef (25% fat)	3 oz (cooked)	6.1	236
• Extra lean ground beef (5% fat)	3 oz (cooked)	2.6	148
Milk			
• Whole milk (3.25%)	1 cup	4.6	146
• Low-fat (1%) milk	1 cup	1.5	102
Breads			
• Croissant (med)	1 medium	6.6	231
• Bagel, oat bran (4")	1 medium	0.2	227
Frozen desserts			
• Regular ice cream	½ cup	4.9	145
• Frozen yogurt, low-fat	½ cup	2.0	110
Table spreads			
• Butter	1 tsp	2.4	34
• Soft margarine with zero *trans fats*	1 tsp	0.7	25
Chicken			
• Fried chicken (leg with skin)	3 oz (cooked)	3.3	212
• Roasted chicken (breast no skin)	3 oz (cooked)	0.9	140
Fish			
• Fried fish	3 oz	2.8	195
• Baked fish	3 oz	1.5	129

Source: Modified from the *Dietary Guidelines for Americans*, 2005. Courtesy of the U.S. Department of Health & Human Services.

Medical News You Can Use

Sugary Drinks Increase Cardiovascular Risk

A study found that even moderate consumption of soda and other sugar-sweetened beverages produces an increase in markers of cardiovascular risk. The study involved interventions that ranged from participants consuming drinks with 40 grams of the sweeteners fructose or glucose to drinks with 80 grams of fructose, glucose, or sucrose. In the 3-week study, adverse effects such as low-density lipoprotein particle size and distribution, waist-to-hip ratio, fasting glucose, and inflammatory markers were observed even in the group that consumed the lower amount of sweeteners.

Source: Data from Aeberli I., et al., Low to moderate sugar-sweetened beverage consumption impairs glucose and lipid metabolism and promotes inflammation in healthy young men: a randomized controlled trial. *American Journal of Clinical Nutrition*, 2011. 94(2):479–485.

Saturated fat intake should be kept as low as possible. It's difficult to completely eliminate them from our diets because they are found in many foods. The main sources of saturated fat in our diets are red meat and dairy products, of which we should limit our consumption.

Trans Fats

What's the word...

trans fatty acids Fats produced by heating liquid vegetable oils in the presence of hydrogen. This process is called hydrogenation.

Trans fats (also known as trans fatty acids), are made by a process called hydrogenation. This process consists of heating liquid vegetable oils in the presence of hydrogen gas. This makes vegetable oils solid, more stable, and less likely to spoil. Turning the oil solid makes them easier to transport. Partially hydrogenated oils are ideal for frying fast foods because they can withstand repeated heating without breaking down, making them attractive for frying fast foods.

Commercially prepared baked goods, margarines, snack foods, and processed foods, along with french fries and other fried foods prepared in restaurants and fast-food franchises are the sources of most of the trans fats in the American diet.

Because they raise bad LDL and lower good HDL, trans fats are worse for cholesterol levels than saturated fats. They also cause inflammation (a main cause of heart disease, stroke, and diabetes). Harmful health effects can result from even small amounts of trans fats.

To help curb the use of these harmful fats, a recent law forces food companies to list trans fats on the label. Consumers can see which products contain trans fats. Also, many companies in the food industry are now promoting their non-use of trans-free oils and fats in their products.

Cholesterol in Food

Decades ago it was discovered that an increased risk for heart disease was related to high blood cholesterol levels. Warnings were issued to avoid foods that contained cholesterol, especially eggs, liver, shrimp, and lobster. However, the advice proved to be wrong. For example, eating shrimp and lobster does not raise LDL cholesterol. Also, most people make more cholesterol than they absorb from their food. Scientific studies show only a weak relationship between the amount of cholesterol a person consumes and his or her blood cholesterol levels.

Only a small part of the cholesterol circulating in the blood comes from the cholesterol we eat. However, for some people, the amount of cholesterol eaten does affect blood

Medical News You Can Use

Dark Chocolate, a Comfort to Early Blood Pressure

Eating dark chocolate may have a small benefit in reducing early hypertension that is equivalent to other non-pharmaceutical interventions. A study compared adults with pre-hypertension of stage 1 high blood pressure who consumed dark or white chocolate daily for 18 weeks. Those who consumed the dark chocolate had significantly lower systolic and diastolic pressures. The blood pressure drop was not accompanied by changes in either body weight or plasma levels of lipids. Among dark chocolate eaters, the prevalence of hypertension also declined from 86% to 68%. These results are not unlike that of sildenafil (Viagra), which also cause relaxation of smooth muscle in the vascular endothelium. The news is good for dark chocolate lovers who worry about their blood pressure.

Source: Data from Taubert D., et al., Effects of low habitual cocoa intake on blood pressure and bioactive nitric oxide: A randomized controlled trial. *Journal of the American Medical Association*, 2007. 298(1):49–60.

cholesterol levels. To avoid a substantial effect on blood cholesterol levels, these people should avoid cholesterol-rich foods. Trial-and-error is the only way to determine if you might be affected by dietary cholesterol.

Fats and Health

Heart disease: Limiting fat intake has often been advocated by various health-oriented organizations. A problem with the message to lower fat intake is that it causes many people to stop eating fats that are good for the heart. These people turn to foods that replace healthful fats with sugar and refined carbohydrates.

Numerous reports have questioned the recommendation of low-fat diets for preventing or retarding heart disease. Studies have found no difference in the heart attack and stroke rates between those who followed a low-fat diet and those who did not.

The *type* of fat in the diet is the important thing. Ounce for ounce, trans fats are worse than saturated fats when it comes to heart disease. Evidence shows that a higher intake of either monounsaturated or polyunsaturated fat (especially the latter) lowers the risk for heart disease.

Breast cancer: Some studies suggest that animal fat intake may be linked to higher risk for breast cancer. Because vegetable fat is not related to risk for breast cancer, these studies suggest that red meat and high-fat dairy products may contain other factors, such as hormones, that increase the risk for breast cancer. Findings from Europe show a lower breast cancer risk among women with a high intake of monounsaturated fats (mainly in the form of olive oil).

Colon cancer: Although fat intake does not seem to increase colon cancer risk, there is strong evidence that high consumption of red meat (i.e., beef, pork, and lamb) and processed meat (i.e., hotdogs, bacon, and deli meats) increases colon cancer risk.

Prostate cancer: The connection between dietary fat and prostate cancer is uncertain. Some evidence shows that diets high in animal fat and saturated fat increase prostate cancer risk. However, other studies have also shown no relationship, while others have pointed to unsaturated fats. Additional research is needed to find the exact links between dietary fat and prostate cancer.

Overweight and obesity: The idea that food fat equals body fat is not completely true. For example, while Americans have gradually decreased the calories they get from fat over the past few decades, the rates of obesity have greatly increased.

Medical News You Can Use

Fish-Heavy Diet May Slow Hardening of Arteries

A diet heavy on omega-3 fatty acids from fish may prevent atherosclerosis over a lifetime. Higher intake of omega-3 fatty acids from fish accounted entirely for the lower intima-media thickness and coronary artery calcification among Japanese men living in Japan compared to Japanese-American and Caucasian-American men. Diet, rather than genetics, appears to account for the two-fold lower coronary heart disease mortality in Japan than in the United States. Japan has one of the highest levels of fish intake in the world. On average, Japanese men consumed 100 grams of fish every day. American men consume 30 grams of fish each day. If the amount of fish could be increased in the United States, there could be a substantial effect on coronary heart disease.

Source: Data from Sekikawa A., et al., Marine-derived n-3 fatty acids and atherosclerosis in Japanese, Japanese-American, and White men: A cross-sectional study. *Journal of the American College of Cardiology,* 2008. 52(6):417–424.

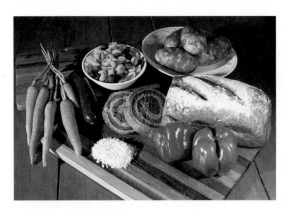

Carbohydrates

Carbohydrates are the main food source of energy for your body. The digestive system breaks all carbohydrates into a simple sugar known as glucose, also called "blood sugar." Glucose is the most important source of energy for your body. It is stored in your liver and muscle as glycogen.

Carbohydrates have been categorized into two groups—simple and complex.

Examples of foods containing simple carbohydrates are table sugar, honey, fruit, milk, maple syrup, and molasses. Examples of foods containing complex carbohydrates are whole grains, fruits, vegetables, and legumes (peas and beans). Complex carbohydrates have been considered to be healthier to eat than simple carbohydrates.

However, fiber is different—it cannot be broken down into glucose, so it passes through the digestive system undigested. Fiber comes in two categories: (1) soluble fiber dissolves in water, whereas (2) insoluble fiber does not. Both promote health. Soluble fiber binds to fatty substances in the intestines and carries them out as waste. This lowers low-density lipoprotein (LDL, or bad cholesterol). Soluble fiber also helps regulate the body's use of sugars, which helps keep hunger and blood sugar in check. Insoluble fiber helps push food through the intestinal tract, which promotes regularity and helps prevent constipation.

Some carbohydrates, when eaten often and in large amounts, can increase the risk for coronary heart disease and diabetes. On the other hand, health benefits can be found with certain carbohydrates.

Carbohydrates from white bread, white rice, pastries, sugared sodas, and other highly processed foods interfere with weight loss and contribute to weight gain. Whole grains, beans, fruits, and vegetables promote health.

What's the word...

glucose Simple sugar circulating in the blood.

glycogen Complex carbohydrates stored primarily in the skeletal muscles and liver. When energy is needed, glycogen is converted to glucose.

Sugar Management for Insulin and Diabetes

The digestive system breaks down digestible carbohydrates into sugar, which then enters the blood. When blood sugar levels rise, special cells in the pancreas produce more insulin, a hormone that signals cells to absorb blood sugar for energy or storage. As cells absorb blood sugar, its levels in the bloodstream begin to fall. That is when other cells in the pancreas start making glucagon, a hormone that tells the liver to start releasing stored sugar. This balancing of insulin and glucagon ensures that cells throughout the body, especially in the brain, have a steady supply of blood sugar.

This process does not work well in some people. People with type 1 diabetes (once called insulin-dependent or juvenile diabetes) do not make enough insulin, so their cells cannot absorb sugar. People with type 2 diabetes (once called non-insulin-dependent, or adult-onset diabetes) have cells that do not respond well to insulin's signal for the cells to absorb sugar from the blood. This condition, known as insulin resistance, causes blood sugar and insulin levels to stay high long after eating. The demands made on the insulin-making cells wears them out over time, and insulin production slows, then stops.

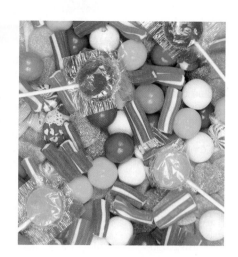

Insulin resistance has also been linked with other problems, such as high blood pressure, high levels of triglycerides, low HDL (good type) cholesterol, and excess weight. The combination of these problems has been given the name metabolic syndrome. Insulin resistance can lead to type 2 diabetes and heart disease.

Insulin resistance is related to genes, a sedentary lifestyle, being overweight, and a diet rich in processed carbohydrates. Note that the more of these conditions exist, the worse the condition. Reducing the intake of refined grains and eating more whole grains in their place can improve insulin sensitivity. The benefit of eating whole grains goes far beyond insulin in helping prevent type 2 diabetes, atherosclerosis (the buildup of cholesterol-filled patches that clog and narrow artery walls), heart disease, and colorectal cancer.

Carbohydrates and the Glycemic Index and Glycemic Load

The glycemic index measures how carbohydrates affect your blood sugar levels. Foods with a high glycemic index, such as white bread and potatoes, cause blood sugar to rise rapidly. Therefore, they are classified as having a high glycemic index. Foods with a low glycemic index, such as whole oats, are digested more slowly and cause a lower and more gradual change in blood sugar. Foods with a score of 70 or higher have a high glycemic index; those with a score of 55 or below have a low glycemic index. See **Table 8.5** for examples. The University of Sydney in Australia maintains an updated searchable database at www.glycemicindex.com.

High-glycemic-index foods have been linked to an increased risk for diabetes, heart disease, and overweight. Foods with a low glycemic index help control type 2 diabetes and help in losing weight. Note, however, that some studies have found that the glycemic index has little effect on weight control. Perhaps the true value of the glycemic index is undetermined. Nevertheless, eating whole grains, beans, fruits, and vegetables—all foods with a low glycemic index—promotes positive health. Processing is an important aspect

Medical News You Can Use

Nuts Lower Lipids

Epidemiological studies have linked eating nuts with a reduced risk of coronary heart disease. Additionally, dietary intervention trials have studied the effects of nut consumption on blood lipid levels. In a recent study, eating an average of 67 grams of nuts a day (2.4 ounces) reduced total cholesterol by 5.9% and LDL cholesterol by 7.4%. These results give further evidence of the relationship that nuts prevent heart disease.

Source: Data from Sabate J., et al., Nut consumption and blood lipid levels: a pooled analysis of 25 intervention trials. *Archives of Internal Medicine,* 2010. 170(9):821–827.

8

Table 8.5 — Glycemic Index

Cereals	GL	GI	Snacks	GL	GI	Pasta	GL	GI	Beans	GL	GI
All Bran	9	51	Chocolate bar	12	46	Cheese tortellini	10	50	Baked	7	44
Bran Buds + psyll	6	45	Corn chips	17	72	Fettucini	15	32	Black, boiled	9	30
Bran Flakes	13	74	Croissant	17	67	Linguini	23	50	Butter, boiled	6	33
Cheerios	15	74	Doughnut	17	76	Macaroni	23	46	Garbanzo, boiled	11	34
Corn Chex	21	83	Graham crackers	14	74	Spaghetti, 5 min. boiled	16	33	Kidney, boiled	7	29
Cornflakes	21	83	Jelly beans	22	80	Spaghetti, 15 min. boiled	21	44	Kidney, canned	9	52
Cream of Wheat	17	66	Life Savers	21	70	Spaghetti, protein-rich	14	28	Lentils, green, brown	5	30
Frosted Flakes	15	55	Oatmeal cookie	9	57	Vermicelli	16	35	Lima, boiled	10	32
Grapenuts	15	67	Pizza, cheese, and tomato sauce	16	60				Navy	12	38
Life	16	66	Pizza Hut, supreme	7	33	**Soups/vegetables**			Pinto, boiled	10	39
Muesli, natural	11	54	Popcorn, light microwave	6	55	Beets, canned	5	64	Red lentils, boiled	5	27
Nutri-grain	10	66	Potato chips	11	56	Black bean soup	17	64	Soy, boiled	1	16
Oatmeal, old-fashioned	11	48	Pound cake	15	54	Carrots, fresh, boiled	3	49			
Puffed Wheat	13	67	Power bars	24	58	Corn, sweet	9	56	**Breads**		
Raisin Bran	12	73	Pretzels	16	83	Green pea, soup	27	66	Bagel, plain	25	72
Rice Chex	23	89	Saltine crackers	12	74	Green pea, frozen	4	47	Baguette, French	15	95
Shredded Wheat	13	67	Shortbread cookies	10	64	Lima beans, frozen	10	32	Croissant	17	67
Special K	11	54	Snickers bar	15	41	Parsnips	12	97	Dark rye	10	76
Total	17	76	Strawberry jam	10	51	Peas, fresh, boiled	7	48	Hamburger bun	9	61
			Vanilla wafers	14	77	Split pea soup w/ham	16	66	Muffin, apple cinnamon	13	44
Fruit						Tomato soup	6	38	Muffin, blueberry	17	59
Apple	6	38	**Crackers**						Pita	10	57
Apricots	5	57	Graham	14	74	**Drinks**			Pizza, cheese	16	60
Banana	12	56	Rice cakes	17	80	Apple juice	12	40	Sourdough	6	54
Cantaloupe	4	65	Rye	11	68	Colas	16	65	Rye	6	64
Cherries	3	22	Soda	13	72	Gatorade	12	78	White	10	70
Dates	42	103				Grapefruit juice	11	48	Wheat	12	68
Grapefruit	3	25	**Cereal grains**			Orange juice	13	46			
Grapes	8	46	Barley	11	25	Pineapple juice	16	46	**Root crops**		
Kiwi	6	52	Basmati white rice	22	58				French fries	22	75
Mango	8	55	Bulgar	16	48	**Milk products**			Potato, new, boiled	12	59
Orange	5	43	Couscous	23	65	Chocolate milk	9	35	Potato, sweet	16	52
Papaya	10	58	Cornmeal	9	68	Custard	7	43	Potato, white, boiled	11	63
Peach	5	42	Millet	25	71	Ice cream, vanilla	8	60	Potato, white, mashed	15	70
Pear	4	40				Skim milk	4	32	Yam	13	54
Pineapple	7	66	**Sugars**			Soy milk	8	31			
Plums	5	39	Fructose	2	22	Whole milk	3	30			
Prunes	10	15	Honey	11	62	Yogurt, fruit	9	36			
Raisins	28	64	Maltose	11	105	Yogurt, plain	3	14			
Watermelon	4	72	Table sugar	7	64						

GL = Glycemic load.
GI = Glycemic index.

in classifying a food's glycemic index. Milling and grinding removes the fiber-rich outer bran and the vitamin- and mineral-rich inner germ.

Another measure, called the glycemic load, takes into account both the impact of a carbohydrate on blood sugar levels and the amount of carbohydrate in the food. A food's glycemic load is determined by multiplying its glycemic index by the amount of carbohydrate it contains. In general, a glycemic load of 20 or more is high, 11 to 19 is medium, and 10 or under is low.

Table 8.6	Sample Substitutions for High-Glycemic-Index Foods		
High-Glycemic-Index Food	Low-Glycemic-Index Alternative	High-Glycemic-Index Food	Low-Glycemic-Index Alternative
Bread, wheat	Oat bran, rye, or pumpernickel bread	Plain cookies and crackers	Cookies made with dried fruits and whole grains such as oats
Processed breakfast cereal	Unrefined cereal such as oats (either muesli or oatmeal)	Cakes and muffins	Cakes and muffins made with fruit, oats, or whole grains
Bananas	Apples	Potatoes	Pasta or legumes

In reviewing the information in Table 8.5, use the following scale to guide you:

Glycemic Load (GL)	Glycemic Index (GI)	Rating
More than 20	More than 70	High
11–19	56–69	Moderate
10 or less	55 or less	Low

Use the glycemic index and glycemic load as a general guide. Whenever possible, try to replace highly processed grains, cereals, and sugars in your diet with minimally processed whole grains (see Table 8.6).

Fiber

Fiber refers to carbohydrates that cannot be digested. A way of categorizing fiber is by how easily it dissolves in water: (1) soluble fiber partially dissolves in water whereas (2) insoluble fiber does not dissolve in water. Though different, these fibers can positively affect your health.

Fiber is found in fruits, vegetables, grains, and legumes. The average American does not eat enough fiber each day. The more calories you eat each day, the more fiber you need (see Table 8.7).

Fiber and Health

Heart Disease: High intake of dietary fiber has been associated with a lower risk for heart disease. Fiber intake has also been associated with the metabolic syndrome that increases the chances of developing heart disease. A higher intake of cereal fiber and whole grains may prevent the metabolic syndrome (combination of high blood pressure, high insulin levels, excess weight, high levels of triglycerides, and low levels of HDL [good type] cholesterol).

Type 2 diabetes: A diet low in cereal fiber and rich in high-glycemic-index foods (which cause big increases in blood sugar) seems to increase the risk of developing diabetes. To protect against heart disease and diabetes, the best advice is to choose whole-grain, high-fiber foods at most meals.

Diverticular disease: Diverticulitis, an inflammation of the intestine, is estimated to occur in one-third of all those over age 45 and in two-thirds of those over age 85. Eating dietary fiber, especially insoluble fiber, is associated with a lower risk for diverticular disease.

Constipation: Constipation is a common gastrointestinal complaint. Fortunately, the consumption of fiber seems to relieve and prevent constipation. Wheat bran and oat bran

The Inside Track

Added Sugars

Added sugars are put into foods and beverages during production (they are not the natural sugars in fruits and milk). Added sugars are found in candy, soft drinks, fruit drinks, pastries, and other manufactured sweets.

Added sugars should account for no more than 25% of your total calories. If your diet is high in added sugars, you will take in fewer essential nutrients.

What's the word...

soluble fiber Partially dissolves in water.

insoluble fiber Does not dissolve in water.

dietary fiber Non-digestible carbohydrates found in plants; two types are soluble and insoluble.

Table 8.7 | Dietary Fiber

The National Academy of Sciences' Institute of Medicine gives the following daily total fiber recommendations for adults:

	Age 50 and younger	Age 51 and older
Men	38 grams	30 grams
Women	25 grams	21 grams

Foods with Soluble and Insoluble Fiber

Soluble Fiber	Insoluble Fiber

• Apples
• Oranges
• Pears
• Peaches
• Grapes
• Prunes
• Blueberries
• Strawberries
• Seeds and Nuts
• Oat bran
• Dried beans
• Oatmeal
• Barley
• Rye
• Vegetables
	• Whole grain
	• Whole wheat breads
	• Barley
	• Brown rice
	• Bulgur
	• Whole-grain breakfast cereals
	• Wheat bran
	• Seeds
	• Vegetables:
	  – Carrots
	  – Cucumbers
	  – Zucchini
	  – Celery
	  – Tomatoes

Foods with High Fiber

Vegetables	Serving Size	Total fiber (grams)
Peas	1 cup	8.8
Potato, baked with skin	1 medium	4.4
Corn	1 cup	4.2
Popcorn, air-popped	3 cups	3.6
Tomato paste	¼ cup	3.0
Carrot	1 medium	2.0

Fruits	Serving Size	Total fiber (grams)
Apple, with skin	1 medium	4.4
Apricots, dried	10 halves	2.6
Raisins	1.5 ounce box	1.6
Orange	1 medium	3.1
Peaches, dried	3 halves	3.2
Blueberries	1 cup	3.5
Pear	1 medium	5.1

Table 8.7	Dietary Fiber, *continued*	

Legumes, Nuts & Seeds	Serving Size	Total Fiber (grams)
Cashews	18 nuts	0.9
Peanuts	28 nuts	2.3
Pistachio nuts	47 nuts	2.9
Almonds	24 nuts	3.3
Baked beans, canned	1 cup	10.4
Lima beans	1 cup	13.2
Black beans	1 cup	15.0
Lentils	1 cup	15.6

Grains, Cereal & Pasta	Serving Size	Total Fiber (grams)
Bread, mixed grain	1 slice	1.7
Bread, whole-wheat	1 slice	1.9
Bread, rye	1 slice	1.9
Oatmeal	1 cup	4.0
Bran flakes	¾ cup	5.1
Spaghetti, whole-wheat	1 cup	6.3

Source: Adapted from the USDA National Nutrient Database for Standard Reference, Release 18. U.S. Department of Agriculture, Agricultural Research Service, 2005.

seem to be more effective than similar amounts of fiber from fruits and vegetables. Be sure to increase fiber intake gradually. As you add more fiber in your diet, you should drink more beverages, because fiber absorbs water.

Fiber is healthy for you, and you should get a least 20 grams or more of it a day. The best sources include whole grain foods, fresh fruits and vegetables, legumes, and nuts.

Medical News You Can Use

Fiber-Full Diet Lengthens Life

In a study of more than 500,000 people, those with the highest dietary fiber intake—an average of 29.4 grams per day for men and 25.8 grams for women—had a 22% lower risk of dying from all causes when compared to those with the lowest dietary fiber intake (average of 12.6 grams per day for men and 10.8 grams for women). The risk of death from cardiovascular disease, infectious, and respiratory diseases was reduced by 24% to 59% in individuals with high fiber consumption. Fiber from grains showed the strongest link to reduced mortality, whereas fiber from beans and vegetables showed only a weak link. U.S. dietary guidelines recommend eating fiber-rich foods to get 14 grams of fiber per 1000 calories.

Source: Data from Park Y., et al. Dietary fiber intake and mortality in the NIH-AARP diet and health study. *Archives of Internal Medicine* 2011; 171(12):1061–1068.

Medical News You Can Use

Dietary Supplements: Unsafe at Certain Doses

About half of Americans take vitamin and mineral supplements as part of their diet. In some cases, taking supplements is advised. For example, the elderly are advised to take calcium and vitamin D supplements to help prevent bone loss. While a daily multi-vitamin supplement can fill nutritional gaps in one's diet, taking high doses of certain vitamins and minerals may be hazardous to one's health. Too much vitamin A may interfere with bone formation and increase the risk of fracture. High levels of folate, found in fortified breads, cereals, and leafy green vegetables, can mask anemia caused by B_{12} deficiency. High doses of vitamin D can result in nausea, vomiting, poor appetite, constipation, and weight loss. Those who take supplements of vitamins and minerals should be aware of the dose levels they take to ensure that adverse health effects do not result.

Source: Data from Johns Hopkins Health Alert: Dietary Supplements—Unsafe at Certain Doses. Johns Hopkins Medicine, March 14 2007.

Ask Yourself

• What types of foods am I eating throughout the day?

• Where do my calories come from?

Vegetables and Fruits and Health

Cardiovascular disease: A diet rich in fruits and vegetables can lower heart disease and stroke risk. Green, leafy vegetables (e.g., lettuce, spinach), cruciferous vegetables (e.g., broccoli, Brussels sprouts), and citrus fruits (e.g., oranges, grapefruit) make important contributions.

Blood pressure: Blood pressure, a main risk factor for heart disease, can be lowered by a proper diet. A fruit-and-vegetable–rich diet lowers blood pressure when some of the carbohydrate is replaced with healthy, unsaturated fat or protein.

Cancer: Non-starchy vegetables—such as lettuce and other leafy greens, broccoli, as well as garlic, onions, and fruits—probably protect against several types of cancers, including those of the mouth, throat, esophagus, and stomach. Fruits probably also protect against lung cancer.

Some fruits and vegetables may have specific components that protect against cancer. Men, for example, may obtain some protection from eating tomatoes. Lycopene, one of the pigments that give tomatoes their red color, could play a part in helping protect men. Therefore, increasing the consumption of tomato-based products (especially cooked tomato products) and other lycopene-containing foods may reduce the occurrence of prostate cancer.

Vitamins

You must get vitamins from food or from a daily multiple-vitamin preparation because your body cannot make them. In the body, vitamins:

- release energy from carbohydrates, lipids, and proteins;
- help grow and repair tissue;
- maintain and support reproductive functions; and
- produce the immune response.

Types of Vitamins

Fat-soluble vitamins dissolve in fat, can be stored in the body, and are not excreted in the urine. They include four vitamins: A, D, E, and K.

Water-soluble vitamins dissolve in water and cannot be stored by the body in significant amounts. They include vitamin C and eight B vitamins: thiamine (B_1), riboflavin

What's the word. . .

vitamin Nutrient necessary for normal functioning of the body; two types are water-soluble and fat-soluble.

(B_2), niacin (B_3), pyridoxine (B_6), cobalamin (B_{12}), folate, pantothenic acid, and biotin. Excess water-soluble vitamins not used in body functions are excreted in the urine.

Vitamin Excesses and Deficiencies

A healthy, balanced diet provides most of the vitamins your body needs. Taking large doses of vitamin supplements can result (if fat-soluble) in an excessive accumulation in the body and cause you harm. Conversely, not getting enough of the right kinds of vitamins in your diet can cause health problems (see **Table 8.8**).

Table 8.8 — Major Vitamins

Vitamin	Major Functions	Rich Food Sources	Deficiency Signs/Symptoms	Toxicity Signs/Symptoms
A and provitamin A (beta-carotene)	Vision in dim light, growth, reproduction, maintains immune system and skin, antioxidant	Liver, milk, dark green and leafy vegetables, carrots, sweet potatoes, mangos, oatmeal, broccoli, apricots, peaches, romaine lettuce	Poor vision in dim light, dry skin, blindness, poor growth, respiratory infections	Intestinal upset, liver damage, hair loss, headache, birth defects, death (beta-carotene is less toxic than vitamin A)
D	Bone and tooth development and growth	Few good food sources other than fortified milk and eggs	Weak, deformed bones (rickets)	Growth failure, loss of appetite, weight loss, death
E	Antioxidant: protects cell membranes	Vegetable oils, whole grains, wheat germ, sunflower seeds, almonds	Anemia (rarely occurs)	Intestinal upset, bleeding problems
C	Scar formation and maintenance, immune system functioning, antioxidant	Citrus fruits, berries, potatoes, broccoli, peppers, cabbage, tomatoes, fortified fruit drinks	Frequent infections, bleeding gums, bruises, poor wound healing, depression (scurvy)	Diarrhea, nosebleeds, headache, weakness, kidney stones, excess iron absorption and storage
Thiamine	Energy metabolism	Pork, liver, nuts, dried beans and peas, whole-grain and enriched breads and cereals	Heart failure, mental confusion, depression, paralysis (beriberi)	No toxicity has been reported
Riboflavin	Energy metabolism	Milk and yogurt, eggs and poultry, meat, liver, whole-grain and enriched breads and cereals	Enlarged, purple tongue; fatigue; oily skin; cracks in the corners of the mouth	No toxicity has been reported
Niacin	Energy metabolism	Protein-rich foods, peanut butter, whole-grain and enriched breads and cereals	Skin rash, diarrhea, weakness, dementia, death (pellagra)	Painful skin flushing, intestinal upset, liver damage
Vitamin B_6	Protein and fat metabolism	Liver, oatmeal, bananas, meat, fish, poultry, whole grains, fortified cereals	Anemia, skin rash, irritability, elevated homocysteine levels	Weakness, depression, permanent nerve damage
Folate (folic acid)	DNA production	Leafy vegetables, oranges, nuts, liver, enriched breads and cereals	Anemia, depression, spina bifida in developing embryo, elevated homocysteine levels	Hides signs of vitamin B_{12} deficiency; may cause allergic response
B_{12}	DNA production	Animal products	Pernicious anemia, fatigue, paralysis, elevated homocysteine levels	No toxicity has been reported

Daily Multivitamin Supplement

Walter Willett (2005) of the Harvard School of Public Health says that most people in the United States get enough vitamins to prevent the classic deficiency diseases. He also states that although we may prevent the classic deficiency diseases, most of us do not get enough of five key vitamins that may be associated with preventing several chronic diseases:

- folic acid;
- vitamin B_6;
- vitamin B_{12};
- vitamin D (see ⬤ Figure 8.1); and
- vitamin E.

A standard, store-brand, 100% RDA-level multivitamin can supply you with enough of these vitamins. Such a supplement cannot replace healthy eating, but it is an inexpensive way of providing a nutritional safety net. See ⬤ Table 8.9 for newly recognized findings on vitamins.

Minerals

Minerals are essential for a variety of important bodily functions. They regulate fluid balance, conduct nerve impulses, and help contract muscles (see ⬤ Table 8.10).

Minerals are classified according to the body's needs. At least 16 minerals are essential to health (e.g., sodium, chloride, potassium, calcium, phosphorus, and magnesium).

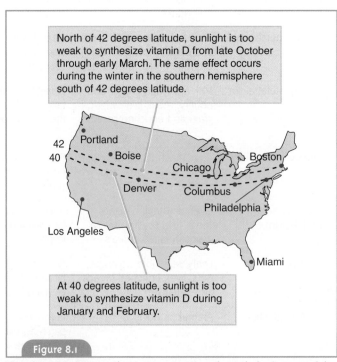

Figure 8.1

Mapping vitamin D synthesis. Vitamin D synthesis halts for part of the winter if sunlight is too weak. In Los Angeles and Miami, the sunlight is strong enough to synthesize vitamin D year-round, even in January.

Table 8.9	Newly Recognized Findings on Vitamins	
Vitamin	**New or Suspected Roles in Health and Disease**	**Daily Optimal Intake**
A	Stimulates production and activity of white blood cells, takes part in remodeling bone, helps maintain health of endothelial cells (those lining the body's interior surfaces), regulates cell growth and division	5000 IU for men; 4000 IU for women
B_6	May help fight heart disease and some types of cancer	1.3 to 1.7 mg
B_{12}	May help fight heart disease and some types of cancer; may help those with dementia or Alzheimer's disease	6 μg
Folic acid	Reduces chances of mothers having children with birth defects (spina bifida or anencephaly); may help fight heart disease and some types of cancer	400 μg
C	Controls infections; neutralizes harmful free radicals; helps make collagen, which is needed for healthy bones, teeth, gums, and blood vessels	90 mg for men; 75 mg for women (add extra 35 mg for smokers); as evidence unfolds, 200 to 300 mg
D	Helps body absorb and retain calcium and phosphorus, both critical for building bone; keeps cancer cells from growing and dividing; prevents risk of fractures; low intake increases risks of prostate, breast, colon, and other cancers	5 μg up to age 50 years; 10 μg between ages 51 and 70 years; 15 μg after age 70 years
E	Thought to prevent heart attacks (further studies are needed)	15 mg from food or 22 IU from natural source or 33 IU of synthetic form; may need 400 IU or more for optimal health
K	Helps make 6 of the 13 proteins needed for blood clotting; involved in building bone; reduces risk of hip fracture	80 μg for men; 65 μg for women

Source: Adapted from Willett W.C. *Eat, Drink, and Be Healthy*, First edition. Fireside, 2005.

Medical News You Can Use

10 Foods That Lower Cholesterol

Changing what you eat can lower your cholesterol just as easily as it is to eat your way to high cholesterol levels. Here are 10 types of food that work to reduce your cholesterol levels.

- Oats such as oatmeal or cold, oat-based cereal like Cheerios;
- Barley and other whole grains;
- Beans;
- Eggplant and okra;
- Nuts;
- Vegetable oils such as canola, sunflower, and safflower;
- Apples, grapes, strawberries, citrus fruits;
- Food fortified with sterols and stanols;
- Soy, such as tofu or soy milk; and
- Fatty fish.

Source: Data from Focus On Cholesterol—10 Foods That Lower Cholesterol And Some That Raise It, Issue #1, Harvard Health Publications, Harvard Medical School, 2011.

8

Table 8.10 Some Essential Minerals

Mineral	Roles	Rich Food Sources	Deficiency Signs/Symptoms	Toxicity Signs/Symptoms
Calcium	Builds and maintains bones and teeth, regulates muscle and nerve function, regulates blood pressure and blood clotting	Milk products; fortified orange juice, tofu, and soy milk; fish with edible small bones such as sardines and salmon; broccoli; hard water	Poor bone growth, weak bones, muscle spasms, convulsions	Kidney stones, calcium deposits in organs, mineral imbalances
Potassium	Maintains fluid balance, necessary for nerve function	Whole grains, fruits and vegetables, yogurt, milk	Muscular weakness, confusion, death	Heart failure
Sodium	Maintains fluid balance, necessary for nerve function	Salt, soy sauce, luncheon meats, processed cheeses, pickled foods, snack foods, canned and dried soups	Muscle cramping, headache, confusion, coma	Hypertension
Magnesium	Regulation of enzyme activity, necessary for nerve function	Green, leafy vegetables, nuts, whole grains, peanut butter	Loss of appetite, muscular weakness, convulsions, confusion, death	Rare
Zinc	Component of many enzymes and the hormone insulin, maintains immune function, necessary for sexual maturation and reproduction	Meats, fish, poultry, whole grains, vegetables	Poor growth, failure to mature sexually, improper healing of wounds	Mineral imbalances, gastrointestinal upsets, anemia, heart disease
Selenium	Component of a group of antioxidant enzymes, immune system function	Seafood, liver, and vegetables and grains grown in selenium-rich soil	May increase risk of heart disease and certain cancers	Hair and nail loss
Iron	Oxygen transport involved in the release of energy	Clams, oysters, liver, red meats, and enriched breads and cereals	Fatigue, weakness, iron-deficiency anemia	Iron poisoning, nausea, vomiting, diarrhea, death

What's the word...

macrominerals Minerals needed by the body in amounts greater than 100 mg.

microminerals (trace minerals) Minerals needed by the body in amounts less than 100 mg.

osteoporosis Disease related to calcium deficiency in which bones become thin and brittle and fracture easily.

anemia A reduction in the number of red blood cells in the blood. Anemia is not a disease but rather a symptom of various diseases, including iron deficiency.

These are known as macrominerals. Microminerals are trace minerals (e.g., iron, zinc, copper, manganese, molybdenum, selenium, iodine, and fluoride).

Two of the most important minerals for keeping yourself healthy are calcium and iron. Calcium is especially important for women, to help them ward off osteoporosis in later life. Iron is important for women to prevent anemia.

Water

Water in the body serves many important purposes:

- Excretes wastes
- Maintains blood circulation throughout the body
- Maintains body temperature
- Digests and absorbs nutrients

Approximately 60% of your total body weight is water. If you lose even 4% of your body weight through sweat, you will lose the ability to make decisions, concentrate, or do physical work. If you lose as much as 20%, you will die.

Water is lost:

- from breathing;
- from sweating; and
- in urine and stool.

Water is taken in from:

- eating food (e.g., fruits, vegetables, soups, meats, and grains);
- water in beverages (e.g., water itself, fruit juices, milk, and sport drinks); and
- the metabolic process or chemical breakdown of foods.

If you lose more water than you drink, you become dehydrated. Dehydration can happen if you are:

- not drinking enough fluids daily;
- working or exercising in a hot or cold environment;
- living at high altitude; and
- drinking too much alcohol.

Clear urine is a sign that you are well-hydrated. The more dehydrated you are, the darker (and smellier) your urine will be, although medications, vitamins, and diet can affect your urine's color.

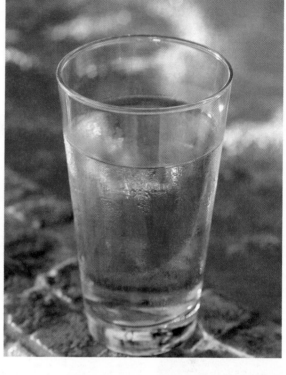

You can restore lost fluids by drinking water. Eating foods high in water content also helps restore fluids (adapted from American College of Sports Medicine position stand).

Before exercise:

- Drink about 16 ounces (2 cups) of fluid about 2 hours before exercise to promote adequate hydration and allow time for excretion of excess water.

During exercise:

- Drink fluids at regular intervals to replace water lost through sweating.
- Drink fluids cooler than the ambient temperature (between 60°F and 72°F) so your body absorbs them better.

During exercise lasting more than 1 hour:

- Consider drinking a sports drink that contains carbohydrates and/or electrolytes.
- If you exercise for less than 1 hour, it does not matter if you drink water or a sports drink.

After exercise:

- Consider weighing yourself before and after exercising to determine how much fluid you have lost—for every pound of weight lost, you should drink at least 16 ounces (2 cups) of fluid.
- If you feel thirsty, chances are dehydration has begun.

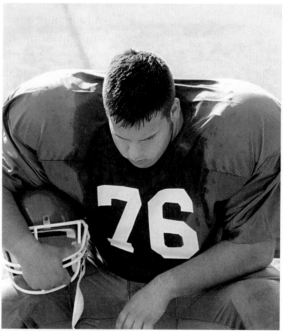

Tipping Point

- Drink 8.5 cups of water each day to stay properly hydrated. Even with all of the coffee and soda we drink, it is still important to drink water.

8

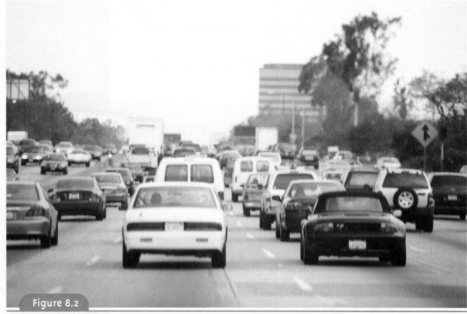

Figure 8.2

Free radical production is increased by exposure to cigarette smoke, exhaust fumes, and radiation.

Free Radicals and Antioxidants

Normal metabolism creates free radicals. Free radicals can damage cell membranes and mutate genes.

Free radical production is increased by cigarette smoke, exhaust fumes, radiation, too much sunlight, some drugs, and too much stress (see **Figure 8.2**).

Antioxidants do battle with free radicals and undo the damage free radicals cause.

Get your antioxidants by eating a variety of fruits and vegetables. If you take antioxidant supplements instead:

- The health benefits of phytochemicals come from working in combination with each other (see **Table 8.11**).
- Isolated phytochemicals may cause more harm than good if taken in high doses.

Put Your Diet into Action

Is your diet meeting your nutrient needs? Answering this question is not an exact science, but useful guidelines are available (see **Lab 8-1**).

Comparison to Dietary Reference Intakes

The Institute of Medicine (IOM) of the National Academies changed the way nutritionists and nutrition scientists evaluate the diets of healthy people by creating the Dietary Reference Intakes (DRIs). See Appendix B.

Comparison to the 2010 Dietary Guidelines for Americans

The *2010 Dietary Guidelines for Americans* provides evidence-based nutrition information and advice for people aged 2 and older. Refer to **Table 8.12** for the "Key Recommendations" for the general public. Due to the overwhelming prevalence of obesity in America, both among children and adults, the *Dietary Guidelines* emphasizes reducing total calorie intake and increasing physical activity. Another big focus of the new

Medical News You Can Use

Periodic Fasting Found to be Good for Health

More than a dozen scientists from the Heart Institute at Intermountain Medical Center in Utah observed an almost 45% lower risk for coronary heart disease and decreased risk for diabetes in cardiac patients who regularly participated in a 24-hour fast. Doctors found that skipping at least two meals on a regular basis led to a dramatic increase in human growth hormone (HGH), which plays a metabolic role in adults by regulating glucose and insulin within the body. Average levels of HGH increase to an average of 1300% in women and nearly 2000% in men. Periodic fasts may serve more than just religious purposes; they also might be a health-conscious and heart-conscious thing to do.

Source: Data from Horne B.D., et al. Usefulness of routine periodic fasting to lower risk of coronary artery disease among patients undergoing coronary angiography. *American Journal of Cardiology* 2008; 102(7):814–819.

Dietary Guidelines is recommending a shift in our food consumption patterns. People are encouraged to consume more of certain foods (and specific nutrients) and less of others (see **Box 8.1**).

Comparison to MyPlate

Built on the *2010 Dietary Guidelines*, MyPlate divides a white plate into four labeled sections that show what a balanced meal should look like. Fruits and vegetables take up half the plate, while the other side offers one section for protein and one section for grains. Dairy is seen to the side in a blue circle much like a cup (see **Figure 8.3**).

Table 8.11	Phytochemicals in Fruits and Vegetables and Their Possible Benefits	
Food	**Phytochemicals**	**Possible Benefits**
Berries Blueberries, strawberries, raspberries, blackberries, currants	Anthocyanides, ellagic acid	Antioxidants, cancer prevention
Chili Peppers	Capsaicin	Possible antioxidant, topical pain relief
Citrus Fruits Oranges, grapefruit, lemons, limes	Flavanones (tangeretic, nobiletin, hesperitin), carotenoids	Antioxidants
Cruciferous Vegetables Broccoli, kale, cauliflower, brussels sprouts, cabbage, mustard greens	Indoles, isothiocyanates, sulphoraphane, carotenoids	Antioxidants, anticancer properties
Garlic Family Garlic, onions, shallots, leeks, chives, scallions	Allylic sulfides, flavonoids (quercetin)	Anticancer properties
Soy	Daidzein, equol, genestein, enterolactone, and other plant estrogens	Reduce risk of breast cancer, prostate cancer, and heart disease

Table 8.12	2010 Dietary Guidelines for Americans: Key Recommendations

Balancing Calories to Manage Weight

- Prevent and/or reduce overweight and obesity through improved eating and physical activity behaviors.
- Control total calorie intake to manage body weight. For people who are overweight or obese, this will mean consuming fewer calories from foods and beverages.
- Increase physical activity and reduce time spent in sedentary behaviors.
- Maintain appropriate calorie balance during each stage of life—childhood, adolescence, adulthood, pregnancy and breastfeeding, and older age.

Foods and Food Components to Reduce

- Reduce daily sodium intake to less than 2,300 milligrams (mg) and further reduce intake to 1,500 mg among persons who are 51 and older and those of any age who are African American or have hypertension, diabetes, or chronic kidney disease. The 1,500 mg recommendation applies to about half of the U.S. population, including children, and the majority of adults.
- Consume less than 10 percent of calories from saturated fatty acids by replacing them with monounsaturated and polyunsaturated fatty acids.
- Consume less than 300 mg per day of dietary cholesterol.
- Keep trans fatty acid consumption as low as possible by limiting foods that contain synthetic sources of trans fats, such as partially hydrogenated oils, and by limiting other solid fats.
- Reduce the intake of calories from solid fats and added sugars.

- Limit the consumption of foods that contain refined grains, especially refined grain foods that contain solid fats, added sugars, and sodium.
- If alcohol is consumed, it should be consumed in moderation—up to one drink per day for women and two drinks per day for men—and only by adults of legal drinking age.

Foods and Nutrients to Increase

Individuals should meet the following recommendations as part of a healthy eating pattern while staying within their calorie needs.

- Increase vegetable and fruit intake.
- Eat a variety of vegetables, especially dark-green and red and orange vegetables, and beans and peas.
- Consume at least half of all grains as whole grains. Increase whole-grain intake by replacing refined grains with whole grains.
- Increase intake of fat-free or low-fat milk and milk products, such as milk, yogurt, cheese, or fortified soy beverages.
- Choose a variety of protein foods, which include seafood, lean meat and poultry, eggs, beans and peas, soy products, and unsalted nuts and seeds.
- Increase the amount and variety of seafood consumed by choosing seafood in place of some meat and poultry.
- Replace protein foods that are higher in solid fats with choices that are lower in solid fats and calories and/or are sources of oils.
- Use oils to replace solid fats where possible.
- Choose foods that provide more potassium, dietary fiber, calcium, and vitamin D, which are nutrients of concern in American diets. These foods include vegetables, fruits, whole grains, and milk and milk products.

Source: Adapted from the *Dietary Guidelines for Americans,* 2010. Courtesy of the U.S. Department of Health & Human Services.

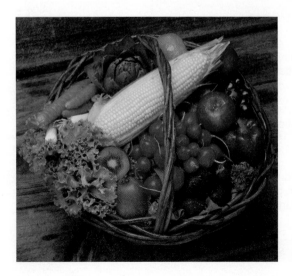

A supporting website, www.ChooseMyPlate.gov, urges portion control and reduced use of sodium. It offers other nutrition tips, such as drinking water instead of sugary drinks, and "how-to" resources. You can also find out how much you need from each food group and what foods are part of each food group.

The new nutrition icon replaces the food pyramid that was introduced by the federal government in 1992. Over the years since its introduction, the food pyramid was criticized for becoming too complicated and confusing for consumers to easily understand. The plate diagram is intended to provide quick information that will help make better food choices.

However, despite being better than the food pyramid, MyPlate has its critics. Harvard School of Public Health nutrition expert Walter C. Willett said that ". . . the most important issues

Box 8.1	New Dietary Guidelines: Which Food to Increase and Which to Reduce

The latest nutrition guidelines from the U.S. Department of Agriculture and the Department of Human Services have a new emphasis: weight control. Previous guidelines focused on nutrients (e.g., fats, proteins, and carbohydrates).

The slogan for the new guidelines is "Calories in, calories out." We should strive to maintain a calorie balance, eating no more calories than we burn each day. With this in mind, the guidelines include these recommendations for foods to cut back on and foods to increase:

7 Foods to Reduce

1. Reduce daily sodium intake to less than 2,300 mg and further reduce intake to 1,500 mg among persons who are 51 and older and those of any age who are African American or have hypertension, diabetes, or chronic kidney disease.
2. Consume less than 10% of calories from saturated fatty acids by replacing them with monounsaturated and polyunsaturated fatty acids.
3. Consume less than 300 mg per day of dietary cholesterol.
4. Keep trans fatty acid consumption as low as possible.
5. Reduce the intake of calories from solid fats and added sugars.
6. Limit the consumption of foods that contain refined grains, especially those with solid fats, added sugars, and sodium.
7. If alcohol is consumed, it should be consumed in moderation—up to one drink per day for women and two drinks per day for men—and only by adults of legal drinking age.

Foods and Nutrients to Increase

Eat more of these foods while staying within your calorie goals.

1. Eat a variety of fruits and vegetables, especially dark green, red, and orange vegetables, fruits, and beans and peas.
2. Consume at least half of all grains as whole grains. Increase whole-grain intake by replacing refined grains with whole grains.
3. Increase intake of fat-free or low-fat milk and milk products, such as milk, yogurt, cheese, or fortified soy beverages.
4. Choose a variety of protein foods, which include seafood, lean meat and poultry, eggs, beans and peas, soy products, and unsalted nuts and seeds.
5. Choose seafood in place of some meat and poultry.
6. Replace protein foods that are high in solid fats with proteins that are low in solid fats and calories.
7. Use healthy vegetable oils to replace solid fats where possible.
8. Choose foods that provide more potassium, dietary fiber, calcium, and vitamin D, which are nutrients of concern in American diets. These foods include vegetables, fruits, whole grains, and milk and milk products.

Source: Data from the *Dietary Guidelines for Americans*, 2010. Courtesy of the U.S. Department of Health & Human Services.

Medical News You Can Use

How to Reduce Salt in Your Diet

For individuals with hypertension, reducing your intake of salt is a lifestyle measure that can help lower your blood pressure. It is recommended to aim for less than 1500 mg of sodium a day. Salt added to food at the table accounts for only 10% of sodium consumed in the American diet. In addition to avoiding the salt shaker, here are other ways to reduce the amount of salt intake in your diet.

- Choose fresh foods over canned or processed items.
- Limit smoked, cured, or processed meats.
- Select canned or processed foods that are sodium-free or low in sodium.
- Try rinsing and draining canned foods.
- Season your foods with herbs and spices instead of salt.

Source: Data from Johns Hopkins Health Alert: Salt Shakedown: How to Reduce Salt in Your Diet. Johns Hopkins Medicine, April 12 2011.

are in the details that are not captured by the icon. What type of grain? What sources of proteins? What fats are used to prepare the vegetables and the grains?"

MyPlate does not show that whole grains are better for you than refined, rapidly digested grains, or that fish and beans are better protein choices than red meat. It does not give any guidance that eating more unsaturated and omega-3 fats is good for health, as is cutting back on saturated fats from meat and dairy. The glass to the side of the plate is deceiving—should we be drinking milk with every meal? Other critics say that MyPlate does not indicate calorie, fat, sodium, or sugar amounts necessary to build that healthy diet nor how to account for mixed dishes or an entire day's eating

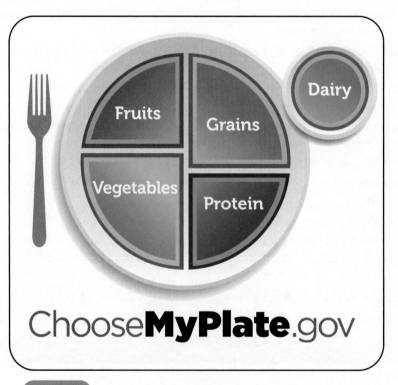

Figure 8.3

MyPlate. (*Source:* Courtesy of the U.S. Department of Agriculture.)

Medical News You Can Use

Exercise Plus DASH Diet Lowers Blood Pressure

Adhering to an exercise and weight loss program along with the DASH (Dietary Approaches to Stop Hypertension) diet may lower blood pressure and markers for cardiovascular disease even further. Among participants in the DASH plus exercise group, systolic blood pressure improved by 16 mm Hg compared to 11 mm Hg for those not in the DASH plus exercise group. Additionally, those in the DASH plus exercise group lost significantly more weight, approximately 19 pounds compared to the control groups, which lost little weight or gained weight in the 4-month study period. If you have high blood pressure and are also overweight, consult with your doctor about how the DASH diet plus exercise can benefit your health.

Source: Data from Blumenthal J.A., et al., Effects of the DASH Diet alone and in combination with exercise and weight loss on blood pressure and cardiovascular biomarkers in men and women with high blood pressure. *Archive of Internal Medicine*, 2010. 170(2):126–135.

pattern. Also, the plate labels types of food (i.e., vegetables, fruits, and grains) except for protein, which is not a type of food but a nutrient. And, there is no mention about the size of the plate, which can affect portion sizes. Despite its shortcomings, MyPlate is better than its prior versions—Food Guide Pyramid and My Pyramid—and is a step in the right direction.

The MyPlate icon is not new. The New American Plate, developed in 1999 by the American Institute for Cancer Research, uses an almost identical plate icon. In the United Kingdom, the Eatwell Plate has served as a pictorial guide to healthy eating. The plate idea has been used as a teaching tool for people with diabetes, called The Idaho Plate Method.

Comparison to the DASH Eating Plan

DASH stands for Dietary Approaches to Stop Hypertension. The DASH diet is an approach to healthy eating that was designed to help treat or prevent high blood pressure (hypertension) but may offer protection against osteoporosis, cancer, heart disease, stroke, and diabetes.

It limits saturated fats and cholesterol, and focuses on increasing the intake of foods rich in potassium, calcium, magnesium, protein, and fiber. The DASH Eating Plan also is consistent with the *Dietary Guidelines* recommendations and with most of the Mediterranean-type of eating (see Box 8.2). It is rich in fruits, vegetables, fat-free or low-fat milk and milk products, whole grains, fish, poultry, and nuts. It contains less sodium, sweets, added sugars, and sugar-containing beverages, fats, and red meats than the typical American diet. The amounts recommended are shown in Table 8.13 .

Fast Food

Fast foods are quick, reasonably priced, and readily available alternatives to home cooking. Although convenient and economical for a busy lifestyle, fast foods are typically high in calories, fat, saturated fat, sugar, and salt (see Table 8.14). To maintain a healthy diet, it is necessary to choose fast foods carefully (see Lab 8-2).

In general, people with high blood pressure, diabetes, and heart disease must be very careful in choosing fast food because of the high content of fat, sodium, and sugar.

Box 8.2 | The Mediterranean Diet

Some experts consider the "Mediterranean diet"—rich in plant foods and monounsaturated fats—to be one of the healthiest in the world. The Mediterranean diet has long been associated with heart health and longevity. Beyond that, it can also be an excellent weight-loss plan, as long as you eat in moderation.

The Mediterranean coastal region stretches across Europe from Spain to the Middle East. Fifty years ago, scientists noticed that people living in this region tended to be healthy and live long lives, primarily because of their diet and lifestyle. Mediterranean cuisine varies by region, but is largely based on vegetables, fruits, olives, beans, whole grains, olive oil, and fish, along with a little dairy and wine. Additionally, the Mediterranean lifestyle includes leisurely dining and regular physical activity.

Studies show that calorie-controlled diets rich in plant foods, healthy fats, and lean protein—like the Mediterranean diet—are a nutritious formula for weight loss. A study in the *New England Journal of Medicine* found that a Mediterranean diet was as effective as a low-fat diet for losing weight and also offered some metabolic benefits.

There is not a single "Mediterranean diet." Instead, it is a dietary pattern of plant foods, monounsaturated fats (mainly olive oil), fish, and limited amounts of animal products.

The basic Mediterranean diet pattern is as follows:

- Legumes: Eat daily.
- Fruit: 2.5 cups daily.
- Vegetables: 2 cups daily.
- Fish: More than twice weekly.
- Nuts: A handful daily.
- Meat/poultry: Less than 4 ounces daily.
- Dairy products: 2 cups of a low-fat variety daily.
- Wine: If you choose to drink alcohol.
- Fats: Use primarily monounsaturated fats.
- Eggs: Less than 4 per week.

Some tips for embracing the Mediterranean style of eating:

- Select whole grains for your breads, cereals, and other starches.
- Choose nuts, seeds, legumes, fish, low-fat dairy, and poultry to satisfy your protein needs (you can include lean meat on occasion as well).
- Most importantly, reduce the amount of saturated and trans fats in your diet. Use olive or canola oil instead of butter or margarine.

The Mediterranean diet mainly emphasizes foods that are low-fat, low-cholesterol, and high-fiber. Reducing total fat is one of the easiest ways to trim calories, because fat is more than twice as caloric as carbs or protein. Furthermore, foods rich in lean protein and fiber (like beans and legumes) are filling and make meals more satisfying.

Nuts, fish, and olive oil provide healthy monounsaturated fats, which also contribute to satisfaction and do not raise cholesterol levels the way saturated fat does.

Most foods included in the Mediterranean diet are fresh and seasonal rather than highly processed. Preparation methods tend to be simple; foods are rarely deep-fried.

And the variety of delicious foods makes it easier to stick to the Mediterranean diet for the long-term. But even on a diet full of healthy foods, it is important to watch portions—especially for higher-calorie foods like nuts and olive oil.

It is important to remember that the Mediterranean diet is not a quick, weight-loss diet, but a way of life. Almost as important as the food is regular physical activity and leisurely dining—taking pleasure and time to savor meals with friends and family.

The Mediterranean diet is free of gimmicks. It has clearly been shown to be a healthy, sustainable diet that can help you trim your waistline in addition to preventing a host of chronic diseases.

Table 8.13	Following the DASH Eating Plan	
Food Group	**Daily Servings**	**Serving Sizes**
Grains*	6–8	1 slice bread 1 oz dry cereal† 1/2 cup cooked rice, pasta, or cereal
Vegetables	4–5	1 cup raw leafy vegetable 1/2 cup cut-up raw or cooked vegetable 1/2 cup vegetable juice
Fruits	4–5	1 medium fruit 1/4 cup dried fruit 1/2 cup fresh, frozen, or canned fruit 1/2 cup fruit juice
Fat-free or low-fat milk and milk products	2–3	1 cup milk or yogurt 1 1/2 oz cheese
Lean meats, poultry, and fish	6 or less	1 oz cooked meats, poultry, or fish 1 egg‡
Nuts, seeds, and legumes	4–5 per week	1/3 cup or 1 1/2 oz nuts 2 Tbsp peanut butter 2 Tbsp or 1/2 oz seeds 1/2 cup cooked legumes (dry beans and peas)
Fats and oils	2–3	1 tsp soft margarine 1 tsp vegetable oil 1 Tbsp mayonnaise 2 Tbsp salad dressing
Sweets and added sugars	5 or less per week	1 Tbsp sugar 1 Tbsp jelly or jam 1/2 cup sorbet, gelatin 1 cup lemonade

* *Whole grains are recommended for most grain servings as a good source of fiber and nutrients.*
† *Serving sizes vary between ½ cup and 1¼ cups, depending on cereal type. Check the product's Nutrition Facts label.*
Source: Courtesy of the U.S. Department of Health & Human Services.

Medical News You Can Use

Burgers, Fries, and Diet Soda are Recipe for Metabolic Syndrome

Middle-aged adults who regularly eat a double burger with fries and a diet soda for lunch or dinner increase their risk of metabolic syndrome by 25%, compared with adults who limit servings of red meat to two servings a week. In fact, eating one serving of french fries each day increased the risk of developing metabolic syndrome by 10%. Other findings of consuming diet sodas showed that soda might reflect poorer glycemic control. Diet sodas may impair the body's ability to predict the caloric content of foods, which may increase intake and body weight.

Source: Data from Lutsey P.L., et al. Dietary intake and the development of the metabolic syndrome: the Atherosclerosis Risk in Communities study. *Circulation* 2008; 117(6):754–761.

Table 8.14 | Partial Composition of Selected Fast-Food Items

Food	Total Calories	Total Fat (grams)	Calories from Fat	Cholesterol (milligrams)	Sodium (milligrams)
Big Mac (beef)	600	33	300	85	1050
Burrito Supreme	440	18	170	45	1220
French fries (medium/salted)	450	22	200	00	290
Turkey sub sandwich	330	5	50	40	1510
Fried chicken breast	380	19	170	145	1150
Pizza (slice)	300	14	120	25	610
Caesar salad (no dressing)	300	26	230	15	690
Caesar salad (with dressing)	450	42	540	55	930
Chocolate shake (medium)	600	18	160	70	470
Starbuck's chocolate Frappuccino Blended Crème, Grande	530	19	170	55	420

Source: Data from Fast Food Facts. Available at http://www.foodfacts.info. Accessed June 6, 2008.

Many fast-food restaurants have switched from beef tallow or lard to hydrogenated vegetable oils for frying. Some restaurants offer low-calorie choices like salads with low-calorie dressing, low-fat milkshakes, whole-grain buns, lean meats, and grilled chicken.

Fast-Food Recommendations

- Choose smaller servings. Consider splitting some items to reduce the amount of calories and fat. Ask for a "doggy bag," or simply leave some food on your plate.
- Pizza: Ask for less cheese and choose low-fat toppings such as onions, mushrooms, green peppers, tomatoes, or other vegetables.

Medical News You Can Use

How Much Weight Would You Gain By Eating an Extra Chocolate Chip Cookie Every Day?

A person eating an extra cookie every day will initially gain weight, but over time more of the cookie's calories go into repairing, replacing, and carrying the extra body tissue. After a few years of daily cookie eating, weight gain will level off at about 6 pounds.

Weight loss happens in a converse fashion: As the body size shrinks, less energy is required to maintain it, so weight loss levels off. To continue losing weight, a stricter diet or more exercise is needed. This explains why small lifestyle changes sometimes have little impact on weight: Walking a mile a day expends about the same amount of energy as is found in one small cookie. Most individuals, after having achieved some weight loss, resume their original diet and exercise habits. Consequently, weight gain recurs rapidly.

Source: Data from Katan M.B. and Ludwig B.S. Extra Calories Cause Weight Gain—But How Much? *Journal of the American Medical Association* 2010; 303(1):65–66.

Medical News You Can Use

Weight Status Is Influenced by Area Restaurants

Researchers found that the mix of restaurants in an area is an important correlate of BMI and the risk of obesity. Overall, the more restaurants in an area, the better the population's weight status. However, people living in areas with a higher ratio of fast-food places were likely to have higher weight status (BMI) and risks of obesity. Those living in areas with a higher ratio of full-service restaurants resisted weight gain and obesity.

Source: Data from Mehta N.K. and Chang V.W., Weight status and restaurant availability—a multilevel analysis. *American Journal of Preventive Medicine*, 2008. 34(2): 127–133.

- Sandwiches: Choose regular- or junior-size lean roast beef, turkey, grilled chicken breast, or lean ham. Extras such as bacon, cheese, or mayonnaise will increase fat and calories. Select whole-grain breads over croissants or biscuits—the latter contain added fat.

- Hamburgers: A single, plain meat patty without cheese and sauces is the best choice. Ask for extra lettuce, tomatoes, and onions. Some restaurants feature hamburgers without buns.

- Meat, Chicken, and Fish: Look for items that are roasted, grilled, baked, or broiled. Avoid meats that are breaded or fried. Use small portions of heavy sauces, such as gravy, if at all.

- Salads: Dressing, bacon bits, and shredded cheese add fat and calories. Choose lettuce and assorted vegetables for most of your salad. Use low-fat or fat-free salad dressings. Ask for the salad dressing on the side.

- Desserts: Choose low-fat frozen yogurt, fruit ices, sorbets, and sherbets. Occasional indulgent desserts can add fun to a carefully selected, well-balanced diet.

Vegetarian Diets

The various classifications of vegetarian include ovo-, lacto-, lacto-ovo-, semi- or partial vegetarian, and vegan.

Nutrients that may be lacking in a vegetarian diet are protein, vitamin B_{12}, vitamin D, riboflavin, calcium, zinc, and iron.

Vegetarians, who limit or omit animal products from their diets, may need to take supplements (e.g., calcium, vitamin B_{12}).

Vegan diets require careful planning to obtain adequate amounts of required nutrients. Obtaining adequate amounts of vitamins D and B_{12} will require supplementation.

Challenges for Special Populations

College Students

College students often eat on the run, eat fast food, and are served from dining hall or cafeteria lines. The circumstances of college life make it all too easy to eat food that is not nutritious or to skip meals, especially breakfast. Think about how, what, and when you eat.

- Don't skip breakfast.
- Take your time when you eat.

What's the word...

lacto-vegetarian Person who includes some or all dairy products in his or her diet.

lacto-ovo-vegetarian Person who includes milk, dairy products, and eggs in his or her diet.

semi- or partial vegetarian Person who eats no red meat but may include chicken or fish, dairy products, and eggs in his or her diet.

vegan Person who eats only foods of plant origin.

vegetarian diet Diet in which vegetables are the foundation and meat products are restricted or eliminated.

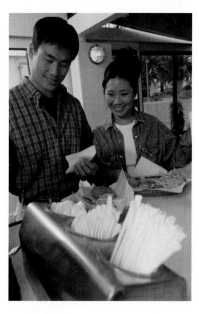

- Be conscious of food choices in the dining hall line or at a fast-food restaurant.
- For snacks, eat granola bars, raw veggies, fruit, low-fat cheese, low-fat yogurt, plain popcorn (no butter!), and soup.
- Drink plenty of water.

Some great ideas for preparing quick, healthy meals can be found at websites such as www.meals.com.

Athletes

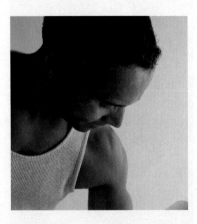

What's the word. . .

carbo loading Stuffing yourself with complex carbohydrates during the days before an endurance event.

Carbo loading builds and maintains stores of glycogen for muscles, which extends endurance and delays fatigue. If you are an endurance athlete:

- A few days before an event, gradually increase the amount of complex carbohydrates you are eating to about 70% of your total calories.
- At the same time, gradually decrease the length of workout time.
- Two to four hours before the event, eat a light meal of bagels, pasta, or breads and cereals.
- Afterward, eat a meal with carbs, protein, and fat to help repair and rebuild muscle.

Everyday exercise rarely requires this dietary pattern. In fact, not all athletes find that carbo loading helps their performance. Test the effects of the carbo-load diet when you are not preparing for competition.

There is no need to take in extra protein; the average American already takes in 50% more calories than needed. As an athlete, you need only 12% protein in your overall daily intake of calories.

Legal supplements (vitamins, minerals, protein, and certain amino acids) most likely do not help.

Women

Because they tend to be smaller than men, women require less protein and fewer calories. Women should concentrate on getting enough of the right nutrients, especially:

- calcium to head off osteoporosis, a special aging hazard for women; and
- iron to avoid anemia, another special hazard for females who menstruate.

Women can get the nutrients they need from nonfat and low-fat dairy; orange juice; fortified cereal; lean, red meat; and green, leafy vegetables.

Men

Men are at risk for heart disease, cancer, and later-life weight gain because they tend to eat more red meat and fewer grains, vegetables, and fruits than recommended. They can get the necessary vitamins, minerals, fiber, and phytochemicals (see Table 8.11) from grains, vegetables, and fruit.

Diabetics

Diabetics must watch their diets very carefully, because they must maintain just the right blood sugar level at all times during the day. If the level falls, they must take immediate remedial action, such as drinking orange juice, to bring it up.

Diabetics must take a blood sugar measurement several times during each day. New instruments that make it easier to do so are now available.

Medical News You Can Use

Potato Chips, a Top Culprit in Gradual Weight Gain

Potato chips may be the most dangerous food for your hips, according to a study that lay out weight-associated foods by pound. Potato chips account for roughly half of the weight gain that a healthy, non-obese American gains over 4 years (1.28 pounds of the 3.35 pounds gained). Other foods strongly associated with weight gain are sugar-sweetened beverages, unprocessed red meats, and processed meats.

Source: Data from Mozaffarian D., et al., Changes in diet and lifestyle and long-term weight gain in women and men. *New England Journal of Medicine*, 2011. 364(25):2392–2404.

A diabetic diet should be low in simple sugars and high in foods with a high glycemic load/index, and should include a reasonable amount of unsaturated fats.

Older People

People older than age 50 are usually less active, so they need to consume fewer calories to balance their calorie output.

The digestive tract of older people is less efficient at absorbing nutrients, so older people need to eat foods fortified with vitamin B_{12} or to take vitamin B_{12} supplements.

Older individuals should also make sure they include foods high in fiber in their diet, because constipation is more of a problem in this age group.

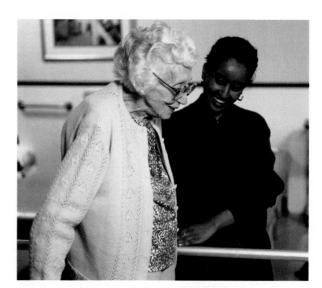

Smart Food Choices

Reading Labels

On a food label's Nutrition Facts panel (see **Labs 8-3 and 8-4**), manufacturers are required to provide information on certain nutrients in a certain order (see **Figure 8.4**):

- If a claim is made about any of the optional components, or if a food is fortified or enriched with any of them, nutrition information for these components is mandatory.
- The required nutrients address today's health concerns. The order in which the information must appear is the priority of current dietary recommendations.

Dietary Supplement Labels

Supplement labels are limited by law in what they can and cannot say (see **Figure 8.5**). They:

- identify the supplement;
- give the quantity (e.g., 40 capsules);
- give directions for using and storing;
- show warnings, if needed;
- list standardization levels, in some cases; and
- list an address from which to obtain more information.

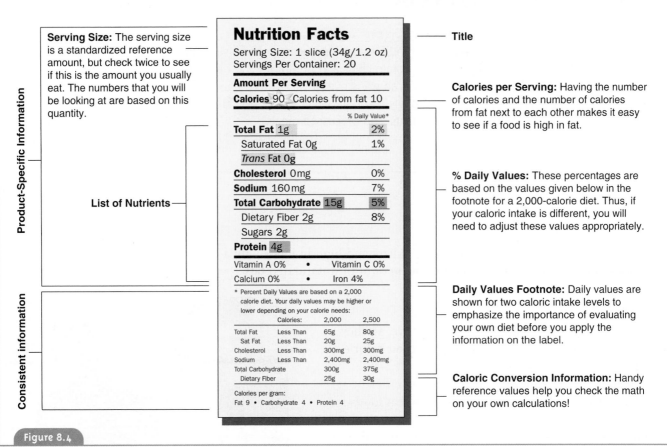

Figure 8.4

The Nutrition Facts panel.

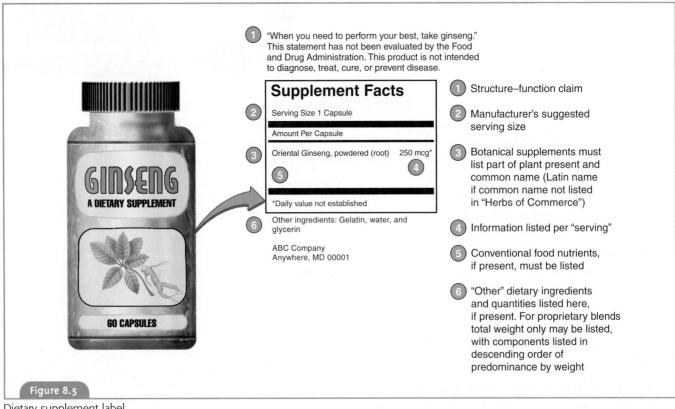

Figure 8.5

Dietary supplement label.

Each product's food label also includes a "supplement facts" box or panel, showing:

- serving size;
- source and amount of ingredients, assigned daily values; and
- name, source, and amount of ingredients not having daily values.

By law, supplements can make only three types of claims:

- Structure–function claims (e.g., "Specially formulated to make you feel on top of the world!") are not reviewed by the FDA, so they must carry a disclaimer: "This statement has not been evaluated by the Food and Drug Administration. This product is not intended to diagnose, treat, cure, or prevent any disease."
- Nutrient content claims must mean the same as they do on food labels. "High potency" may be applied only to single-ingredient supplements with 100% of the daily value and only to a multi-ingredient supplement if it has a minimum of two-thirds of the combined daily values.
- Disease claims may be made only if authorized by the FDA or some other such body. A calcium supplement is allowed to say that it will help prevent osteoporosis, for example.

Food Additives

Additives—mainly sugar, salt, and corn syrup, along with citric acid, baking soda, vegetable colors, mustard, and pepper—are added to food to:

- enhance taste or change appearance;
- help process the food;
- keep the food fresh; and
- boost nutritional value.

Possible health problems from consuming food with additives include:

- spells of sweating and a rise in blood pressure for some people after eating food in which monosodium glutamate is used as a flavor enhancer;
- possibly increased (but still low) risk for certain cancers from the additives butylated hydroxyanisole and butylated hydroxytoluene, which are used to keep foods fresh (the FDA is reviewing the use of these additives, and some manufacturers have stopped using them);
- a (usually low) risk for cancer-causing agents in the stomach from consuming the small amounts of nitrates and nitrites added to protect meats from botulism; and
- severe reactions in some people to sulfites, which are used to keep vegetables from turning brown (the FDA strictly limits the use of sulfites and requires such foods to be clearly labeled).

If you are sensitive to an additive, check food labels when you shop and ask questions when you eat out.

Irradiated Foods

Irradiation has been used for a long time to sterilize plastic wrap, milk cartons, teething rings, contact lenses, and medical supplies. Newer methods of irradiation using electricity and X-rays do not require radioactive materials.

Since 1963, the federal government has allowed, one food group at a time, the irradiation of:

- pork;
- raw poultry;

> **What's the word...**
> **irradiation** Treatment with gamma rays, X-rays, or high-voltage electrons to kill pathogens and, in the case of food, to increase shelf life.

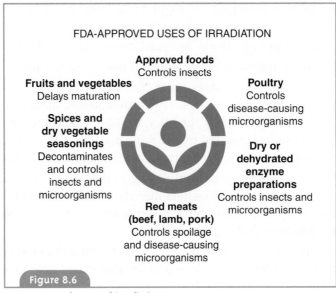

Figure 8.6

FDA-approved uses of irradiation.

- red meat;
- fruits;
- vegetables;
- wheat and flour;
- white potatoes; and
- herbs and spices.

All primary irradiated foods have the Radura symbol (see **Figure 8.6**) and a brief information label. Irradiation kills most pathogens but does not completely sterilize a product. Proper handling is still necessary.

Not many irradiated foods are available because consumers are skeptical or fearful of them. But when consumers have information about irradiation and its benefits, most want to purchase these products (Insel et al. 2007).

Genetically Modified Foods

How do you modify an organism genetically? You insert genes from one organism into another to introduce new traits or enhance existing ones. Why would you do this? Well, for one thing, it makes crops:

- more resistant to disease, heat, and frost;
- last longer;
- better tasting and more nutritious; and
- require less fertilizer and pesticides.

This process could save billions in costs, because such crops are more productive. This would help feed the hungry in the developing world.

What is the downside? We do not know if genetic modification of food crops will:

- create previously unknown "transgenic" organisms that might have adverse effects on us and our environment;
- cross-pollinate and destroy other plants; and
- create superweeds that resist herbicides.

What's the word...

genetic modification Manipulating the DNA of an organism to change some of its characteristics.

transgenic An organism into which hereditary (i.e., genetic) material from another organism has been introduced.

Whether you know it or not, you have been eating genetically modified foods since 1996, if what you eat comes from a supermarket. So far, such modification seems to be benign and helpful. Only time will tell.

Organic Foods

Concerned about Frankenfood? Do not want to eat meat from cattle fed with growth hormone, or vegetables and fruit sprayed with so many pesticides that even bugs will not eat them? Look for the USDA organic label (see Figure 8.7). Foodstuffs cannot carry it, unless the following conditions are met in their production:

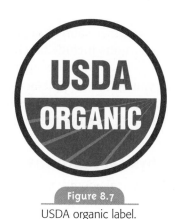

Figure 8.7

USDA organic label.

- crops meet strict limits on pesticide spraying;
- no sewage sludge is mixed into the soil;
- cattle are allowed outdoors and fed only organic feed;
- no antibiotics or growth hormones are used; and
- no genetic engineering or ionizing radiation takes place.

There are degrees of organic, however, so check the small print:

- "100% organic" means all organic ingredients: can carry USDA label;
- "Organic" means 95% organic ingredients: can still carry label; or
- "Made with organic ingredients" means 70% organic: no label allowed.

Assessing and Changing Your Diet

How can you tell whether you are getting the right amounts of the essential nutrients to meet your needs? Complete Lab 8-1 to find out.

Stay on the Healthy Path

Now you know what and how to eat so as to keep yourself healthy. Help yourself stay on the right path: Dust off and apply the self-management skills you learned from the beginning of this text.

Use the MyPyramid and the *Dietary Guidelines* to help you figure out what is good to eat and what to avoid. Then, follow these tips:

- Cook at home.
- Plan ahead when you shop for food.
- Consume only small amounts of red meat; eat fish and poultry at least one to two times a week.
- Have a few meatless meals each week.

Benefits of Food

If you think you should take supplements to get the vitamins you need, think again. You lose out on other essential nutrients if you eat a diet high in calories, fat, and sodium and think you can make up for it with supplements.

Fruits and vegetables also have a lot more antioxidants and phytochemicals than supplements:

- Three-fourths of a cup of cooked kale (with a lot less of vitamins E and C) will neutralize as many free radicals as approximately 80 times as much vitamin E or more than 50 times as much vitamin C in supplement form.

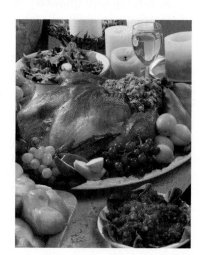

- Other sources of antioxidants high in oxygen radical absorbance capacity (ORAC) units include blueberries, blackberries, strawberries, prunes, plums, raisins, beets, and red bell peppers—even brussels sprouts, if you like them.

If you do take supplements, look for the U.S. Pharmacopoeia symbol on the bottle. The supplement should dissolve completely in less than 45 minutes. Supplements that take longer to dissolve will not go into the bloodstream and cannot do you any good.

Physical Performance

If physical activity is your thing—especially if you are a competitive athlete—you are always looking for an edge. Our advice? Skip the supplements and do this instead:

- Drink enough water.
- Know and consume a well-balanced diet, with enough fruits and vegetables and variety, and you will get all the vitamins and minerals you need without taking supplements.
- Skip the protein-rich diet. It is unlikely to build bigger muscles. Even worse, it may dehydrate you and take away calcium.
- Limit the calories you get from fat to no more than 30% of your total calories.
- Starchy foods high in complex carbohydrates are what your body prefers for fuel.
- Avoid sugary foods.

Nutritional Quackery

If you read a typical fitness magazine, you will see no shortage of nutrition advertisements. Popular claims by nutrition quacks (pretenders to medical skill) are that their products and services will:

- take off body fat and lower weight;
- build muscle;
- boost energy;
- enhance endurance;
- fight fatigue; and
- relieve muscle soreness.

How Is Nutritional Quackery Harmful?

- Buying into quackery may increase health risks by preventing you from seeking adequate medical care.
- Products and services by quacks are usually expensive.
- Products and services may detract from scientific nutrition recommendations.
- False claims may promote distrust of the medical community.

Fad Diets

Billions of dollars are made annually in the sale and promotion of fad diets. What is a fad diet? It is a dietary plan that is more trend than science; a dietary plan that attempts to convince a consumer that one particular food is to blame for his or her weight problem; a dietary plan that promotes "fast and simple" weight loss.

The truth is, people do not become overweight in a short time, and they can't return to good form in a short time. Diets do not work for the long term, but lifestyle changes do! You must be willing to persist. If it sounds too good to be true, it probably is. See the Time Out feature for a summary of the most popular fad diets, their claims, and the pros and cons for each approach.

Dietary Supplements

Just about anything can be sold as long as it is called a "dietary supplement." The FDA considers dietary supplements to be food, so they are not evaluated for safety and effectiveness. People tend to believe that the products on the market have been researched, tested, and inspected.

Avoid buying products with claims like "fat burner," "fat metabolizer," "energy enhancer," "performance booster," "strength booster," "ergogenic aid," "anabolic optimizer," or "genetic optimizer."

Reflect >>>> Reinforce >>>> Reinvigorate

Knowledge Check

Answers in Appendix D

1. Anyone vigorously exercising for more than 1 hour should:
   A. Consider drinking an electrolyte/carbohydrate drink
   B. Drink only water
   C. Feel it is fine to drink soda pop to replace fluids
   D. Tough it out

2. For best absorption of fluids by the body, which temperature is best?
   A. Cooler than ambient temperature
   B. Warmer than ambient temperature
   C. Same as ambient temperature
   D. Temperature does not matter

3. Susan lives a very busy life and is on the go most waking hours of the day. Her three children seem to be involved in every sport and activity available through their school and community. Susan exercises daily. She belongs to a book club, volunteers at the local hospital, and is active in her church's programs. She brings home fast-food meals several times each week. She is considering giving vitamin supplements to her family, because she has little time to prepare well-balanced meals at home. Which is the recommended method for Susan to determine whether she needs to give her family a vitamin supplement?
   A. Compare the foods eaten by her family to dietary standards—namely, the Dietary Reference Intakes (DRIs)
   B. Have anthropometric measures made
   C. Obtain a biochemical assessment of their body fluids (e.g., blood, urine)
   D. Have a clinical nutrition examination of their hair, nails, and skin

4. Which vegetarian diet contains no animal products?
   A. Lacto-vegetarian
   B. Lacto-ovo-vegetarian
   C. Vegan
   D. Semi-vegetarian

5. Vegetarians limiting or omitting animal products from their diets may need to take:
   A. Vitamin B_{12}
   B. Calcium supplements
   C. Iron supplements
   D. All of the above

6. What is the difference between complete and incomplete proteins?
   A. Only complete proteins assist in body structure.
   B. Only complete proteins possess all the essential amino acids.
   C. Only incomplete proteins build red blood cells.
   D. Only incomplete proteins are found in animal products.

7. The numerical value given to a food to indicate how quickly the body turns it into sugar based on the number of carbohydrates in one serving, is called its:
   A. Vitamin output
   B. Glycemic index
   C. Nutritional content
   D. Glycemic load

8. Which of the following, if taken in excess, will the body retain?

   A. Vitamin B_2
   B. Vitamin B_{12}
   C. Vitamin C
   D. Vitamin E

9. Which of the following nutrients is known for fighting osteoporosis?

   A. Calcium
   B. Iron
   C. Sodium
   D. Magnesium

10. Which of the following is the USDA's calorie recommendation for active men and women?

    A. 1600 calories
    B. 2200 calories
    C. 2800 calories
    D. 3200 calories

Modern Modifications

- Try granola bars, raw vegetables, fruit, and plain popcorn (no butter) for snacks.
- Drink plenty of water.
- Try to stick with meat dishes that are grilled, baked, roasted, or broiled.
- Have your salad dressing in a separate dish and dip your fork in it before the salad.
- Have sorbet or frozen yogurt instead of ice cream.
- Have a sandwich on whole-grain bread.

Critical Thinking

Abby is a 20-year-old sophomore at State College. She has been making statements for some time regarding being "unhappy" about her weight but has yet to take any action on it. She has been thinking about her diet, but she is unsure what to change. Yesterday, her intake was as follows:

- Breakfast: 2 eggs scrambled, 3 slices of bacon, 2 pieces of toast with butter
- Lunch: peanut butter sandwich, Big Grab bag of Doritos, milk
- Dinner: spaghetti with meat sauce, 4 bread sticks with butter and garlic, Coke, pie slice
- Other: chocolate granola bar, 2 more Cokes, hot wings with friends, "a couple" of beers

Based on this menu, what areas of Abby's diet would you characterize as nutritionally adequate? Excessive? Lacking? How would you adapt Abby's diet to better conform to the Food Guide Pyramid (MyPyramidPlan.com)? The Healthy Eating Pyramid?

Going Above and Beyond

Websites

American Dietetic Association
http://www.eatright.org
Mayo Clinic Diet and Nutrition Resource Center
http://www.mayoclinic.com

Federal Citizen Information Center: Food
http://www.pueblo.gsa.gov/food.htm

Gateways to Government Nutrition Information
http://www.nutrition.gov or http://www.foodsafety.gov

MedlinePlus: Nutrition
http://www.nlm.nih.gov/medlineplus/nutrition.html

National Cancer Institute 5-a-Day Program
http://cancercontrol.cancer.gov/5ad_exec.html

U.S. Food and Drug Administration
http://www.fda.gov/Food/default.htm

USDA Food and Nutrition Information Center
http://www.nal.usda.gov/fnic

Nutrition Analysis Tool, University of Illinois, Urbana/Champaign
http://www.myfoodrecord.com/mainnat.html

Center for Science in the Public Interest
http://cspinet.org

Office of Dietary Supplements
http://dietary-supplements.info.nih.gov

Fast Food Finder
http://www.all-weightloss.net/fastfood.htm

Glycemic Index Foundation—University of Sydney
http://www.glycemicindex.com

References and Suggested Readings

————. Multivitamins. September 2010. www.ConsumerReports.org

————. Nutrition. Sudbury, MA: Jones & Bartlett, 2007.

————. Vitamins and minerals, part II: Who needs supplements? *ACSM Health and Fitness Journal* 2001; 5:33–36.

————. Vitamins and minerals, part III: Can you get too much? *ACSM Health and Fitness Journal* 2001; 5:26–28.

American Dietetics Association (ADA). Vegetarian diets: Position of the American Dietetics Association. *Journal of the American Dietetics Association* 1997; 7:1317–1321.

Clark K. Water, sports drinks, juice, or soda? *ACSM Health and Fitness Journal* 1998; 2:41.

Connor S. L., Gustafson J. R., and Artaud-Wild, S. M. The Cholesterol-saturated fat index for coronary prevention: Background, use, and a comprehensive table of foods. *Journal of the American Dietetic Association* 1989; 89:807–816.

Connor S. L., Gustafson J. R., Artaud-Wild S. M., Classick-Kohn C. J., Connor W. E. The cholesterol-saturated fat index for coronary prevention: background, use, and a comprehensive table of foods. *Journal of the American Dietetic Association* 1989; 89:807–816.

Foster-Powell K., et al. International table of glycemic index and glycemic load values: 2002. *American Journal of Clinical Nutrition* 2002; 76:5–56.

Fuchs C. S., Giovannucci E. L., Colditz G. A., Hunter D. J., Stampfer M. J., Rosner B., Speizer F. E., and Willett W. Dietary fiber and the risk of colorectal cancer and adenoma in women. *New England Journal of Medicine* 1999; 340:169–176.

Gardner C. D., Kiazand A., Alhassan S., et al. Comparison of the Atkins, Zone, Ornish, and LEARN diets for change in weight and related risk factors among overweight premenopausal women: The A to Z Weight Loss Study, a Randomized Trial. *Journal of the American Medical Association* 2007; 297(9):969–977.

Insel P., Turner R. E., and Ross D. Discovering Nutrition. Sudbury, MA: Jones and Bartlett, 2006.

Manner M. M. Vitamins and minerals, part I: How much do you need? *ACSM Health and Fitness Journal* 2001; 5:33–36.

Mendosa D. Revised international table of glycemic index (GI) and glycemic load (GL) values—2002. http://diabetes.about.com/ [October 2, 2008].

USDA and USDHHS. *Dietary Guidelines for Americans, 2010.* 7th edition, Washington, DC: U.S. Government Printing Office, 2010.

Willett W. C. *Eat, Drink, and Be Healthy.* New York: Fireside, 2005.

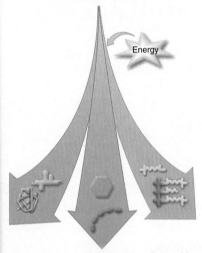

EXTRACTION OF ENERGY

Protein
(amino acids)

Carbohydrates
(sugars)

Fats
(fatty acids)

Molecular building blocks

Energy

Amino acids and
body protein

Glucose and
glycogen

Fatty acids and
lipids

BIOSYNTHESIS

Cells use metabolic reactions to extract
energy from food and to form building blocks
for biosynthesis.

What's the word...

metabolism The rate
at which your body
uses energy.

**adenosine triphos-
phate (ATP)** The only
form of energy used in
the human body.

aerobic Using oxygen.

anaerobic Without
using oxygen.

Energy Production

You need energy to move. When you are doing nothing, your metabolic rate is low. If you start moving, your metabolism increases.

How do you get the energy to move around—or run a marathon? You get it from the carbohydrates, fats, and proteins in food.

During digestion, most carbohydrates are converted to glucose. Some glucose remains in the blood, where it can be used as a quick source of energy. The rest of the glucose is converted to glycogen and stored in the liver, muscles, and kidneys. When glycogen stores are full, leftover glucose is converted to body fat (Figure TO1.1).

Protein is used mainly to build tissue. But some protein may also be stored as body fat. When other energy fuels run out, the body uses the protein in body fat for energy.

Your body cells convert glucose, glycogen, and fat to adenosine triphosphate (ATP). When a cell needs energy, it breaks down ATP.

When you exercise, your body mobilizes its stores of fat to increase ATP production.

ATP can be used in two ways: with oxygen (aerobic) or without oxygen (anaerobic).

ATP contracts your muscles during exercise. The amount of ATP needed depends on how long and how hard your body works.

Aerobic and Anaerobic Activity

If a movement is quick, occurring at the beginning of exercise and at high points of exercise intensity, the body uses the small amount of ATP in the cells (e.g., sprinting; a clean-and-jerk weight lift).

If the movement must be sustained over time, during prolonged but low to relatively moderate exercise (e.g., jogging or running for a distance), the body must create the supply of ATP.

The Energy Systems

Three different energy systems create energy: immediate energy system, anaerobic energy system, and aerobic energy system. Each system is defined by the way it produces and uses ATP (Table TO1.1)

Immediate Energy System

ATP is the immediate source of energy within all cells of our body for activities such as sprinting. There are small stores of ATP within skeletal muscle, and these energy stores provide immediate energy to sustain physical activities for a short time. Once the ATP is used, it breaks down into adenosine diphosphate (ADP). For regeneration of ADP into ATP for more energy, creatine phosphate (CP) is needed. CP regenerates ATP. Without CP, ATP could provide energy for only a few seconds. With CP, the ATP-CP system can provide energy for about 10 seconds before other energy systems must take over.

Anaerobic Energy System

When vigorous-intensity exercise continues beyond 30 seconds, the only way to continue providing ATP to the exercising muscle is by using glucose in the muscle. Glucose is obtained from glycogen. However, in the process of generating ATP from glucose, lactic

Table TO1.1	Characteristics of the Body's Energy Systems		
	ENERGY SYSTEM*		
	Immediate	Nonoxidative	Oxidative
Duration of activity for which system predominates	0–10 seconds	10 seconds–2 minutes	>2 minutes
Intensity of activity for which system predominates	High	High	Low to moderately high
Rate of ATP production	Immediate, very rapid	Rapid	Slower but prolonged
Fuel	Adenosine triphosphate (ATP), creatine phosphate (CP)	Muscle stores of glycogen and glucose	Body stores of glycogen, glucose, fat, and protein
Oxygen used?	No	No	Yes
Sample activities	Weight lifting, picking up a bag of groceries	400-meter run, running up several flights of stairs	1500-meter run, 30-minute walk, standing in line for a long time

*For most activities, all three systems contribute to energy production; the duration and intensity of the activity determine which system predominates.

Source: Adapted from Brooks G. A., et al. *Exercise Physiology: Human Bioenergetics and Its Application,* 3rd ed. McGraw-Hill, 2000.

acid is formed. Normally, only a small amount of lactic acid is present in the blood and muscle. When lactic acid begins to accumulate in the muscle and then blood, it is a sign of muscular fatigue.

Aerobic Energy System

The aerobic system provides energy to support long-term steady-state exercise, such as long-distance running or swimming. Muscles can use both glucose and fatty acids for energy. These fuel sources can be taken from the circulating blood and from stores within the muscle. Glucose is stored as glycogen and fatty acids are stored as triglycerides in the muscle. When long-duration activities are performed at a slow pace, more "fat," in the form of fatty acids, is used for energy than muscle glycogen.

Role of Energy Systems in Exercise

All three energy systems are involved during most types of exercise. When exercise duration increases, a shift occurs from anaerobic energy to aerobic energy.

Fit individuals use more stored fat than persons who are less active, so they can exercise longer.

As the intensity and duration of your workout increases, more energy is needed to sustain that level of activity, so more oxygen is required.

The more aerobically fit you are, the higher your VO_{2max}, and the more energy you produce. This increases your ability to exercise at a higher level of intensity and for longer periods.

Being aware of how your body produces and uses energy helps you make the connection between nutrition and exercise.

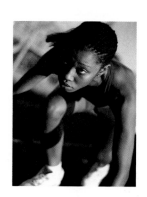

Fad Diets

Have you ever heard the saying, "If it sounds too good to be true, then it probably is"? When it comes to dieting, you can count on it. Fad diets have been around for as long as people have been eating, but now they represent a formidable industry. Billions of dollars are made every year on products designed to help people lose weight.

Most of the diet plans on the market fail to actually teach people how to eat correctly. They promise fast weight loss, and sometimes even deliver on that claim. Of course as soon as the individual stops the diet, he or she invariably returns to the old dietary patterns and the weight piles on again.

In general, fad diets are flawed in the following ways:

- Many propose a diet that places people at risk for coronary heart disease.
- Most describe some specific food or combination of foods as "fat-burning" foods. No scientific evidence exists to support this claim.
- Most fad diets require extremely restrictive dietary patterns—patterns that most people cannot maintain for long periods of time. Significant restrictions on the consumption of macronutrients (fats, carbohydrates, proteins) tend to trigger strong cravings for the missing component.
- Highly imbalanced diets can eventually lead to ketosis, a state where the body believes it is starving and begins to metabolize muscle mass instead of fat.
- Almost none of the fad diets encourage physical activity or even discuss the importance of physical activity in weight management.

Table TO2.1 lists some of the more popular diets and offers a brief analysis of their content.

Table TO2.1	Criticisms of Popular Weight Loss Diets
Diet	**Criticisms**
Low Carbohydrate	
South Beach	• May be deficient in fiber and calcium due to limited amount of whole grains and dairy products • May be difficult to follow due to limited amounts of whole grains and restriction of sweets • Restricts some good foods such as carrots, bananas, pineapple, and watermelon • Needs more research
Atkins	• Deficient in certain nutrients such as vitamin D, calcium, and folate due to elimination of fruits and grains, most vegetable and dairy products. Can lead to osteoporosis • No fiber and health-promoting phytochemicals from fruits, vegetables, whole grains, and other plan foods • Long term intake of excess of dietary fat, especially saturated fat can raise total blood cholesterol and LDL-cholesterol levels • Must purchase Atkins foods • High protein amounts uric acid levels and possible gout • Kidney stone formation is also associated with excess protein intake • Short-term weight loss can occur, but the potential for heart disease worsens. Initial weight loss is mostly water weight • Needs more research

Table TO2.1 | Criticisms of Popular Weight Loss Diets, *continued*

Diet	Criticisms
Low Carbohydrate	
The Zone	• May be deficient in certain vitamins and minerals such as vitamins D and E, iron, magnesium, calcium, and fiber • Complicated calculating protein and carbohydrates before eating especially when eating out • Not supported by scientific research
Moderate Carbohydrate	
Weight Watchers	• Participants must pay a sign-up fee plus a monthly fee • Weekly meetings increases dieter's weight loss success • Men may feel uncomfortable in weekly meetings since most participants are female
Jenny Craig	• Requires packaged meals—not conducive for teaching how to shop, cook and eat own meals. After the program weight gain is likely • Cost of ready-made meals can be expensive for some dieters • May have difficulty eating meals long-term, especially when traveling, socially dining, or during illness • Men may feel uncomfortable in the program since most participants are female
High Carbohydrate	
Volumetrics	• Balanced eating plan promoting healthy food choices and portion-control • High volume of fiber-rich foods for meals and snacks may cause gastrointestinal distress for some dieters
Dean Ornish	• Potential nutritional problems: – Inadequate calcium and vitamin D increases risk of osteoporosis – Deficient in zinc and vitamin B_{12} due to infrequent meat consumption – Inadequate in vitamin E which is found in oils, nuts, and other foods rich in fat • High volume of fiber-rich foods for meals and snacks may cause gastrointestinal distress for some dieters • Emphasis on a very low-fat vegetarian diet can be a challenge for those who have little time to cook, are traveling, or dining out.
Slim Fast	• Expected to purchase Slim-Fast products for breakfast and lunch meals which becomes expensive, "burnout," and limits the dieter's ability to select healthy options (e.g., whole grain cereals, nonfat milk) • May be deficient in calcium, iron, vitamin E, and other nutrients • Recommends exercise • Research suggests that weight loss for up to two years can be obtained—beyond that, data is lacking

Ethnic Diets
Mediterranean and Ethnic Diets

The Mediterranean diet is based on the dietary traditions of the countries surrounding the Mediterranean Sea (Crete, Greece, southern Italy, and North Africa). The people who live there exhibit strikingly lower rates of chronic disease.

The traditional diets of the Mediterranean region are mainly based on the foods from a rich diversity of plant sources and include fruits, vegetables, whole grains, beans, nuts, and seeds. Fruits and vegetables are locally grown and often consumed raw or processed very little. This factor may be significant in determining their potential value for fiber and antioxidants.

- In North Africa, couscous, vegetables, and legumes are the core of the diet.
- In southern Europe, the diet includes rice, polenta, pasta, and potatoes, along with vegetables and legumes.
- In the eastern Mediterranean, bulgur and rice, together with vegetables and legumes such as chickpeas, are the main part of many meals.
- Throughout the Mediterranean, bread is a staple eaten without butter or margarine.

Characteristics of the Mediterranean Diet

Fish, Poultry, and Red Meat
Red meat (associated with colon cancer, prostate cancer, and heart disease) is eaten sparingly. In addition to poultry, only about 15 ounces of red meat per week are consumed. Fish consumption varies from one country to another but averages 5 to 15 ounces per week.

Dairy Products
Cheese and yogurt from goats, sheep, buffalo, cows, and camels are traditionally consumed in low to moderate amounts. In the entire region, very little fresh milk is drunk. Butter and cream are used only on special occasions. The bacterial cultures of yogurt may contribute to good health.

Wine with Meals
Throughout the Mediterranean, wine is consumed in moderation and is usually taken with meals. For men, moderation is two glasses per day, for women one glass per day.

Olive Oil and Total Fat
Olive oil, which is high in monounsaturated fat, is a good source of antioxidants. It is the main source of fat in the Mediterranean diet. Current research suggests that olive oil may actually increase HDL (good) cholesterol but has little effect on LDL (bad) cholesterol.

Physical Activity
The people of the Mediterranean engage in physical activity in their everyday lives and consider it vital to maintaining good health and proper weight.

Other Ethnic Diets

Every ethnic diet has its healthy and unhealthy foods, sauces, and preparation. The guidelines for healthy eating given in this chapter can be applied to any diet.

The suggestions that follow are based on recommendations from the National Institutes of Health and the American Dietetic Association (**Table TO3.1**).

Table TO3.1	Ethnic Diet Recommendations
Good	**Not as Good**
Chinese	
Steamed, poached, boiled, roasted, barbecued, or lightly stir-fried fresh fish and seafood, skinless chicken, or tofu; with mixed vegetables, Chinese greens, steamed rice, steamed spring rolls, or soft noodles; with hoisin sauce, oyster sauce, wine sauce, plum sauce, velvet sauce, or hot mustard	Crab Rangoon, crispy duck or chicken, or anything breaded or deep-fried, including fried rice, fried wontons, egg rolls, and fried or crispy noodles
Thai	
Dishes barbecued, sautéed, broiled, boiled, steamed, braised, or marinated; skewered and grilled meats; with fish sauce, basil sauce, or hot sauces; bean thread noodles; Thai salad	Coconut milk soup; peanut sauce or dishes topped with nuts; crispy noodles; red, green, and yellow curries containing coconut milk
Japanese	
Dishes boiled or made in boiling broth, steamed, simmered, broiled, or grilled; with mixed rice, steamed rice, or buckwheat, wheat, or rice noodles	Dishes battered and fried or deep-fried; fried pork cutlet, fried tofu
Mexican	
Fish marinated in lime juice; soft corn or wheat tortillas, burritos, fajitas, enchiladas, soft tacos, tamales filled with beans, vegetables, or lean meats; with refried beans, nonfat or low-fat rice and beans; with salsa, enchilada sauce, or picante sauce; gazpacho, menudo, or black bean soup; fruit or flan	Crispy fried tortillas; fried dishes such as chile rellenos, chimichangas, flautas, or tostadas; nachos and cheese, chili con queso, and other dishes made with cheese or cheese sauce; guacamole, sour cream; refried beans made with lard; fried ice cream
Italian	
Pasta primavera or pasta, polenta, risotto, or gnocchi; with marinara, red or white wine sauce, red or white clam sauce, light mushroom sauce; dishes grilled or made with tomato-based sauce, broth and wine sauce, or lemon sauce; seafood stew; vegetable, minestrone, or bean soups	Cheese or smoked meats; dishes prepared alfredo, carbonara, fried, creamed, or with cream; veal scallopini; chicken, veal, or eggplant parmigiana; Italian sausage, salami, or prosciutto; buttered garlic bread; cannoli
French	
Fresh fish, shrimp, scallops, mussels, or skinless chicken, steamed, skewered, and broiled or grilled; without sauces; clear soups	Dishes prepared in cream sauce, baked with cream and cheese, or in a pastry crust; drawn butter, hollandaise sauce, or mayonnaise-based sauce
Indian	
Dishes prepared with curry and roasted in a clay oven or pan-roasted; kabobs; yogurt and cucumber salad, and other yogurt-based dishes and sauces; lentils and basmati rice; baked bread	Any fried or coconut-milk–based dishes; meat in cream sauce; clarified butter; fried breads

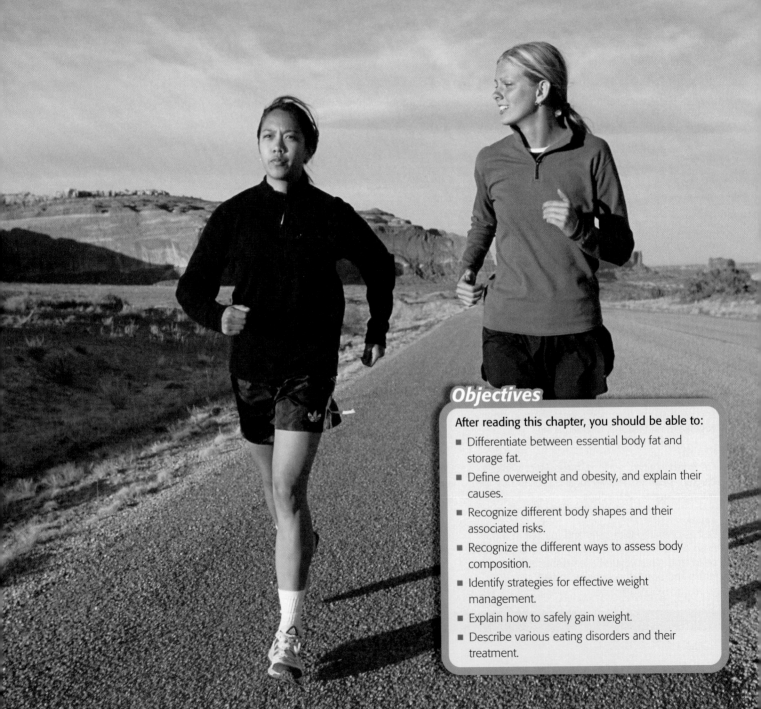

 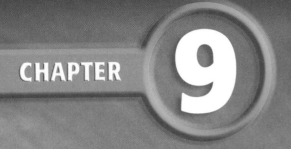

Body Composition and Body Weight

Objectives

After reading this chapter, you should be able to:

- Differentiate between essential body fat and storage fat.
- Define overweight and obesity, and explain their causes.
- Recognize different body shapes and their associated risks.
- Recognize the different ways to assess body composition.
- Identify strategies for effective weight management.
- Explain how to safely gain weight.
- Describe various eating disorders and their treatment.

What Is Body Composition?

Nothing is more personal than your own body. And nothing has a greater influence over how long that body functions properly than its composition. **Body composition** is the ratio of muscle mass to fat mass. *Muscle mass* is composed of muscle, bone, organs, and other tissues of the body. *Fat mass* is the total amount of essential and storage fat in the body.

Essential Body Fat

Your essential body fat resides in your nerve cells, muscles, and bone marrow, as well as in your lungs, heart, liver, and intestines. It has many important functions:

- Keeps your physiological activity normal (e.g., nerve conduction)
- Helps keep your body warm
- Protects your organs from injury
- Stores energy needed when your body is active or when you are injured or ill

The desirable amount of essential fat for a healthy person is:

- Adult women: 8% to 12% of total body weight
- Adult men: 3% to 5% of total body weight

Women have more essential body fat in their hips, thighs, breasts, and uterus.

Storage Fat

Some fat beyond what is essential is also desirable. Besides organ protection and body insulation, **storage fat** supplies energy: 3500 calories per pound of adipose tissue
 Figure 9.1 . A variety of methods exist for determining whether body composition places a person at risk for disease (see Lab 9-1 for instructions on how to assess your body composition). Some methods are simple calculations and are based on the relationship between the person's height and weight. Other methods look specifically at the fat contained in the body.

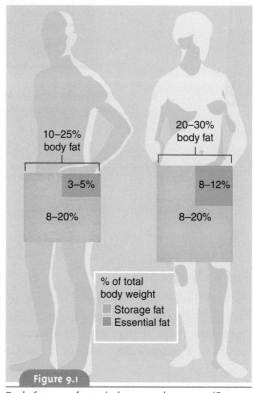

10–25% body fat

3–5%

8–20%

20–30% body fat

8–12%

8–20%

% of total body weight
▢ Storage fat
▢ Essential fat

Figure 9.1

Body fatness of a typical man and woman. (*Source:* Data from Position of The American Dietetic Association and The Canadian Dietetic Association: Nutrition for physical fitness and athletic performance for adults. *Journal of the American Dietetic Association* 1993; 93(6): 691–696.)

What's the word...

body composition Proportion of fat, muscle, bone, and other tissues in the body.

essential body fat Minimum amount of body fat needed for good health.

storage fat Excess fat deposited in adipose tissue (fat cells) that protects organs and insulates the body.

What Causes Weight Gain?

Your weight changes depend on a simple rule:

When the number of calories consumed is not equal to the number of calories used, the following occurs:

Calories Consumed > Calories Used = **Weight Gain**
Calories Consumed < Calories Used = **Weight Loss**
Calories Consumed = Calories Used = **No Weight Gain**

See Figure 9.2 .

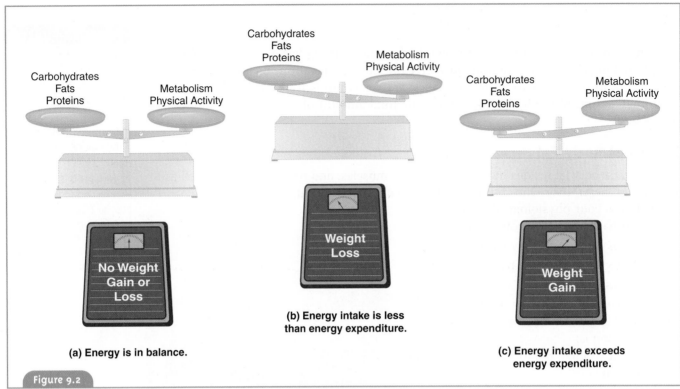

(a) Energy is in balance.

(b) Energy intake is less than energy expenditure.

(c) Energy intake exceeds energy expenditure.

Figure 9.2

The balance between energy intake and expenditure controls weight management.

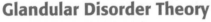

Theories of Weight Gain

Fat Cell Theory

Fat cell theory says that obesity is related to too many fat cells and enlarged fat cells (see **Figure 9.3**). People with an above-average number of fat cells may have been born with them or may have developed them at certain times because of overeating. Restricting calories decreases only the size of fat cells, not the number.

Set Point Theory

Set point theory states that obese individuals are "programmed" to carry a certain amount of weight. This programming originates from a weight regulatory mechanism in the brain's hypothalamus. Even if you lose weight, your body strives to get back to its set point. To lose weight, you must change the set point.

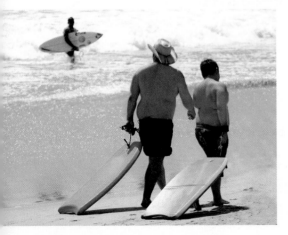

Glandular Disorder Theory

Hypothyroidism is seldom the main reason for overweight or obesity. Treatment with thyroid hormone, although medically unnecessary, does not usually cause a significant weight reduction.

Genetics

More than 400 different genes have been implicated in the development of overweight or obesity, although only a handful appear to be major players. Genes contribute to obesity in many ways, such as by affecting appetite, satiety (the sense of fullness), metabolism, food cravings, body fat distribution, and the tendency to use eating as a way to cope with stress.

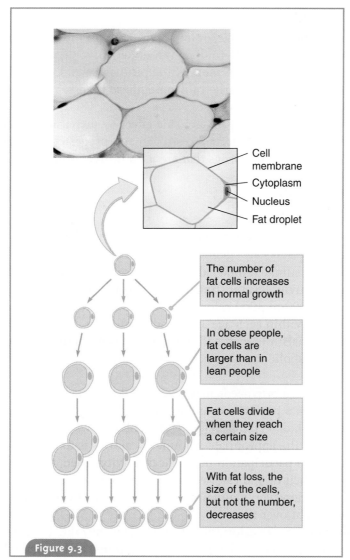

Cell
membrane
Cytoplasm
Nucleus
Fat droplet

The number of
fat cells increases
in normal growth

In obese people,
fat cells are
larger than in
lean people

Fat cells divide
when they reach
a certain size

With fat loss, the
size of the cells,
but not the number,
decreases

Figure 9.3

The formation of fat cells.

The strength of the genetic influence on weight disorders varies quite a bit from person to person. For some people, genes account for just 25% of the predisposition to be overweight, while for others the genetic influence is as high as 70% to 80%.

Genes are probably a significant contributor to your obesity if you have most or all of the following characteristics:

- You have been overweight for much of your life.

- One or both of your parents or several other blood relatives are significantly overweight. If both of your parents have obesity, your likelihood of developing obesity is as high as 80%.

- You can't lose weight even when you increase your physical activity and stick to a low-calorie diet for many months.

People with a moderate genetic predisposition to be overweight have a good chance of losing weight on their own by eating fewer calories and getting more vigorous exercise. However, those with a strong genetic predisposition to obesity may not be able to lose weight with the usual forms of diet and exercise. These people can maintain weight loss only under a doctor's guidance. They are also the most likely to require weight loss drugs or surgery.

9

Diseases and Drugs

A few illnesses involving an imbalance or an abnormality in the endocrine glands can also affect weight. These include hypothyroidism (an underactive thyroid), polycystic ovarian syndrome, and certain unusual tumors of the pituitary gland, adrenal glands, or the pancreas. However, in the vast majority of people, these illnesses are not responsible for weight gain. Most are extremely rare.

Several drugs can cause weight gain as a side effect by increasing appetite or slowing metabolism. These include corticosteroids, estrogen and progesterone, certain anti-cancer medications, antidepressants, and drugs that are used to treat other psychiatric conditions.

Calorie Consumption

Understanding Calorie Needs

The total number of calories a person needs each day varies depending on a number of factors, including the person's age, gender, height, weight, and level of physical activity. **Table 9.1** provides estimated total calorie needs for weight maintenance based on age, gender, and physical activity level. Estimates range from 1600 to 2400 calories per day for adult women and 2000 to 3000 calories per day for adult men, depending on age and physical activity level. Within each age and gender category, the low end of the range is for sedentary individuals; the high end of the range is for active individuals. Due to reductions in basal metabolic rate that occur with aging, calorie needs generally decrease for adults as they age.

Knowing one's daily calorie needs may be a useful reference point for determining whether the calories that a person eats and drinks are appropriate to the number of calories he or she needs each day (see **Lab 9-2**). The best way for people to assess whether they are eating the appropriate amount of calories is to monitor body weight and adjust calorie intake and participation in physical activity based on changes in weight over time. A calorie deficit of 500 calories or more per day is a common initial goal for weight loss for adults. However, maintaining a smaller deficit can have a meaningful influence on body weight over time.

Americans are eating more calories on average than they did 40 years ago. Experts say it's a combination of increased availability, bigger portions, and more high-calorie foods. Almost everywhere we go, food is readily available. Grocery stores stock their shelves with a greater selection of products. Prepackaged foods, fast-food restaurants, and soft drinks are readily accessible. While such foods are fast and convenient, they tend to be high in fat, sugar, and calories (see **Box 9.1**). Choosing many foods from these categories can contribute to an excessive calorie intake. Some foods are marketed as healthy, low fat, or fat free but may contain a lot of calories. It is important to read food labels for nutritional information and to eat in moderation.

Portion size has also increased. People may be eating more during a meal or snack because of larger portion sizes **Figure 9.4**. This results in increased calorie consumption. If the body does not burn off the extra calories consumed from larger portions, fast-food, or soft drinks, weight gain can occur.

A single "super-sized" meal at a fast-food restaurant may contain 1,500–2,000 calories—almost all the calories that most people need for an entire day. People will often eat what's in front of them, even if they are already full. How do portions today compare to portion sizes 20 years ago? They are larger! The National Institutes of Health (NIH) has developed a website (see Figure 9.4) to inform people about the increasing portion sizes.

Americans are also eating more high-calorie foods (especially salty snacks, soft drinks, and pizza), which are much more readily available than lower-calorie choices

Table 9.1	Estimated Calorie Needs per Day by Age, Gender, and Physical Acitvity Level[a]

Estimated amounts of calories needed to maintain calorie balance for various gender and age groups at three different levels of physical activity. The estimates are rounded to the nearest 200 calories. An individual's calorie needs may be higher or lower than these average estimates.

		Physical Activity Level[b]		
Gender	Age (years)	Sedentary	Moderately Active	Active
Child (female and male)	2–3	1,000–1,200[c]	1,000–1,400[c]	1,000–1,400[c]
Female[d]	4–8	1,200–1,400	1,400–1,600	1,400–1,800
	9–13	1,400–1,600	1,600–2,000	1,800–2,200
	14–18	1,800	2,000	2,400
	19–30	1,800–2,000	2,000–2,200	2,400
	31–50	1,800	2,000	2,200
	51+	1,600	1,800	2,000–2,200
Male	4–8	1,200–1,400	1,400–1,600	1,600–2,000
	9–13	1,600–2,000	1,800–2,200	2,000–2,600
	14–18	2,000–2,400	2,400–2,800	2,800–3,200
	19–30	2,400–2,600	2,600–2,800	3,000
	31–50	2,200–2,400	2,400–2,600	2,800–3,000
	51+	2,000–2,200	2,200–2,400	2,400–2,800

a. Based on Estimated Energy Requirements (EER) equations, using reference heights (average) and reference weights (healthy) for each age/gender group. For children and adolescents, reference height and weight vary. For adults, the reference man is 5 feet 10 inches tall and weighs 154 pounds. The reference woman is 5 feet 4 inches tall and weighs 126 pounds. EER equations are from the Institute of Medicine. Dietary Reference Intakes for Energy, Carbohydrate, Fiber, Fat, Fatty Acids, Cholesterol, Protein, and Amino Acids. Washington (DC): The National Academies Press, 2002.

b. Sedentary means a lifestyle that includes only the light physical activity associated with typical day-to-day life. Moderately active means a lifestyle that includes physical activity equivalent to walking about 1.5 to 3 miles per day at 3 to 4 miles per hour, in addition to the light physical activity associated with typical day-to-day life. Active means a lifestyle that includes physical activity equivalent to walking more than 3 miles per day at 3 to 4 miles per hour, in addition to the light physical activity associated with typical day-to-day life.

c. The calorie ranges shown are to accommodate needs of different ages within the group. For children and adolescents, more calories are needed at older ages. For adults, fewer calories are needed at older ages.

d. Estimates for females do not include women who are pregnant or breastfeeding.

Source: Reproduced from the Dietary Guidelines for Americans, 2010. Courtesy of the U.S. Department of Health & Human Services.

Box 9.1 Why Americans Are Fat: Another Point of View

Science journalist Gary Taubes has written a provocative book *Why We Get Fat: And What to Do About It.* He does not accept conventional wisdom. His basic thesis is that:

- The calories-in/calories-out model is wrong.
- Carbohydrates are *the* cause of obesity and are also important causes of heart disease, type 2 diabetes, cancer, Alzheimer's, and most of the so-called diseases of civilization.
- A low-fat diet is not healthy.
- A low-carb diet is essential both for weight loss and for health.
- Dieters can satisfy their hunger pangs and eat as much as they want and still lose weight as long as they restrict carbohydrates.

Mr. Taubes supports his thesis with data from the scientific literature and with persuasive arguments about insulin, blood sugar levels, glycemic index, insulin resistance, fat storage, inflammation, the metabolic syndrome, and other details of metabolism. Many readers will come away convinced that all we need to do to eliminate obesity, heart disease, and many other diseases is to get people to limit carbohydrates in their diet.

Rather than jumping on the low-carb bandwagon before his ideas are properly tested, the precautionary principle suggests that it might be more reasonable to follow a moderate diet like the Mediterranean diet, to limit "empty calories" from simple carbohydrates like sugar, to eat a variety of vegetables and fruits, to choose low-calorie density foods that are more filling, to limit meat intake, and to limit salt.

What's Wrong with Low-Carb Diets

The most extreme low-carb diet was pioneered by the late Robert Atkins, M.D. It promised a quick and long-lasting weight loss and prevention of chronic disease, all while allowing high-fat steak and bacon. Since then, other, more moderate low-carb diets have allowed small amounts of carbohydrate-rich foods, but they still cut out most grains as well as starchy vegetables and even fruit.

These diets have turned out to be less effective and less healthy than originally claimed. Often, the weight returned and as it did, problems such as high cholesterol and high blood pressure came back.

Low-carb diets usually begin with an "induction" phase that eliminates nearly every source of carbohydrate. Often, you'll consume as few as 20 grams of carbohydrate a day.

When carbohydrate consumption falls below 100 grams, the body usually responds by burning muscle tissue for the glycogen (stored glucose) it contains. When those glycogen stores start to run out, the body resorts to burning body fat. But that is an inefficient, complicated way to produce blood sugar. The body tries to do it only when it absolutely has to (such as when it's starving)—and for a good reason. Turning fat into blood sugar comes at a price in the form of by-products called ketones. They make your breath smell funny. They can also make you tired, lightheaded, headachy, and nauseated. Feeling lousy is certainly one way to dampen the appetite.

With virtually no carbs in your system, you may even have trouble concentrating. According to the Institute of Medicine of the National Academy of Sciences, the human brain requires the equivalent of 130 grams of carbohydrate a day to function optimally—and that is a minimum.

Box 9.1	Why Americans Are Fat: Another Point of View, *continued*

If you are overweight or obese and you have insulin resistance—and especially if you have prediabetes or diabetes—cutting way back on carbohydrates can have immediate health benefits. Your blood sugar and insulin levels will go down, your triglycerides and blood pressure may fall, and your levels of "good" HDL cholesterol may rise.

But the low-carb diet will also wreak some havoc. When your body breaks down lean body mass—muscle—for energy, your metabolism slows because muscle tissue burns up a lot of calories. This may be one reason that the weight often comes back after you have been avoiding carbs for a while.

The alleged effects on your heart are also questionable. Especially if you switch to a high-saturated-fat diet, as people do when they start eating mainly steak and bacon, your "bad" LDL cholesterol will go up. Levels of homocysteine, an amino acid that increases the risk of heart disease, may also rise if you eat a lot of meat and too few vegetables. And to get rid of the ketones produced when your body burns fat for energy, your kidneys need to work overtime, which raises your risk for kidney stones.

Ironically, low-carb diets may even interfere with insulin sensitivity; a certain amount of carbohydrate in your diet may be needed for the pancreas, which produces the insulin that keeps blood sugar in check, to work well.

such as salads and whole fruits. Fat isn't necessarily the problem; in fact, the fat content of our diet has actually gone down in the past 25 years. But many low-fat foods are very high in calories because they contain large amounts of sugar to improve their taste and palatability. In fact, many low-fat foods are actually higher in calories than foods that are not low fat.

Calories Expended

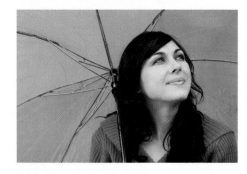

Our bodies need calories for functions such as breathing, digestion, and daily activities. Weight gain occurs when calories consumed exceed this need. For example, to lose 1 pound, you must decrease caloric intake by 3500 calories and maintain the same amount of activity, or increase physical activity so that it burns 3500 calories. Physical activity plays a key role in energy balance because it uses up calories consumed. See page 199 for why exercise is important in losing weight.

Despite all the benefits of being physically active, most Americans are sedentary. Technology has created many time- and labor-saving products. Some examples include cars, elevators, computers, dishwashers, and televisions. Cars are used to run short-distance errands instead of walking or riding a bicycle. As a result, these recent lifestyle changes have reduced the overall amount of energy expended in our daily lives, in recent years 25% of adults reported no leisure-time physical activity.

The belief that physical activity is limited to exercise or sports may keep people from being active. Another myth is that physical activity must be vigorous to achieve health benefits. Physical activity is any bodily movement that results in an expenditure of energy. Moderate-intensity activities such as household chores, gardening, and walking can also provide health benefits.

Portion Distortion

As portions have grown larger over the past 40 years, so have North Americans. Studies show that the more food put in front of people, the more they eat.

Since the 1960s, the serving sizes of foods sold in stores and restaurants—from candy bars to burgers and soda—have become much bigger. For example, bagels used to be 2 to 3 ounces (about 200 calories); today they are 5 to 6 ounces (more than 400 calories, depending on the type and equivalent to five pieces of bread).

"Super-size" portions are partially to blame for Americans' overweight explosion. It could also be that many people are innocently overeating. Nutritionists observe that most Americans overestimate how much food makes up a serving size.

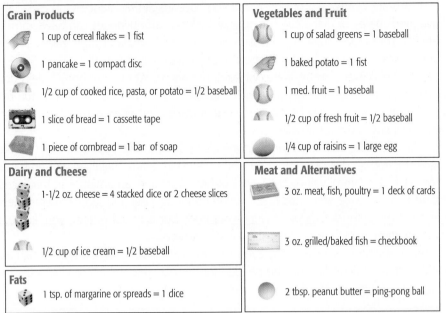

1 Serving Looks Like . . .

Grain Products
- 1 cup of cereal flakes = 1 fist
- 1 pancake = 1 compact disc
- 1/2 cup of cooked rice, pasta, or potato = 1/2 baseball
- 1 slice of bread = 1 cassette tape
- 1 piece of cornbread = 1 bar of soap

Vegetables and Fruit
- 1 cup of salad greens = 1 baseball
- 1 baked potato = 1 fist
- 1 med. fruit = 1 baseball
- 1/2 cup of fresh fruit = 1/2 baseball
- 1/4 cup of raisins = 1 large egg

Dairy and Cheese
- 1-1/2 oz. cheese = 4 stacked dice or 2 cheese slices
- 1/2 cup of ice cream = 1/2 baseball

Meat and Alternatives
- 3 oz. meat, fish, poultry = 1 deck of cards
- 3 oz. grilled/baked fish = checkbook
- 2 tbsp. peanut butter = ping-pong ball

Fats
- 1 tsp. of margarine or spreads = 1 dice

Source: Department of Health and Human Services/National Institutes of Health, 2005.

A "portion" is the amount of a specific food you **choose** to eat for a meal or snack. Portions can be bigger or smaller than the recommended food servings.

A "serving" is a unit of measure used to describe the amount of food **recommended** from each food group. It is the amount of food listed on the Nutrition Facts panel on packaged food or the amount of food recommended in the *Dietary Guidelines for Americans.*

Healthy eating plans use certain numbers of servings of fruits, vegetables, carbohydrates, etc. But exactly how much is a serving of broccoli or a serving of cheese?

Estimating serving sizes is easier than you think—just use a familiar object for a reference. At **http://hp2010.nhlbihin.net/portion /servingcard7.pdf** you can download a Serving Size card shown here to help you recall what a standard food serving looks like. Print and cut out the card and laminate it for longtime use.

Rather than cutting carbs, fats, or proteins, using the familiar objects helps you become aware of how much you are eating. For example, a 3-ounce serving of meat is the size of a deck of cards.

There is no need to go hungry; you can increase the portions of some foods such as fruits and vegetables. You can eat lots of broccoli, green beans, deep-green lettuce, apples, and strawberries without eating too many additional calories. Besides, most people do not eat enough fruits and vegetables to meet the dietary guidelines.

Figure 9.4

Portion distortion. (*Source:* Courtesy of the U.S. Department of Health & Human Services/National Institutes of Health.)

Socioeconomic, Age, and Gender Factors

- **Age:** Fatness increases during adulthood and declines in the elderly.
- **Gender:** Obesity is more prevalent in women than men.
- **Culture:** People in developed countries have more body fat than those in developing societies.
- **Race/ethnicity:** Obesity is more prevalent in African-American, Hispanic, Native American, and Pacific Islander people.
- **Income:** Obesity is more prevalent in lower-income women.
- **Education:** Less-educated women have a higher incidence of obesity.

Medical News You Can Use

Half of Americans Projected to Be Obese in 2030

If the current "obesity epidemic" continues unchecked, 50% of the US adult population will be obese—with body mass index values of 30 or higher—by 2030.

Researchers projected that, as a result of the burgeoning obese population, the United States will see the following health impacts:

- 6 to 8.5 million more people with diabetes
- 5.7 to 7.3 million more cases of heart disease and stroke
- 490,000 to 670,000 additional cancers
- 26 to 55 million quality-adjusted life-years lost

The economic burden of these increasing morbidities will be substantial.

The researchers also calculated what would happen if everyone's BMI was 1% lower—about 2 lb (1 kg) in an average adult. In the United States, more than 2 million cases of diabetes, about 1.5 million cardiovascular disease diagnoses, and about 100,000 cancers would be avoided.

Source: Wang Y, et.al. Health and economic burden of the projected obesity trends in the USA and the UK. *Lancet* 2011; 378:815–825.

- Employment: Unemployed women have a higher incidence of obesity.
- Marriage: Married men have a higher incidence of obesity.
- Residence: Rural women have a higher incidence of obesity.
- Region: People living in the Southern states have a higher incidence of obesity.

Psychological Factors

- Weight cycling: This is a pattern of losing and regaining weight, over and over again (yo-yo dieting). Experts believe that despite potential risks, any successful effort to lose pounds, even if temporary, can have potential benefits.
- Restrained eaters: This involves trying to reduce food intake by fasting or avoiding food as long as possible, usually by skipping meals or delaying eating. When emotionally stressed, the restrained eater overeats without realizing it.
- Binge eaters: This involves compulsive overeating, sometimes for days. Such behavior is common among people in weight-loss programs.

Determining Recommended Body Composition

Using weight as the primary determinant is not necessarily a good indicator of how healthy you are. What is important is the ratio of body fat to lean body mass in your body composition.

For instance, a female bodybuilder may weigh more than a standard chart says she should. But she may have only about 8% to 13% of her body weight in total fat. This is probably the least amount of body fat a woman can have and still be healthy.

What society deems as a desirable or ideal body differs in different time periods, usually depending on trends in fashion. It used to be—and still is in some cultures—that women with a good bit of nonessential fat were considered physically attractive and sexually desirable. Today the skinny fashion-model body type is "in" Figure 9.5 .

Methods exist for determining body composition by using both weight and body fat.

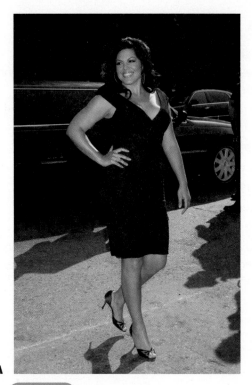
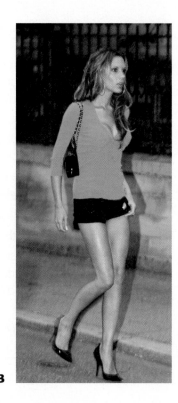

A   B

Figure 9.5

Voluptuous women were once considered the female ideal **(A)**; in today's society Victoria Beckham embodies a popular standard **(B)**.

Assessing Body Composition Using Weight

You can assess your body composition by comparing yourself to a weight-to-height table or by measuring your body mass index.

- Use a scale to measure your weight.
- Use a tape measure to measure your height.

Height–Weight Tables

Many versions of height–weight tables are available, all with different weight ranges. Some tables take into account a person's frame size and age; others do not.

Body composition measured on a table does not show the proportion of body fat to lean muscle mass. Athletes may be overweight as measured by the table, but not unhealthy.

Height–weight tables may serve as an excellent way for doctors to make sure babies are growing normally, but are not generally useful for adults as a measure of personal health. The use of the height–weight table is not recommended.

Body Mass Index

The body mass index (BMI), based on an individual's height and weight (see **Table 9.2**), is a simple estimate of body composition (see **Lab 9-1**, Activity 3). A BMI number is *not* a certain percentage of body fat.

The BMI determines whether a person's weight falls within a healthy range. You can look up your BMI in Table 9.2, or use an Internet calculator at http://nhlbisupport.com/bmi, or you can calculate your BMI by following these four steps:

1. Measure your height in inches (without shoes) and your weight in pounds (without clothing).

What's the word...

body mass index (BMI)

1. Measure your height in inches (without shoes) and your weight in pounds (without clothing).
2. Multiply your weight by 703.
3. Divide that number by your height.
4. Divide again by your height.

Table 9.2 Body Mass Index Table

Height (inches)	Normal						Overweight					Obese										Extreme Obesity														
BMI	19	20	21	22	23	24	25	26	27	28	29	30	31	32	33	34	35	36	37	38	39	40	41	42	43	44	45	46	47	48	49	50	51	52	53	54
																Body Weight (pounds)																				
58	91	96	100	105	110	115	119	124	129	134	138	143	148	153	158	162	167	172	177	181	186	191	196	201	205	210	215	220	224	229	234	239	244	248	253	258
59	94	99	104	109	114	119	124	128	133	138	143	148	153	158	163	168	173	178	183	188	193	198	203	208	212	217	222	227	232	237	242	247	252	257	262	267
60	97	102	107	112	118	123	128	133	138	143	148	153	158	163	168	174	179	184	189	194	199	204	209	215	220	225	230	235	240	245	250	255	261	266	271	276
61	100	106	111	116	122	127	132	137	143	148	153	158	164	169	174	180	185	190	195	201	206	211	217	222	227	232	238	243	248	254	259	264	269	275	280	285
62	104	109	115	120	126	131	136	142	147	153	158	164	169	175	180	186	191	196	202	207	213	218	224	229	235	240	246	251	256	262	267	273	278	284	289	295
63	107	113	118	124	130	135	141	146	152	158	163	169	175	180	186	191	197	203	208	214	220	225	231	237	242	248	254	259	265	270	278	282	287	293	299	304
64	110	116	122	128	134	140	145	151	157	163	169	174	180	186	192	197	204	209	215	221	227	232	238	244	250	256	262	267	273	279	285	291	296	302	308	314
65	114	120	126	132	138	144	150	156	162	168	174	180	186	192	198	204	210	216	222	228	234	240	246	252	258	264	270	276	282	288	294	300	306	312	318	324
66	118	124	130	136	142	148	155	161	167	173	179	186	192	198	204	210	216	223	229	235	241	247	253	260	266	272	278	284	291	297	303	309	315	322	328	334
67	121	127	134	140	146	153	159	166	172	178	185	191	198	204	211	217	223	230	236	242	249	255	261	268	274	280	287	293	299	306	312	319	325	331	338	344
68	125	131	138	144	151	158	164	171	177	184	190	197	203	210	216	223	230	236	243	249	256	262	269	276	282	289	295	302	308	315	322	328	335	341	348	354
69	128	135	142	149	155	162	169	176	182	189	196	203	209	216	223	230	236	243	250	257	263	270	277	284	291	297	304	311	318	324	331	338	345	351	358	365
70	132	139	146	153	160	167	174	181	188	195	202	209	216	222	229	236	243	250	257	264	271	278	285	292	299	306	313	320	327	334	341	348	355	362	369	376
71	136	143	150	157	165	172	179	186	193	200	208	215	222	229	236	243	250	257	265	272	279	286	293	301	308	315	322	329	338	343	351	358	365	372	379	386
72	140	147	154	162	169	177	184	191	199	206	213	221	228	235	242	250	258	265	272	279	287	294	302	309	316	324	333	338	346	353	361	368	375	383	390	397
73	144	151	159	166	174	182	189	197	204	212	219	227	235	242	250	257	265	272	280	288	295	302	310	318	325	333	340	348	355	363	371	378	386	393	401	408
74	148	155	163	171	179	186	194	202	210	218	225	233	241	249	256	264	272	280	287	295	303	311	319	326	334	342	350	358	365	373	381	389	396	404	412	420
75	152	160	168	176	184	192	200	208	216	224	232	240	248	256	264	272	279	287	295	303	311	319	327	335	343	351	359	367	375	383	391	399	407	415	423	431
76	156	164	172	180	189	197	205	213	221	230	238	246	254	263	271	279	287	295	304	312	320	328	336	344	353	361	369	377	385	394	402	410	418	426	435	443

Source: Courtesy of the National Heart, Lung, and Blood Institute.

2. Multiply your weight by 703.
3. Divide that number by your height.
4. Divide again by your height.

What Does BMI Mean?

You can interpret BMI values for adults with one fixed number, regardless of age or gender, using the guidelines in Table 9.3 . The BMI range associated with the lowest rate of illness and death is about 19–25 in men and 18–25 in women, so people with BMIs in this healthiest range are considered to be of normal weight. Higher BMIs are associated with higher rates of illness and death (see Figure 9.6). People with BMIs of 25–30 are considered overweight, and those with BMIs of 30 or higher are considered to have obesity. Obesity has been further subdivided into mild (BMI of 30–35), moderate (35–40), and severe (BMI of 40 and above).

People with a BMI lower than 18 are considered underweight. Underweight people also have higher death rates than people of normal weight do, but many people in this category are underweight because they already have a severe illness, such as cancer, chronic infections, or anorexia.

Table 9.3	Classification of BMI Values
BMI	**Classification**
Less than 18.5	Underweight
18.5–24.9	Normal
25–29.9	Overweight
30–34.9	Mildly Obese
35.0–39.9	Moderately Obese
40 or greater	Severely Obese

A problem with using BMI for body composition is that any weight loss or gain is difficult to interpret. The BMI does not differentiate fat weight from muscle weight. Examples of this occur in football players and bodybuilders with a large muscle mass and who also have a BMI greater than 30 but are not overfat.

Using the BMI alone leads to two forms of misclassification: (1) judging highly muscular individuals with a high BMI as being "overfat" when they are not. The disease risk faced by these individuals is significantly lower than BMI would indicate. (2) The BMI can fail to identify people at increased risk who are in the "healthy" BMI zone but have an elevated body fat content.

BMI measurements should be used cautiously for people who are petite, have large body frames, or are highly muscular.

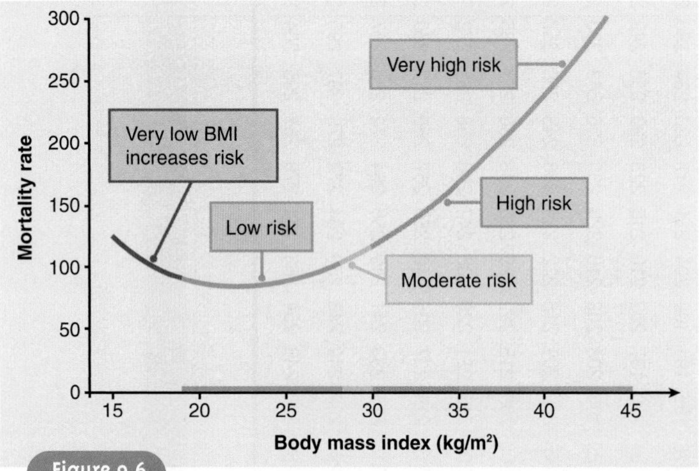

Figure 9.6

BMI and mortality.

Assessing Body Fatness

A certain amount of fat is essential to bodily functions. Fat regulates body temperature, cushions and insulates organs and tissues, and is the main form of the body's energy storage.

Your body fat percentage is simply the percentage of fat your body contains. If you are 150 pounds and 10% fat, it means that your body consists of 15 pounds fat and 135 pounds lean body mass (bone, muscle, organ tissue, blood, and everything else).

If you look around the Internet, you will see a lot of different recommendations for body fat percentages. However, a study (Gallagher et al., 2000) converted BMI

Table 9.4	Body Fat Ranges for Adults			
Adult Females				
Age	Increased Risk	Healthy	Increased Risk	Greatly Increased Risk
20–39	Less than 21%	21% to 32%	33% to 38%	Over 39%
40–59	Less than 23%	23% to 33%	34% to 39%	Over 40%
60–79	Less than 24%	24% to 35%	36% to 41%	Over 42%
Adult Males				
Age	Increased Risk	Healthy	Increased Risk	Greatly Increased Risk
20–39	Less than 8%	8% to 19%	20% to 24%	Over 25%
40–59	Less than 11%	11% to 21%	22% to 27%	Over 28%
60–79	Less than 13%	13% to 24%	24% to 29%	Over 30%

Source: Adapted from Gallagher D. G., et al. Healthy percentage body fat ranges: an approach for developing guidelines based on body mass index. *American Journal of Clinical Nutrition* 2000; 72(3):694–701.

guidelines established by the NIH and the World Health Organization into body fat percentages in adults (see   Table 9.4). These are the best available recommended body fat percentages.

Body fatness can be estimated by several methods, with each having some disadvantages.

Skinfold Measurements

Because half of your body's fat is located under your skin, you can estimate your percentage of body fat by measuring skinfold thickness (see   Lab 9-1 , Activity 5). This requires some skill. A technician or health professional uses calipers, a measuring instrument, to gauge the thickness of a fold of skin on the body at several different sites (e.g., upper arm, waist, and thigh). The keys for accuracy are locating the specific sites and then applying the calipers correctly.

The measurements are entered into a formula to produce an estimate of body fat percentage, or you can simply look up the total sum for the three skinfold sites (upper arm, waist, thigh) in the Lab Manual's table for men or for women.

This method gives a reasonable estimate, but the results often vary when different people take the measurements, making this test not very reliable. Another potential problem may be that the person feels a lack of privacy if certain body areas are pinched.

Bioelectrical Impedance

This test uses a small, harmless, electrical current to measure the electrical resistance of the body. Electrodes are attached to the wrist and ankle, and a small electrical impulse is sent through the body.

It is based on the principle that current flows more easily and faster through the parts of the body composed mostly of water (blood, urine, and muscle) than it does through bone, fat, or air. Special "body fat" scales that use this principle in combination with the height and weight can calculate a body's fat percentage. Results can vary with the amount of water in the body and are considered unreliable in people with obesity. This method is more costly than the skinfold method.

Bioelectrical impedance

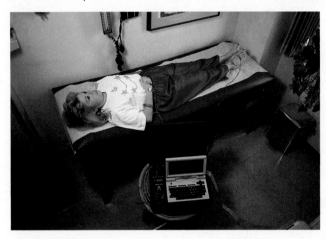

Procedure

1. You stand with bare feet on a device resembling a conventional bathroom scale with two built-in footpad electrodes.

   OR

   You lie on a cot and spot electrodes are placed on your hands and bare feet and connected to a bioelectrical impedance machine.
2. A built-in computer measures your bioelectrical impedance and then uses this number and your gender, height, fitness level, weight, and in some cases your age to assess your percentage of body fat.

Caution

- You need to be adequately hydrated.
- If you are dehydrated, the amount of fat will likely be underestimated.
- People with pacemakers are not candidates for this method.

Disadvantages

- Tends to overestimate your body fat if you are lean and athletic, unless the machine is equipped with an "athlete" mode.
- Does not take into account the location of body fat.

Hydrostatic (Underwater) Weighing

Hydrostatic (underwater) weighing is another method to measure body fat percentage.

This test, based on the principle that fat tissue is less dense than muscle and bone, uses a special bathtub-sized tank to weigh a person underwater. That weight is then compared to the person's weight on land; a formula identifies the percentage of body fat that would account for the difference. Underwater weighing is considered the most accurate method, but it is generally available only at universities and research facilities.

Procedure

1. You are weighed while suspended on a trapeze in the air.
2. You are then seated on a special scale and totally submerged in a pool or tank.
3. You exhale as much air as possible and remain motionless as your weight is recorded.
4. The procedure is repeated two to five times to get a dependable weight number.
- Because fat floats, an overweight person will weigh less underwater than a lean person of the same body weight.
- Your percentage of body fat is calculated from equations based on density of body composition.

Disadvantages

- Underwater weighing requires expensive equipment.
- The procedure requires a well-trained technician.

- The calculation of body fat percentage is based on studies of young Caucasians. The formula may not fit all cases.
- Some people feel uncomfortable when they are fully submerged, leading to incorrect readings.
- There is always air left in the lungs. It is difficult to accurately correct for this.
- This method does not take into account the location of body fat.

Densitometry (Air Displacement)

Air displacement is more practical to use as a measure of body fat than water displacement. A new device, the Bod Pod, allows an individual to sit in a sealed chamber of known volume and displace a certain volume of air.

Body Fat Distribution

It is not only how much fat an individual has, but where the fat is on the body that affects a person's health (Figure 9.7). Women usually collect fat in their hips and buttocks, giving their figures a "pear" shape. Men typically build up fat around their bellies, giving them more of an "apple" shape. This is not a hard-and-fast rule. Some men are pear shaped and some women become apple shaped, especially after menopause. Most people have a combination of both characteristics. It's healthier not to develop a beer belly. If you carry fat mainly around the middle ("apple-shaped"), you are more likely to develop diabetes and related health problems than if you tend to be heavier around your hips and thighs ("pear-shaped").

Underwater weighing

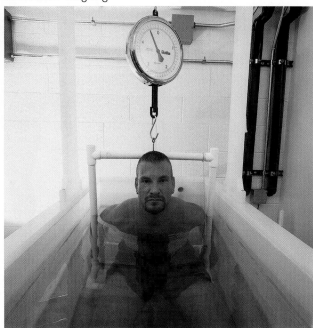

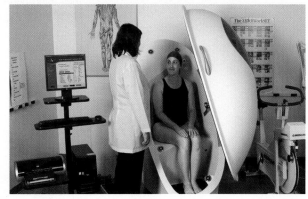

Bod Pod

Waist-to-Hip Ratio

Your waist-to-hip ratio (WHR) tells you where you store body fat (Figure 9.8) and (Lab 9-1), Activity 2.

WHR = Waist Circumference (inches) ÷ Hip Circumference (inches)
Standard WHRs for:
- Men should be less than 0.95
- Women should be no more than 0.8

Ratios greater than these indicate a tendency toward central (torso) obesity. People who store excess fat centrally, as opposed to in their extremities, are at an increased risk for cardiorespiratory diseases and diabetes.

Waist Circumference

Some experts believe that measuring your waist is as good as the WHR and is easier to do.
- See (Lab 9-1), Activity 1 for detailed instructions on how to measure your waist circumference.
- Note that if an individual is less than 5 feet in height or has a BMI of 35 or greater, waist circumference standards used for the general population may not apply.

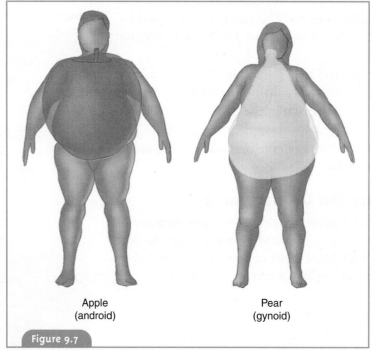

Apple
(android)

Pear
(gynoid)

Figure 9.7

Differences in body fat distribution. Men tend to carry excess fat around their abdomen ("apple" shape). Women tend to accumulate excess fat in their hips, buttocks, and thighs ("pear" shape).

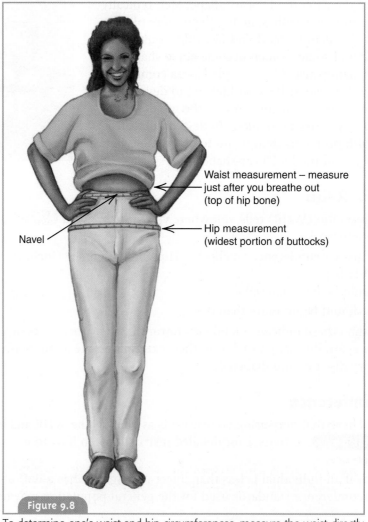

Waist measurement – measure just after you breathe out (top of hip bone)

Hip measurement (widest portion of buttocks)

Navel

Figure 9.8

To determine one's waist and hip circumferences, measure the waist directly above the hip bone; measure the hips at the widest point of the buttocks.

Waist-to-Height Ratio (WHtR)

Recent research shows that the waist-to-height ratio (WHtR) is a much better measure than BMI, waist-to-hip ratio, and waist circumference for assessing obesity, cardiovascular risk, and other health risks associated with excess body fat. Despite the superiority of WHtR, however, the other measures should all be combined for a better predictor of cardiovascular disease (**Figure 9.9**).

Many male and female athletes, who often have a higher percentage of muscle and a lower percentage of body fat, have relatively high BMIs, but their WHTRs are within a healthy range. This also holds true for women who have a "pear" rather than an "apple" shape. A general suggestion is that regardless of your weight, age, or gender, maintaining a waist circumference that is less than half of your height is an easy way to reduce your risk for cardiovascular disease.

The WHtR is calculated by dividing waist size by height, and takes gender into account (see **Lab 9-1** , Activity 4). For example, a male with a 32-inch waist who is 5'10" (70 inches) would divide 32 by 70 to get a WHtR of 45.7%.

The following chart (see **Table 9.5**) helps determine if your WHtR falls in a healthy range (the ratios are percentages).

Importance of Regular Assessment of Body Composition

As most people age, they lose lean body mass and gain body fat.

From about the age of 25 years until 65 years, most people gain about 40 pounds. They also lose about 20 pounds of lean tissue mass.

That means they have actually gained 60 pounds of fat!

It is important, especially if you are undertaking a weight-loss program of diet and exercise, to reassess and record your body composition about once a month **Lab 9-3** .

Combine exercise with dieting, because, as stated earlier, dieting alone can cost you lean body mass. This is not a healthy change in your body composition.

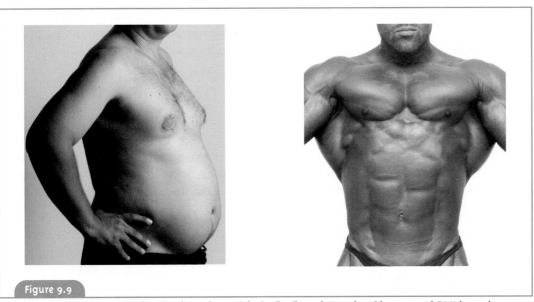

Figure 9.9

BMI does not take into consideration how the weight is distributed. People with a normal BMI but a large waist circumference and with a WHtR of over 0.55 have a 20% higher mortality risk than persons with a normal waist size.

Table 9.5	Waist-to-Height Ratio
Women (the ratios are percentages)	
Ratio less than 35	Abnormally underweight to underweight
Ratio 35 to 42	Underweight
Ratio 42 to 46	Slightly underweight to healthy
Ratio 46 to 49	Healthy
Ratio 49 to 54	Overweight
Ratio 54 to 58	Seriously overweight
Ratio over 58	Highly obese
Men (the ratios are percentages)	
Ratio less than 35	Extremely underweight to underweight
Ratio 35 to 43	Underweight
Ratio 43 to 46	Slightly underweight to healthy
Ratio 46 to 53	Healthy
Ratio 53 to 58	Overweight
Ratio 58 to 63	Extremely overweight to obese
Ratio over 63	Highly obese

You will be surprised to find that, as a result of the exercise, you have gained more lean mass and lost body fat. If you lost 4 pounds, you may have gained 4 pounds of lean mass, meaning you lost 8 pounds of fat! Isn't that pretty encouraging?

Health Risks of Overweight and Obesity

Obesity

More than 60% of adults in the United States are either overweight or obese (NCHS, 2004). The obesity epidemic covered on television and in newspapers did not occur overnight, of course. Obesity and overweight are chronic conditions. Indeed, a variety of factors play a role in obesity.

Health Risks of Too Much Body Fat

The main concern about overweight and obesity is one of health and not appearance. Too much storage fat is unhealthy.

Obese people are at a higher risk for diabetes, heart disease, stroke, high blood pressure, and premature death. They are also prone to gallbladder disease, arthritis, varicose veins, and shortness of breath   Table 9.6 .

Table 9.6	Health Risks Associated with Obesity
Obesity is associated with an increased risk of:	
▪ Premature death ▪ Type 2 diabetes ▪ Heart disease ▪ Stroke ▪ Hypertension ▪ Gallbladder disease ▪ Osteoarthritis (degeneration of cartilage and bone in joints) ▪ Sleep apnea ▪ Asthma ▪ Breathing problems ▪ Cancer (endometrial, colon, kidney, gallbladder, and postmenopausal breast cancer)	▪ High blood cholesterol ▪ Complications of pregnancy ▪ Menstrual irregularities ▪ Hirsutism (presence of excess body and facial hair) ▪ Stress incontinence (urine leakage caused by weak pelvic-floor muscles) ▪ Increased surgical risk ▪ Psychological disorders, such as depression ▪ Psychological difficulties due to social stigmatization

Source: Modified from Pollock M. L., Schmidt D. H., and Jackson A. S. Measurement of cardio-respiratory fitness and body composition in the clinical setting. *Comprehensive Therapy* 1980; 6(9):12–27. Reprinted with kind permission of Springer Science and Business Media.

Premature Death

Because excess weight plays a role in so many common and deadly diseases, overweight and obesity can cut years off your life. Severe obesity can lower life expectancy by an estimated 5 to 20 years.

Heart Disease

- Heart disease (heart attack, congestive heart failure, sudden cardiac death, chest pain, and abnormal heart rhythm) is increased in those who are overweight or obese.
- Obesity is associated with elevated triglycerides (blood fat) and decreased HDL (good) cholesterol.
- High blood pressure is about six times more common in obese people than those who are lean.

Diabetes

- More than 80% of people with type 2 diabetes are overweight or obese.
- A weight gain of 11 to 18 pounds increases a person's risk of developing type 2 diabetes to twice that of individuals who have not gained weight.

Cancer

- Overweight and obesity are associated with an increased risk for some types of cancer, including endometrial (cancer of the lining of the uterus), colon, gallbladder, prostate, kidney, and postmenopausal breast cancer.
- Women gaining more than 20 pounds from age 18 to midlife double their risk of postmenopausal breast cancer.

Breathing Problems

- Sleep apnea (interrupted breathing while sleeping) is more common in obese persons.
- Obesity is associated with a higher prevalence of asthma.

Medical News You Can Use

Using a Tape Measure to Predict Your Heart Attack Risk

Abdominal fat is a strong risk factor for heart attacks. Waist size may even be more important than body mass index in predicting heart disease. Measuring hip size to the equation may make the prediction even more accurate. In a study that examined 27,000 people from 52 countries, as waist circumference increased, so did the risk of heart attack. Men and women with the largest waist circumference had almost double the risk of heart attack than those with the smallest waist sizes. Measuring your waist-to-hip ratio is another way to estimate heart disease risk. A more even distribution of fat between the waist and hips is less risky than fat predominantly in the abdomen.

To determine your risk, measure your bare midriff just above the hipbones with a standard tape measure. The measurement should be taken right after exhaling normally. Your waist measurement should be below 40 inches if you are a man and below 35 inches if you are a woman. Because Asians have smaller builds, measurements should be below 37 inches and below 31 inches, respectively, for men and women. To find your waist-to-hip ratio, divide your waist measurement by the measurement of your hips at their widest point. Men with a ratio greater than 1.0 and women with a ratio greater than 0.8 are at greatest risk for heart disease.

Source: Data from *Weight and Waist Measurement: Tools for Adults.* National Institute of Diabetes and Digestive and Kidney Diseases (NIDDK), 2008. NIH Publication No. 04–5283.

Arthritis

For every 2-pound increase in weight, the risk of developing arthritis increases by 9% to 13%. However, symptoms of arthritis can improve with weight loss.

Additional Health Consequences

The Inside Track

Risk of chronic disease rises when:

- Body fat in adult women exceeds 30%
- Body fat in adult men exceeds 25%

- Overweight and obesity are associated with increased risks of gallbladder disease, incontinence, surgical complications, and depression.
- Obesity can affect the quality of life through limited mobility and decreased physical endurance, as well as through social, academic, and job discrimination.
- Obesity in premenopausal women is associated with irregular menstrual cycles and infertility.

Pregnancy and Childbirth

- Obesity during pregnancy is associated with increased risk of death in both the baby and the mother, and a tenfold increase in the risk of maternal high blood pressure.
- Obese women are more likely to have gestational diabetes and problems with labor and delivery.
- Infants born to women who are obese during pregnancy are more likely to have a high birth weight and low blood sugar (associated with brain damage and seizures).
- Obesity during pregnancy is associated with increased risk of birth defects, particularly neural tube defects such as spina bifida.

Children and Adolescents

- The Centers for Disease Control and Prevention estimates that 16% of all children 6 to 19 years old are overweight. That is a 45% increase in the last 10 years.

- Risk factors for heart disease, such as high cholesterol and high blood pressure, occur with increased frequency in overweight children and adolescents compared to those with a healthy weight.

- The incidence of type 2 diabetes (non-insulin-dependent), previously considered an adult disease, has increased dramatically in children and adolescents. Overweight and obesity are closely linked to type 2 diabetes.

- Overweight adolescents have a 70% chance of becoming overweight or obese adults. This risk increases to 80% if one or more parent is overweight or obese.

- Obese people are more likely to have accidents, because they can't move easily.

- Obese people are socially and occupationally stigmatized, and generally have lower self-esteem.

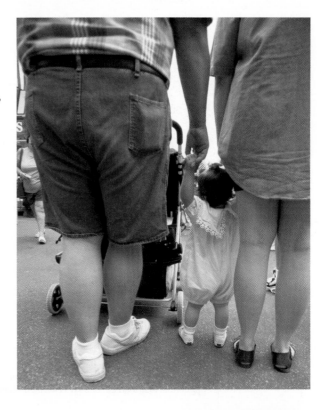

Weight Management

Overweight and obesity are common, serious, and costly. Weight-related conditions include heart disease, stroke, type 2 diabetes, and certain types of cancer—some of the leading causes of death.

Using measured heights and weights, an estimated 34.2% of US adults aged 20 years and over are overweight, 33.8% are obese, and 5.7% are extremely obese, as shown in Figure 9.10.

Obesity prevalence varies across states and regions. Percentages of obese adults range from 21% in Colorado to 34% in Mississippi. Twelve states had a prevalence of 30% or more. Figure 9.11 shows how the states' obesity rates compare with one another.

Losing weight permanently is difficult. Studies show that 95% of all dieters regain their lost weight and go on to add more pounds. However, lessons can be learned from those who have been successful. Their successes prove that anyone can lose weight.

A *Consumer Reports* (2002) survey of more than 32,000 dieters on long-term weight-loss maintenance found that ordinary people can be successful without using expensive commercial diet programs, special foods, dietary supplements, or drugs. Long-term weight loss is a result of lifetime healthful living.

Most successful long-term dieters chose walking, and a sizable number added weight lifting. They also consumed lean protein with judicious amounts of healthful fats.

Where to Begin?

- Complete the body composition assessments in Lab 9-1. Take your photo in tight-fitting clothes. Attach a date to it. Keep this on hand as motivation.

- Set a realistic weight-loss goal. Most experts say it is reasonable to lose half a pound to 2 pounds per week. Some people lose more; some lose less. You have to burn 3500 calories more than you consume to lose 1 pound.

Studies show that dieters lose about 10% of their starting weight in the first 3 to 6 months (ACSM, 2001; NHLBI, 1998). For those who weigh 200 pounds, that is about 20 pounds.

- Keep a food diary. Write down what you ate, how much you ate, when you ate, and whether you think you were overeating. Dieters who keep a daily food record usually lose more weight.

> **What's the word...**
>
> **weight management**
> The adoption of healthful and sustainable eating and exercise behaviors indicated for reduced disease risk and improved feelings of energy and well-being.

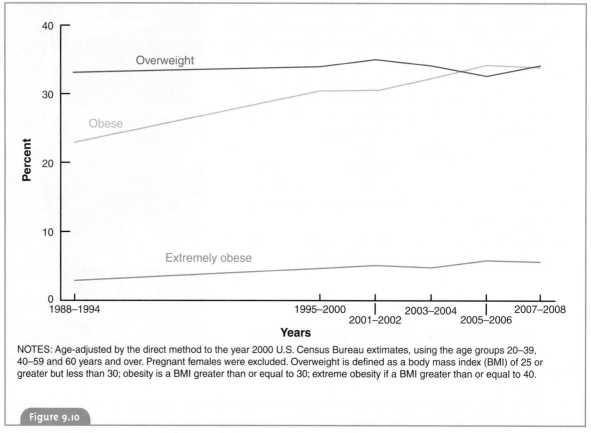

NOTES: Age-adjusted by the direct method to the year 2000 U.S. Census Bureau extimates, using the age groups 20–39, 40–59 and 60 years and over. Pregnant females were excluded. Overweight is defined as a body mass index (BMI) of 25 or greater but less than 30; obesity is a BMI greater than or equal to 30; extreme obesity if a BMI greater than or equal to 40.

Figure 9.10

Trends in overweight, obesity, and extreme obesity among adults aged 20–74 years: United States, 1960–2008. (*Source:* Reproduced from Ogden C.L. and Carroll M.D. *Prevalence of Overweight, Obesity, and Extreme Obesity Among Adults: United States, Trends 1960-1962 Through 2007-2008.* National Health and Nutrition Examination Survey, National Center for Health Statistics. 2007–2008. Courtesy of the Centers for Disease Control and Prevention.)

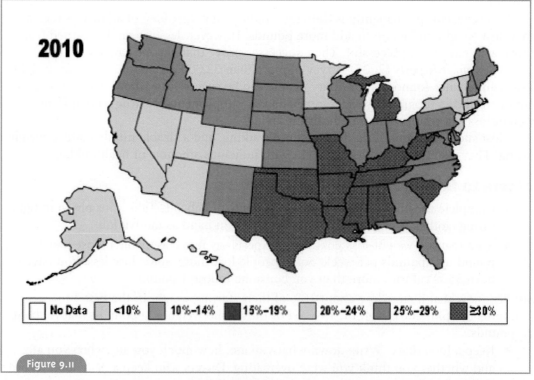

Figure 9.11

Prevalence of obesity (BMI > 30) among U.S. Adults. (*Source:* Reproduced from the Centers for Disease Control and Prevention.)

Exercise

If one person cuts back on calories without exercising and another person increases exercise without cutting back on calories, the first person would lose weight more quickly. That's because it's easier to cut 500 calories a day from your diet than it is to burn 500 extra calories through exercise.

If you only cut back on calories, you are more likely to regain the weight you lost. Why? The body reacts to weight loss as if it is starving and, in response, slows its metabolism. When your metabolism slows, you burn fewer calories—even at rest. When you burn fewer calories, several things can happen. If you continue eating fewer calories, you will either stop losing weight as quickly as you have been, or you will stop losing weight altogether. If you increase your calorie consumption, you may actually gain weight more quickly than you have in the past. The solution is to increase your physical activity because doing so will counteract the metabolic slowdown caused by reducing calories.

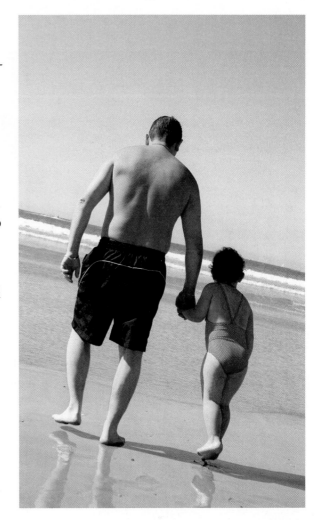

A regular schedule of exercise raises not only your energy expenditure while you are exercising but also your resting energy expenditure—that is, the rate at which you burn calories even when the workout is over and you are resting.

- Increasing exercise while eating the same number of calories is not very effective for losing weight in the short term. To lose even a small amount of weight just by exercising, you have to exercise a lot. For example, to burn 1 pound of fat, you have to briskly walk or run 35 miles.

- The National Academies' Institute of Medicine's activity guideline (2002) says that, although health benefits are achieved from 30 minutes of activities, it takes 1 hour or more to prevent weight gain. Sedentary individuals can meet this goal by using moderate-intensity activity (e.g., walking at 4 miles per hour) for a total of 60 minutes on most days of the week, or engaging in a high-intensity activity (e.g., jogging, running) for 20 to 30 minutes 4 to 7 days per week.

Medical News You Can Use

Calories Burn Long After Intense Workout

People who exercise vigorously get a bonus for their hard work: They continue to burn extra calories long after they are finished working out. Researchers found that men who biked intensely on a stationary bike for 45 minutes burned an extra 190 calories over the 14 hours after their workout. This is in addition to the calories they used while exercising. To get the extra calorie-burning benefits, the workout needs to be intense enough that you are sweating, your body temperature is up, and your heart beats fast. The results may also apply to women and to other high-intensity, sweat-producing activities such as running, jogging, and playing intense games of basketball and soccer.

Source: Data from Knab A. M., et al. A 45-minute vigorous exercise bout increases metabolic rate for 14 Hours. *Medicine and Science in Sports and Exercise* 2011; 43(9); 1643–1648.

9

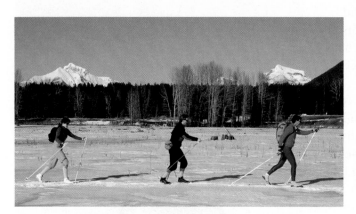
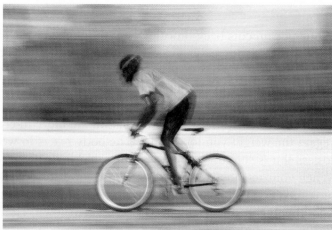

- While vigorous exercise uses calories at a higher rate, any physical activity burns calories. For example, a 140-pound person can burn 175 calories in 30 minutes of moderate bicycling, and 322 calories in 30 minutes of moderate jogging. The same person can also burn 105 calories by vacuuming or raking leaves for the same amount of time.

- Evidence clearly shows the need for activity in a weight-reduction program. Dieting can lead to weight loss, but the loss accompanies a greater loss of protein (lean tissue) and water. When lean tissue is lost, the body becomes less able to burn calories and more fat weight is eventually gained.

- Studies show that weight loss with exercise maximizes the removal of fat, minimizes the loss of protein, and helps maintain the metabolic rate. Dieting alone is seldom effective over the long term. Most weight-loss diets fail and the person has more weight and fat than before the dieting began.

Certain cautions should be taken by overweight and obese persons during exercising:

- For maximum benefit and minimum risk, choose low- to moderate-intensity activities.

- Ease into an exercise program. Increase the duration and frequency of exercise before increasing the intensity.

- Include strength training to build or maintain lean muscle.

Eat Fewer Calories

Your diet should be low in calories, but not too low (1,200 calories a day for women or 1,500 a day for men, except under the supervision of a health professional). Diets lower than 800 kcal/day have been found to be no more effective than low-calorie diets in producing weight loss. They can endanger your health by depriving you of necessary nutrients.

To lose weight, try to eat 300 to 500 fewer calories than you need and to exercise 30 to 60 minutes on most days of the week. This is a general guide to the number of calories you might want to consume if you are trying to lose 0.5 to 2 pounds per week.

How can you meet your daily calorie target? One approach is to add up the number of calories per serving of all the foods that you eat, and then plan your food intake accordingly. You can buy books or a smart phone app that list calories per serving for many foods. In addition, the nutrition labels on all packaged foods and beverages provide calories per serving information.

Some people focus on reducing the fat in their diet because, at nine calories per gram, fat by weight contains more than twice as many calories as carbohydrates or protein (four calories per gram). Don't be mistaken in believing that cutting fat always means cutting calories. Some fat-free foods actually contain more calories than the regular versions because manufacturers use extra sugar to make up for the flavor lost in removing the fat. Moreover, low-fat or nonfat foods are not low-calorie if you consume them in large quantities.

Cut Back on Simple Sugars (Carbohydrates)

The body's use of carbohydrates seems to be the key to weight mangement. Eating foods that make your blood sugar and insulin levels shoot up and then crash may contribute to weight gain. Such foods include white bread, white rice, other highly processed grain products, and potatoes. As an alternative, choose foods that have a gentler effect on blood sugar (refer to the discussion of glycemic load in Chapter 6 for more information). These include whole grains such as whole-grain breads and pasta, oats, as well as beans, nuts, fruits, and vegetables.

Eat Lean Protein

Eating lean protein includes reduced-fat dairy products, egg whites, fish, chicken, and lean cuts of beef and pork. Adding protein to the diet slows the absorption of food—blood sugar will rise more slowly. You will not be as hungry.

Eating more protein and fewer carbohydrates has become a popular dieting approach. The long-term effects of eating this way on weight and overall health need further study. Such a diet might cause kidney damage in some people and rob bones of calcium. Avoid protein containing saturated and trans fats.

Eat Fruits and Vegetables

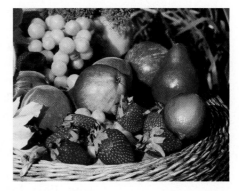

Fruits and vegetables are clearly an important part of a good diet. Almost everyone can benefit from eating more of them. They also provide fiber. Some experts recommend at least nine servings per day rather than the often-recommended five servings. Choose a variety that includes dark-green, leafy vegetables; yellow, orange, and red fruits and vegetables; cooked tomatoes; and citrus fruits. Try to avoid fruit drinks because they are high in calories.

Eat High-Fiber Grains and Legumes

This type of eating includes oatmeal, brown rice, whole-wheat bread, and lentils. You can trick your stomach into feeling full before you have eaten too many calories. Examples of foods with the lowest energy density include water-rich fruits and vegetables, whole grains, and lean meats.

Include Small Amounts of Healthful Fats

Examples of healthful fats are olive oil, avocadoes, nuts, olives, and fatty fish (e.g., salmon). Fat in a meal or in snacks such as nuts helps you feel full. Actually, eating certain healthful kinds of fats—mono- and polyunsaturated vegetable oils, nuts, and fish oil—seems to protect people against heart disease. Once again, avoid saturated and trans fats.

Eat Slowly—Enjoy Your Food

It takes about 20 minutes for your brain to "tell" you when you feel full. Until then, you continue to feel hungry and want to eat. If you eat quickly, you will end up consuming more than you need to feel full. But eating slowly gives your brain the time it needs to signal that you have had enough.

Other Strategies

Avoid overeating by using these tactics:

- Limit or avoid desserts—anything with simple sugars and/or refined carbohydrates, because they are all calories and not much nutrition.
- Eat smaller portions; use small plates and bowls.
- Keep a food log—know how many calories you are eating.
- Eat a healthy snack before mealtime to curb your appetite.
- Stop eating before you feel full; you do not have to eat everything.
- Keep tempting food out of sight.
- When eating out order a small-sized portion, share a meal, or take home part of the meal.
- Eat a nutrient-dense breakfast.

Weight-Loss Options to Avoid

Using a Diet Book

Be wary of diet books, especially those recommending a single food, such as grapefruit or cabbage, or an imbalance of foods. The problem with following a special diet of the kind usually found in popular diet books is that it is difficult to stay with it. Once you backslide, you regain weight, and that can be really discouraging.

It is better to permanently change the way you eat, with balance and good sense. That is the kind of diet you are most likely to stay with, and be happy about your success.

Diet Supplements

Diet supplements are the new snake oil. They promise the easy way out, but cannot guarantee success. In fact, they are sold as supplements precisely so that they can steer clear of government regulation, and some are unsafe.

Can you live the rest of your life on a diet drink? Not likely. To get a quick weight loss (mainly muscle mass), you are substituting a diet supplement for the range of nutrients you need and can get from a healthy, balanced diet.

There is no good shortcut to healthy and sustainable weight loss.

Medical Help

Not everyone needs to see a doctor to lose weight, but some might want to for two reasons. First, for professional guidance, if you have not been able to lose weight on your own by dieting and exercising. Second, to obtain a doctor's evaluation for health complications that might be associated with your excess weight.

Prescription Drugs

There are prescription drugs available that can help people lose weight. Only a few are approved by the Food and Drug Administration: either to suppress appetite, or to block fat absorption in the small intestines. However, they are not intended to be taken for a lifetime. You'll still need to learn a positive way to eat! Drugs should be used only as a part of a comprehensive program that includes behavior therapy, diet changes, and physical activity. Medical monitoring for side effects must be continued while using the drugs.

Other drugs, such as those that increase the metabolic rate, are not recommended and may even be unsafe: Some weight-loss drugs have been found to cause potentially fatal heart problems. Even if safe, it is not a good idea to depend on drugs alone. Proper diet and exercise are still the real answer.

Weight-loss drugs do not do the job by themselves. But for people whose health is at risk and who are struggling to reduce their weight through diet and exercise, drug therapy may increase the odds of success. Experts agree that weight-loss drugs, which all have side effects, are not for the mildly overweight or those who just want to lose a few pounds to improve their appearance.

Weight-loss drugs are not for everyone. If the person hasn't lost at least a pound a week in the first month on a weight-loss medication, he or she is unlikely to benefit from the drug.

Surgery

A growing number of people who find it impossible to change their eating and non-exercise habits have turned to surgery to change their bodies. The very obese who cannot control their appetites are often candidates. Due to the frequency and significance of complications, surgical approaches to weight control should be considered only as a last resort for the obese.

A popular but potentially risky procedure is gastric bypass (Figure 9.12). The stomach is divided into two parts, using staples, and one part is used as a small pouch for digesting food. The patient feels full after eating only a small amount and cannot eat more without getting sick.

A related surgical technique is resectioning the intestines so that only a small amount of food is digested.

A third method is liposuction, in which subcutaneous fat is suctioned away (Figure 9.12B). It is intended for body reshaping, not weight loss.

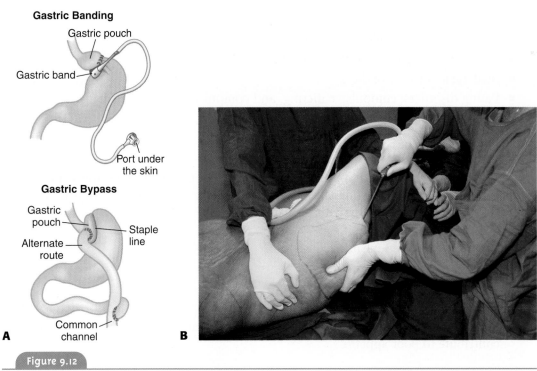

Figure 9.12

A. Gastric bypass surgery is a surgical procedure used to treat obesity. After surgery, the obese person experiences discomfort after overeating and is less likely to overeat. (*Source:* Reprinted with permission from Steinbrook R. Surgery for severe obesity. *New England Journal of Medicine* 2004; 350(11):1075–1079.) **B**. Liposuction has gained popularity in recent years.

9

Health Risks of Being Underweight

Dieting (or more simply, a change in your eating habits) should be combined with exercise to balance the intake and output of calories.

Another major reason to include exercise with dieting or controlled eating is to preserve and build lean body mass, essential for good health. Dieting alone to lose weight often results in unhealthy loss of lean body mass. Weight loss with exercise maximizes the removal of fat, minimizes the loss of protein, and helps maintain the metabolic rate.

It is easier to reduce caloric intake (refusing to eat a piece of cake with 250 calories) than it is to burn off the calories (jogging more than 2 miles at 110 calories per mile). Dieting alone uses deprivation to achieve weight loss, but with a greater loss of protein (lean tissue) and water. The body becomes less able to burn calories and more fat is eventually gained.

Dieting alone is seldom effective over the long term. Most weight-loss diets fail and the person ends up with more weight and fat than before dieting began.

Underweight

Underweight is not as common as overweight. When being underweight is part of one's genetic make-up, and diet and other health behaviors are fine, the health risk is not a problem.

If the cause is not hereditary, and underweight is the result of undernutrition, deficits in protein and other energy-producing nutrients can cause disorders such as fatigue, reproduction problems in women, and susceptibility to disease.

Causes of Underweight

- Hereditary and metabolic factors
- Prolonged psychological and emotional stress
- Addiction to alcohol and illicit drugs
- Inadequate or bizarre diets
- Eating disorders, compulsive dieting, and compulsive overexercising
- An underlying disease (e.g., cancer) (Insel, Turner, and Ross, 2006)

How to Gain Weight

Gaining weight can be difficult, but the basic concepts of energy balance apply. For example, to gain 1 pound, you must increase daily caloric intake by 3500 calories and maintain the same amount of activity.

- Eat small frequent meals.
- Eat snacks between meals.
- Eat high-calorie foods and drinks.
- Eat extra servings of nutritious carbohydrates.
- Exercise to increase muscle mass.
- Use a balanced vitamin/mineral supplement to ensure that a deficiency does not contribute to poor appetite.

Eating Disorders

Eating disorders are a severe psychological response to body image issues Figure 9.13 . They occur mainly among high-achievement–oriented girls and young women.

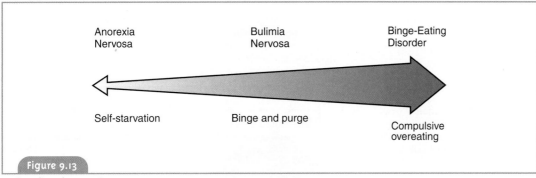

Figure 9.13

Eating disorder continuum.

Affected individuals see themselves as overweight even though they are not. Unusual eating habits develop: avoiding food and meals, and picking out a few foods and eating these in small quantities.

Anorexia Nervosa

Anorexia nervosa is an obsession for thinness manifested in self-imposed starvation. Those suffering from anorexia nervosa develop emaciated bodies. This condition can be fatal if left untreated. Also, about 25% of anorexics exercise compulsively to stay lean (Figure 9.14).

Related to anorexia is female athlete triad, an increasingly common condition among female athletes (Figure 9.15). The symptoms and results include amenorrhea and osteoporosis.

Bulimia

Bulimics engage in binge-eating episodes at least twice a week for three months, followed by behaviors that compensate for the binges, such as severe dieting, purging, or a combination of dieting and purging. The body weights of bulimics are close to or slightly above that considered healthy for their heights.

What's the word...

anorexia nervosa Extreme restriction of food intake.

female athlete triad Combination of eating disorders, amenorrhea, and osteoporosis.

amenorrhea Absence of normal menstruation.

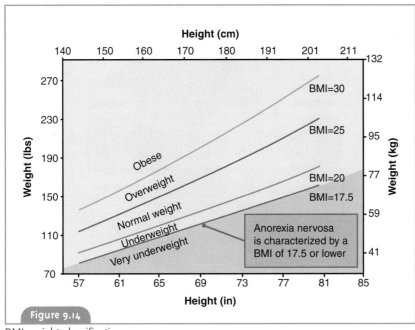

Figure 9.14

BMI weight classification.

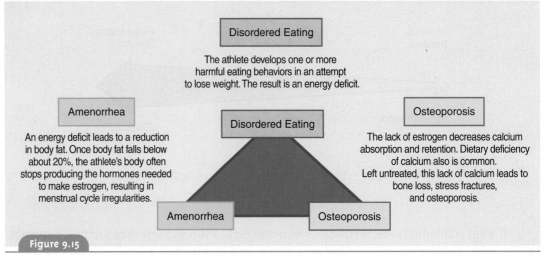

Figure 9.15
Red flags for female athlete triad.

Binge-Eating Disorder

Binge-eating disorder is the most common eating disorder seen in people of all ages and backgrounds. Like people with bulimia, those with binge-eating disorder consume significantly more food than is typically eaten in a given period of time. Not all binge-eaters are obese, although many obese people binge (**Figure 9.16**).

Treating Eating Disorders

Eating disorders (see **Table 9.7**), such as anorexia and bulimia, are very difficult to treat successfully. People with eating disorders deny them and are secretive about them. If you are a friend or family member who wants to help, here is where to start:

- Tell the person you are concerned about their weight loss.
- Encourage the person to discuss with you any problems or anxieties.

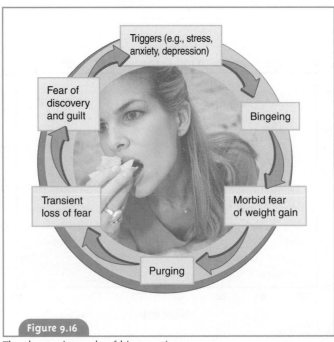

Figure 9.16
The destructive cycle of binge eating.

Table 9.7	Eating Disorders		
	Characteristics	**Related Health Issues**	**Treatment**
Anorexia	Intense fear of weight gain Strict dietary restriction Significant weight loss Possible excessive exercise	Slow the heart rate Lower blood pressure Increasing risk of heart failure Starvation Damage to the brain Hair and nails grow brittle Skin may dry out, become yellow Develop covering of soft hair Anemia Swollen joints Reduced muscle mass Light-headedness Brittle bones	Restoring weight lost Treating psychological disturbances such as distortion of body image, low self-esteem, and interpersonal conflicts Achieving long-term remission and rehabilitation
Bulimia	Intense fear of weight gain Consumption of large quantity of calories in single episode (binge) Consumption followed by elimination of food from body (purge) Guilt and shame associated with behavior	Acid in vomit can wear down the outer layer of the teeth Inflame and damage the glands near the cheeks Damage to the stomach Irregular heartbeat Heart failure Chemical imbalances Peptic ulcers Pancreatitis Long-term constipation	Reduce or eliminate binge-eating and purging behavior Nutritional rehabilitation Psychosocial intervention Establish a pattern of regular, non-binge meals Improvement of attitudes related to the eating disorder Encouragement of healthy exercise Resolution of mood or anxiety disorders
Binge eating	Frequent compulsive overeating No purge cycle Eating occurs whether hungry or full Guilt and shame associated with behavior	High blood pressure High cholesterol level Fatigue Joint pain Type 2 diabetes Gallbladder disease Heart disease	Similar to bulimia Research is under way to study the effectiveness of different interventions

Source: Modified from Pollock M.L., Schmidt D.H., and Jackson A.S. Measurement of cardio-respiratory fitness and body composition in the clinical setting. Comprehensive Therapy 1980; 6(9):12–27. Reprinted with kind permission of Springer Science and Business Media.

- Make no judgments.
- Urge the person to see a professional—counselor, doctor, or psychologist.
- Talk to a counselor to see if intervention is possible—and about your own feelings, if you are very distressed yourself over the situation.

Professional treatment for eating disorders is a must. Usually a combination of overall supervision by a physician, medication such as an antidepressant, and psychotherapy are required.

Reflect >>>> Reinforce >>>> Reinvigorate

Knowledge Check

Answers in Appendix D

1. Body composition consists of:

    A. Fat, muscle, bone, and other body tissues

    B. Storage fat

    C. Essential fat and muscle mass only

2. The risk of chronic disease rises when your body fat:

    A. Is found only in your legs

    B. Exceeds 12% (men) and 20% (women)

    C. Exceeds 25% (men) and 30% (women)

3. You are healthy only if:

    A. You are a bodybuilder whose weight matches your height on a standard chart

    B. Your body shape matches the ideal

    C. You have the right amount of body fat and lean body mass

Scenario One: During Megan's first year in college she gained 12 pounds. Because she didn't like the cafeteria food in her dorm, she ate one or more meals at various fast-food restaurants each day. Moreover, her college did not require a physical education class, so her physical activity involved walking to classes and little else.

4. Which is the most practical method for Megan to assess her *body weight*?

    A. Body mass index (BMI)

    B. Weight-to-height tables

    C. Underwater weighing

5. Which is the most practical method for Megan to assess her *body fat*?

    A. Underwater weighing

    B. Skinfold measurements

    C. Bioelectrical impedance analysis

Scenario Two: Patti has just discovered that her BMI is 27, which means she is considered overweight. She has decided that she will lose the necessary weight to lower her BMI to the healthy score of 23.

6. What is the most effective and healthy way for Patti to lower her BMI score?

    A. Exercising 3 times a week without changing her eating habits

    B. Going on a strict diet with no exercise

    C. Combining regular exercise and a healthy diet

7. How often should Patti be reassessing her body composition?

    A. Every 2 weeks

    B. Every 3 months

    C. Every month

8. When you are trying to lose weight, which of the following is the most effective way to shed unwanted pounds?

    A. Cut out all of the empty calories in your diet (candy, white bread, soda) and be involved in moderate activity (walking for 30 minutes 4 days per week)

    B. Exercise 4 days per week very intensely (30-minute jog) while keeping the same diet

    C. Do more household chores, such as vacuuming, raking, and washing dishes, while maintaining the same diet

9. While reading about the different reasons for weight gain, you learned about three different theories on excessive weight gain. Which theory says that everyone has a set number of fat cells and that when you lose weight you are not decreasing the number of fat cells, but the actual size of the fat cell?

A. Glandular disorder theory

B. Set point theory

C. Fat cell theory

10. Diet books seem to come and go. You see people on talk shows talking about one fad diet or another, and that is exactly what they are: fads. Which of the following reasons is why most of these fad diets do not work?

A. These diets do not generate the results that they claim they can.

B. They often involve extreme changes to your lifestyle that are difficult (and possibly unsafe) to maintain.

C. They don't take into account your caloric intake.

Modern Modifications

How many times have you vowed to eat better and exercise more? Right. And how long did that effort last? Right again. Is there a way to keep yourself on track to shape up? Yes, there is: Use proven techniques to modify your behavior.

Monitor yourself by observing and recording each aspect of what you do:

- Amount of sedentary time spent per day
- Calories taken in each time you eat something
- Frequency, duration, and intensity of each exercise you do
- Changes in your body shape, composition, and weight as your program progresses

Monitoring is a continuous process of self-motivation. Focus on what matters. Keep records. Use the charts in the lab manual to track your progress.

Keep a Food Diary

Track your eating habits for the next few days. Record:

- What you eat
- How much you eat
- When you eat: Try to associate it with an event (i.e., 3 PM break between classes)
- Why you eat: Was it lunch time? Were you just hungry? Were you stressed or bored?
- How did you feel after? Satisfied? Still hungry? Guilty?

Critical Thinking

1. Paul is in his first year at State College. He has gained 17 pounds during the year. Paul carries 17 credit hours, and he works 20 to 25 hours each week. He does not believe he has enough time for exercise. Because of the hectic nature of his schedule and his dislike of residence hall food, Paul eats at least one meal at a fast-food restaurant each day. He has tried two popular magazine diets during the year but has not kept the weight off. What is the most significant issue Paul faces? What is the most likely

explanation for his weight gain? Describe a strategy for Paul to lose and keep off the extra weight. What are the long-term risks facing Paul if he continues this pattern?

2. Lateisha has decided to lose some extra body fat. What would be the most reasonable way for Lateisha to track her body fat? Where, in the university community, can she get this procedure done? How often should she have her body fat checked?

Going Above and Beyond

Websites

The Obesity Society
http://www.obesity.org

American Dietetic Association
http://www.eatright.org

Center for Science in the Public Interest
http://www.cspinet.org

Centers for Disease Control and Prevention, Obesity and Genetics
www.cdc.gov/genomics/training/perspectives/obesity.htm

Fast Food Facts: Interactive Food Finder
http://www.all-weightloss.net/fastfood.htm

Frontline on Fat
http://www.pbs.org/wgbh/pages/frontline/shows/fat

MedlinePlus on Obesity and Weight Control
http://www.nlm.nih.gov/medlineplus/obesity.html
http://www.nlm.nih.gov/medlineplus/weightcontrol.html

National Association of Anorexia Nervosa and Associated Disorders (ANAD)
http://www.anad.org

National Eating Disorders Association
http://www.nationaleatingdisorders.org

National Heart Lung and Blood Institute Portion Distortion
http://hp2010.nhlbihin.net/portion/

Office of Dietary Supplements
http://ods.od.nih.gov/

Shape Up America!
http://shapeup.org

USDA Food and Nutrition Information Center
http://www.nal.usda.gov/fnic

Weight-Control Information Network
http://publications.usa.gov/USAPubs.php

Weight Loss 2000
http://www.weightloss2000.com

References and Suggested Readings

ACSM. Position stand: Appropriate intervention strategies for weight loss and prevention of weight regain for adults. *Medicine and Science in Sports and Exercise* 2001; 33:2145–2156.

ADA. Weight management: Position of the American Dietetics Association. *Journal of the American Dietetics Association* 1997; 97:71–74.

Anderson R. E. Exercise, active lifestyle, and obesity: Making an exercise prescription work. *Physician and Sports Medicine* 1999; 27:41–50.

Foreyt J. P. An etiological approach to obesity. *Hospital Practice* 1997; 123–148.

Gallagher, D., et al., Healthy percentage body fat ranges. *American Journal of Clinical Nutrition* 2000; 72(3):694–701.

Hill J. O., et al. *The Step Diet Book.* New York: Workman Publishing Company, 2004.

Insel P., Turner R. E., and Ross D. *Discovering Nutrition.* Sudbury, MA: Jones and Bartlett, 2006.

———. *Nutrition.* Sudbury, MA: Jones and Bartlett, 2007.

Institute of Medicine. *Dietary Reference Intakes for Energy, Carbohydrate, Fiber, Fat, Fatty Acids, Cholesterol, Protein, and Amino Acids.* Washington, D.C.: National Academies Press, 2005.

Klem M. L., et al. A descriptive study of individuals successful at long-term maintenance of substantial weight loss. *American Journal of Clinical Nutrition* 1997; 66:239–249.

NCCDPHP. *Defining Overweight and Obesity.* Atlanta, GA: NCCDPHP, 2004. http://www.cdc.gov/obesity/defining.html [October 19, 2004].

———. *Factors Contributing to Obesity.* Atlanta, GA: NCCDPHP, 2001. http://www.cdc.gov/obesity/causes/index.html [October 19, 2004].

NCHS. *Prevalence of Overweight and Obesity Among Adults:* United States, 1999–2002. Hyattsville, MD: NCHS, 2004. http://www.cdc.gov/nchs/products/hestats.htm [October 19, 2004].

NHLBI. Clinical guidelines on the identification, evaluation, and treatment of overweight and obesity in adults. NIH Publication No. 98-4083 (1998). http://www.nhlbi.nih.gov/guidelines/obesity/practgde.htm.

Rubinstein S. and Caballero B. Is Miss America an undernourished role model? *Journal of the American Medical Association* 2000; 283:1569.

The truth about dieting. *Consumer Reports* 2002; 67:26–31.

Stevens J., et al. The effect of age on the association between body-mass index and mortality. *New England Journal of Medicine* 1998; 338:1–7.

Taubes, G. *Why We Get Fat: And What to Do About It.* New York: Alfred A. Knopf, 2011.

Wickelgren I. Obesity: How big a problem? *Science* 1998; 280:1364–1376.

Willett W. C. *Eat, Drink, and Be Healthy.* New York: Fireside, 2005.

———. Guidelines for healthy weight. *New England Journal of Medicine* 1999; 341:427–434.

———. Is dietary fat a major determinant of body fat? *American Journal of Clinical Nutrition* 1998; 76(suppl):556s–562s.

USDA and USDHHS. *Dietary Guidelines for Americans, 2010,* 7th edition, Washington, DC: U.S. Government Printing Office, 2010.

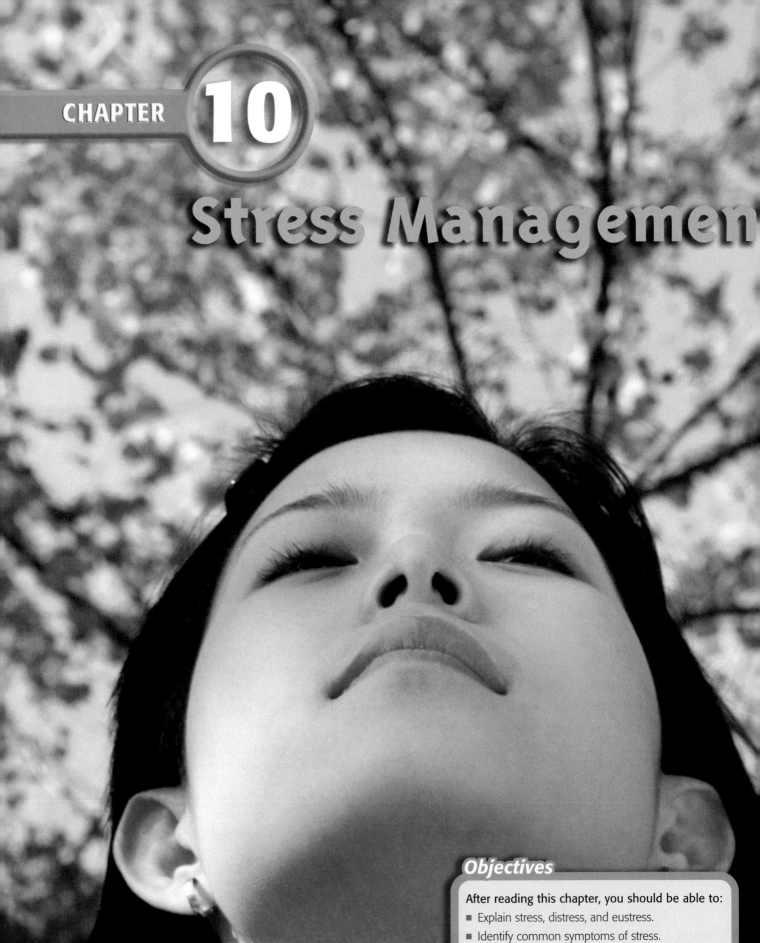

CHAPTER 10

Stress Managemen

Objectives

After reading this chapter, you should be able to:

- Explain stress, distress, and eustress.
- Identify common symptoms of stress.
- Describe common sources of stress.
- Describe strategies useful in coping with stress.

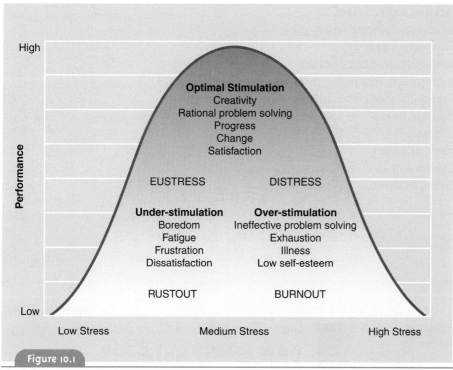

Figure 10.1

The stress continuum showing the effects of stress on performance.

What Is Stress?

Stress can be broadly defined as an automatic physical response to any stimulus that requires you to adjust to change. Good stress (eustress) helps you perform better and overcome obstacles. Bad stress (distress) upsets you and makes you sick. Chronic or overabundant stress wears down the ability to adapt and cope **Figure 10.1**.

You feel distressed if you believe that:

- You have more problems than you can handle.
- You don't feel up to a task.

Exercising until you are exhausted is a physical **stressor**. Taking a tough exam is a mental stressor. Giving an in-class report is a social stressor. Being in a room filled with loud music is an environmental stressor. How you respond to the stressor is known as your stress response.

Stress and College

There is no avoiding it: College students experience significant stress. How many of the following daily hassles are you confronted with? An article in the *College Student Journal* (1999) stated that students are more often challenged by daily hassles than by major life events, with the top five sources of stress being changes in sleeping habits, vacations/breaks, changes in eating habits, increased workload, and new responsibilities.

Sources of Stress in Daily College Life

- Financial aid and school loans
- Budgeting money

What's the word...

stress The automatic physical response of the body to any stimulus that requires adjusting to change.

eustress Helpful or good response to a stressor.

distress Harmful or bad response to a stressor.

stressor A source or cause of stress; may be physical, mental, social, or environmental.

10

- Parental expectations
- Roommate compatibility
- Choosing a major
- Academic deadlines (exams, papers, projects)
- Peer groups and peer pressures (drugs and alcohol)
- Decisions about sexuality
- Homesickness
- Grades
- Medical issues
- Changes in sleep patterns
- Transportation

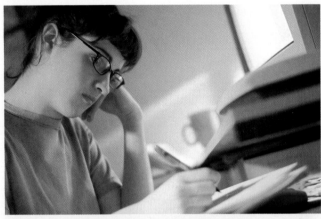

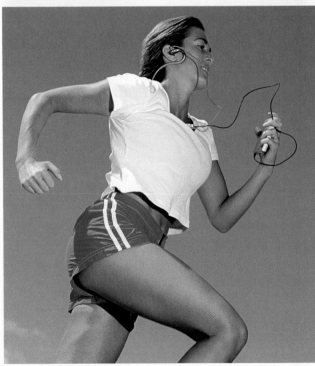

How Does Your Body Respond to Stress?

In response to stress, your body pours stimulant hormones, such as adrenaline, into your bloodstream. The effects are:

- You sweat to cool the extra body heat.
- You hear and see better, to assess the situation and act quickly.
- Your heart speeds up, to get more blood to the muscles, brain, and heart.
- Blood flow increases to your brain, heart, and muscles—most important in dealing with danger.
- Your muscles tense to prepare for action.
- Less blood flows to your skin, digestive tract, kidneys and liver—least needed in times of crisis.
- You breathe faster, to take in more oxygen.
- Your liver dumps extra sugar and fats into your bloodstream for quick energy.
- Platelets and blood-clotting factors rise to prevent hemorrhage in case of injury.

Endorphins are believed to be a source of "runner's high," an example of eustress.

How Does Your Nervous System React to Stress?

The sympathetic nervous subsystem of the autonomic nervous system triggers energy output to handle a crisis, including stress. It acts on many parts of the body, such as sweat glands, blood vessels, and muscles.

How Does Your Endocrine System React to Stress?

The endocrine system releases hormones to control body functions. In response to a stressor, it releases extra hormones from the adrenal glands and pituitary gland, giving rise to the stress response.

What Is the Fight-or-Flight Response?

The stress hormones (epinephrine, norepinephrine, cortisol) secreted into the bloodstream prepare the body for quick action during times of stress. The stress response is often called "fight-or-flight" because it gets you ready to take action either by staying and fighting or by running away from danger. Even in situations not requiring a physical response (e.g., being late for an in-class exam, having to stop at three red lights in a row, being unable to find a parking space), the fight-or-flight response may be activated.

How Do You Return to Normal?

Once you have stopped stressing over something, the parasympathetic subsystem of your autonomic nervous system takes over and calms you down. It takes you back to homeostasis by bringing down your blood pressure, heart rate, and hormone levels; drying your sweaty palms; and slowing your breathing back to a normal pace.

Personality Types and Stress

Certain kinds of behavior can aggravate the effects of stress. Extreme type-A people are at risk of coronary problems, unless they are able to channel their drive in constructive ways and keep themselves in good physical shape.

Type-B people take things easy, do not respond to pressure or hurry, and do not set deadlines for themselves. They have a secure sense of self-esteem. However, an extreme type-B person may be avoiding life's challenges and as a result may not accomplish much.

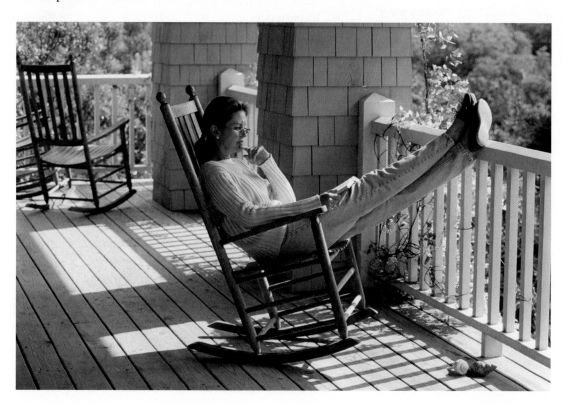

What's the word...

endocrine system Consists of glands that produce hormones that control body functions.

hormone Chemical messenger released into the bloodstream that controls many body activities.

gland A group of cells that secretes hormones.

stress hormones (e.g., epinephrine) A hormone that prepares the body to react during times of stress or in an emergency.

homeostasis Stability and consistency of a person's physiology.

type A An individual exhibiting a sense of time urgency ("hurry sickness"), aggressiveness, and competitiveness, usually combined with hostility. Describes a great majority of Americans.

type B An individual displaying no sense of time urgency, no hostility, noncompetitiveness, patience, and a secure sense of self-esteem.

10

Unhealthy Responses to Stress

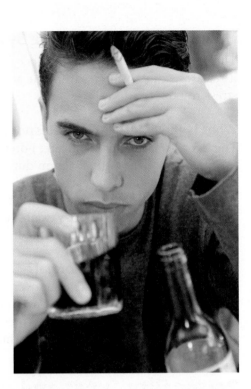

Behavioral Responses

- Pacing and fidgeting, nail-biting, foot-tapping
- Overeating or weight gain, insufficient food, or underweight
- Smoking, drinking too much, taking illegal or unsafe drugs
- Taking prescription or over-the-counter drugs that promise some form of relief such as muscle relaxants, sleeping pills, or anti-anxiety pills
- Crying, yelling, swearing, blaming other people and things
- Throwing things or hitting someone
- Watching endless hours of TV
- Sleeping too much

What's the word...

general adaptation syndrome A series of body changes that result from stress. The syndrome occurs in three stages: alarm, resistance, and exhaustion.

Mental Responses

- Decreased concentration and memory
- Mind racing or going blank, confusion, indecisiveness
- Loss of sense of humor

Emotional Responses

- Anger and frustration, short temper, irritability, impatience
- Anxiety, nervousness, worry, fear
- Boredom, general fatigue, depression, low self-esteem

Stress and Disease

Of all illnesses, 50% to 80% relate to stress. The top-selling drugs in the United States are for stress-related disorders. According to the American Academy of Family Physicians, two-thirds of all medical office visits are for stress-related illnesses Figure 10.2 .

General Adaptation Syndrome

The general adaptation syndrome to stress (alarm, resistance, exhaustion) was first described by Dr. Hans Selye, a biologist Figure 10.3 .

In the *alarm* stage, the first stage, the body prepares for quick action. The adrenal glands secrete stress hormones into the bloodstream, which prepares

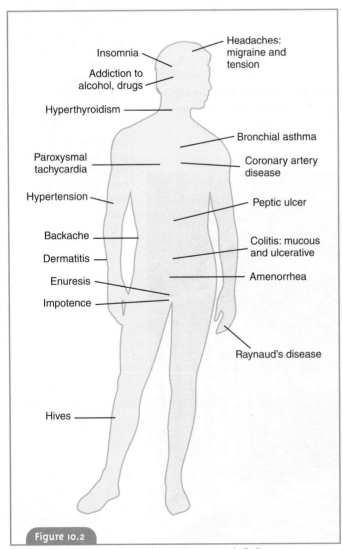

Insomnia

Addiction to alcohol, drugs

Hyperthyroidism

Paroxysmal tachycardia

Hypertension

Backache

Dermatitis

Enuresis

Impotence

Hives

Headaches: migraine and tension

Bronchial asthma

Coronary artery disease

Peptic ulcer

Colitis: mucous and ulcerative

Amenorrhea

Raynaud's disease

Figure 10.2

Stress relates to an estimated 50% to 80% of all diseases.

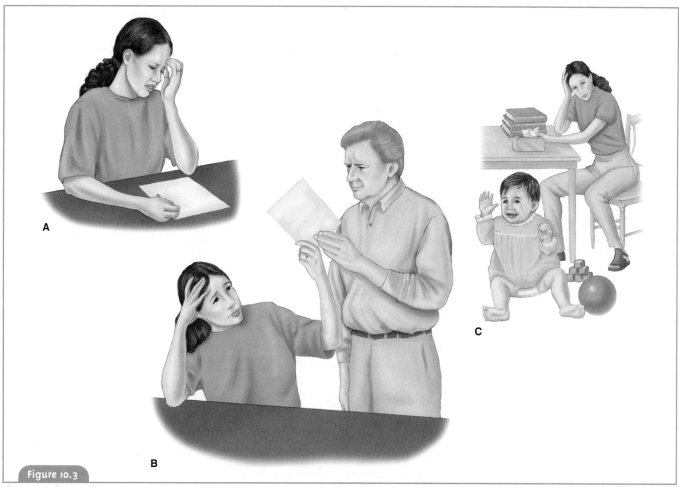

Figure 10.3

There are three stages of general adaptation syndrome. (a) In the alarm stage, the body's normal resistance to stress is lowered from the first interaction with the stressor. (b) In the resistance stage, the body adapts to the continued presence of the stressor and resistance increases. (c) In the exhaustion stage, the body loses its ability to resist the stressor any longer and becomes exhausted. The body's defenses are also weakened.

the body to deal physically with the stressor. This stage is where the fight-or-flight reaction occurs.

In the *resistance* stage, the second stage, the body attempts to regain internal balance. The body is no longer in the emergency state but continues to fight off unresolved stress in the individual. Adrenaline is no longer secreted, relieving the person's sense of urgency to respond to the stressor, but other stress-related hormones remain present, breaking down the body's ability to fight off disease. The longer one retains stress, the more damage occurs.

The *exhaustion* stage, the third stage, represents the wearing on the body that increases the risk of illness and premature death. Experts call the long-term wear of the stress response the **allostatic load**. When you are unable to cope with stress due to the allostatic load, you become more susceptible to illnesses.

Psychoneuroimmunology

Depending on your body's and mind's ability to cope with stress, you can develop some serious health problems as a result of chronic stress, especially in your circulatory and immune systems:

- High blood pressure and arteriosclerosis leading to stroke or heart attack
- Increased susceptibility to colds, infections, rheumatoid arthritis, cancer, herpes, HIV

What's the word...

allostatic load The ongoing demand on the body from long-term exposure to stress hormones.

psychoneuroimmunology Study of nervous, endocrine, and immune systems interaction.

10

Other health problems from poor response to stress can include:

- Rapid or irregular heart rate, chest pains
- Muscle aches or stiffness (especially in neck, shoulders, and low back)
- Temporomandibular joint dysfunction
- Tension or migraine headaches
- Flushing or sweating, trembling, fatigue, cold extremities
- Nausea, abdominal cramps, irritable bowel syndrome, ulcers, and colitis
- Bronchial asthma, allergies, insomnia

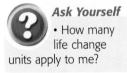

Ask Yourself
• How many life change units apply to me?

Sources of Stress

There are many negative and positive sources of stress in your life. They can be especially stressful if they come in clusters.

- *Life changes:* Experiencing multiple life changes within 1 year shows a high degree of recent life stress. Examples include death of a family member, laid off from work, divorce, and engagement to marry.
- *Daily hassles:* Commuting, misplacing keys, mechanical breakdowns, money worries, arguments, lousy weather, waiting in long or slow lines, noise, bright lights, heat, violence, confined spaces. (See **Lab 10-1**, Activity 1.)
- *College-life stress:* Adjusting to a new locale, making new friends, keeping up with tougher academic work, taking exams, meeting deadlines, too much caffeine, not enough sleep, overloaded schedule, worry about earning money to live on or taking on loans to pay expenses. (See Lab 10-1, Activity 2.)
- *Job stress:* Rushed by tight schedules and deadlines; too much overtime taking away from personal life; concerns about job performance, job security, or money earned; interactions with co-workers, bosses, or customers; no input on how work is done; dealing with bureaucratic rules and regulations **Figure 10.4**.

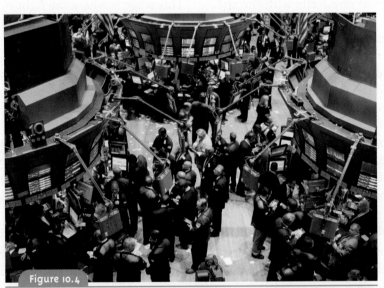

Figure 10.4

An extreme example of job-related stress is working on the New York Stock Exchange. So many people have heart attacks there every year that the exchange has installed a defibrillator near the phone banks.

- *Social stress:* Changes in relationships with family and old friends, aggressive behavior from others, negative community pressures from ethnic or lifestyle prejudice and discrimination, difficulties in using English as a second language.
- *Negative thought patterns:* Pessimistic thinking, self-criticism, over-analyzing situations and relationships.
- *Personality difficulties:* Unrealistic expectations, taking things too personally, exaggerating, all-or-nothing or rigid thinking.

Key Strategies for Coping with Stress Effectively

Effective coping strategies are anything that helps change or reduce the stress or the perception of stress.

Of course, if you treat only the symptoms of your stress, you'll simply develop other symptoms. For example, if you get headaches when stressed, and your method of dealing with the stress is to take ibuprofin, you haven't addressed the cause of the stress. Odds are that you'll experience the headaches again. Over time, the continued exposure to unaddressed stress may lead to ulcers, depression, or even some forms of coronary artery disease or cancer.

Time Management

- Rank tasks in order of importance. (See **Lab 10-2**, Activity 1 on time ranking.)
- Schedule tasks with a time period for each. Break your day into quarter-hour or half-hour segments. (See Lab 10-2, Activity 2 on scheduling.)
- List your deadlines on a calendar or daily planner so that you can allow time to meet them.
- Delegate. Ask for help. Involve others in doing your low-priority tasks.
- Say "no" if demands seem unreasonable or you do not have time for them.
- Have a place for everything and put everything in its place.
- Schedule personal time each day for exercise, a hobby, meditation, or some other activity that improves your quality of life.
- Watch less television (limit yourself to 1 hour each night).

Healthy Diet

What you eat plays a big role in your risk of developing many illnesses, including hypertension, heart disease, diabetes, and cancer, which in turn affect your overall stress level. Obesity caused by overeating is linked with many ailments, too. It is also a source of stress for those who are continually reminded of their failure to achieve the slim look desired in America.

- Eat a well-balanced diet of milk, whole grains, fruits, vegetables, fish, and poultry; eat slowly; eat less junk food.
- Take in less caffeine (e.g., coffee, tea, colas, too much chocolate). Caffeine generates a stress reaction in the body.
- Avoid "stress-reducing" supplements, such as those containing vitamins and amino acid compounds. They do not help reduce the effects of stress.

The Inside Track

Roadblocks to Effective Time Management

- *Time urgency:* Rushing to meet deadlines
- *Time juggling:* Trying to do more than one thing at a time
- *Procrastination:* Avoiding or putting off what should be done, from apathy or fear of failure
- *Perfectionism:* Being obsessed with doing everything perfectly; getting caught up in details and not seeing the whole picture
- *Workaholism:* Spending too much time at work
- *Can't say "no":* Taking on responsibilities you don't have time for or can't handle in a bid to get approval or acceptance
- *Polyphasic thinking:* Being preoccupied with many thoughts at one time

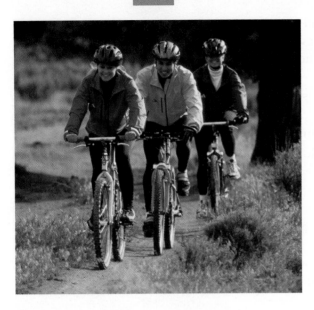

Exercise

Exercise is a good way to dissipate stress. Get regular exercise (at least 30 minutes, three times per week). Take a brisk walk, a run, or a bike ride.

Cardiovascular exercise flushes stress hormones out of the body. Otherwise, they pool in the body and cause havoc (e.g., cortisol destroys white blood cells). Regular cardiovascular exercise may contribute to an overall sense of relaxation.

Exercise may also combat emotional problems, such as depression, by increasing the level of endorphins, chemicals in the brain that seem to enhance a sense of well-being and relieve anxiety.

Sleep

Sleep reduces stress. Tired people do not cope well with stressful situations. If you get enough sleep, you feel better and are more resilient and adaptable.

Successful sleep is:

- Waking naturally
- Waking refreshed
- Having plenty of daytime energy

The "power nap" or catnap is short (5 to 20 minutes) and can be rejuvenating. Many people don't get enough sleep, some by choice. But bad things happen when you are sleep deprived:

- You doze off in class.
- You can't focus on an exam.
- You risk serious injury by dozing off while driving or working.

Lack of sleep also adversely affects your health:

- You are at a greater risk of infection.
- You become moody.
- You have problems with memory.

When are you getting enough sleep? When you wake up naturally without an alarm clock and feel alert during the day.

Medical News You Can Use

Yoga Reduces Atrial Fibrillation Episodes

Taking a 45-minute yoga class three times a week was associated with halving of atrial fibrillation (AF) episodes. The number of AF episodes in the small study was significantly reduced from 3.8 to 2.1 during the 3-month study period. Although it is not known how yoga helps the reduction, it appears that yoga has a significant impact on regulating patients' heartbeat and improves overall quality of life. Clinicians are advising that yoga does not fix everything and patients should continue to take their medication. However, the effects of regular yoga exercises have positive effects.

Source: Data from Lakkireddy D., et al. Impact of yoga on arrhythmia burden and quality of life (QoL) in patients with symptomatic paroxysmal atrial fibrillation: The Yoga My Heart Study. *Journal of the American College of Cardiology* 2011; 57:129.

Social Support

Social ties—at least those representing positive relationships—significantly protect health and well-being. Support from friends, co-workers, relatives, and spouses may provide outright assistance or may be largely emotional. Those who have greater social support fare better when faced with stressors such as surgery, exams, and job strain. Negative relationships such as an embattled marriage or a draining caretaking arrangement can be more harmful than helpful.

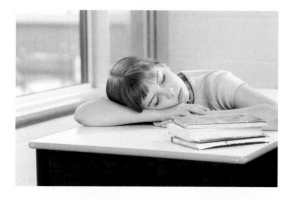

Some ways of strengthening social ties include the following:

- Don't wait for others to call; phone and propose an activity.
- Volunteer your talents to serve others.
- Find people similar to yourself through classes, organizations, and special interest groups.
- Attend religious services.
- Offer to help friends, family, and neighbors. Also accept help when it is offered to you.

Keep your connections to family and friends strong. When you are feeling stressed, talk to a family member, friend, counselor, school advisor, teacher, or someone else whom you respect and trust. You'll be surprised how much better you feel after talking to someone.

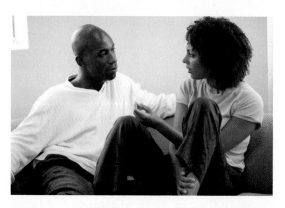

Healthy Thought Patterns

Attitude is crucial to stress management. In sailing terms, *attitude* is how sails are set to take advantage of prevailing winds. Thus, what we believe determines how we react to stress.

Positive thinking can help you manage stress. If you say to yourself, "I will ace that exam," you are more likely to do well and feel less stressed.

Anger Management

Anger creates physical symptoms similar to stress: faster heartbeat and breathing, muscle tension, flushed face, and trembling. Out-of-control anger is bad for you. It hurts you and your relationships with others.

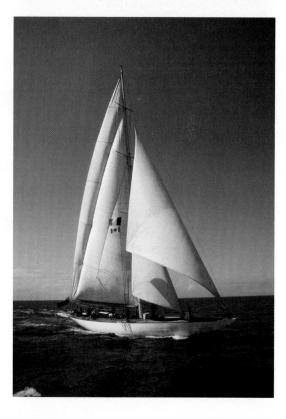

If you are angry:

- Reframe the situation. Maybe the cause isn't directed at you.
- Distract yourself. Count to 10. Imagine yourself in a peaceful place.
- Analyze the conflict. Listen to the other person's point of view. Negotiate a constructive solution.

If the other person is angry at you:

- Respond to conflict calmly.
- Ask why the person is angry.
- Focus on resolving the cause of the anger.
- If all else fails, disengage and try again later.

Table 10.1	Defense Mechanisms		
Defense Mechanism	**Positive or Negative?**	**Definition**	**Simple Example**
Affiliation	Positive	Sharing your feelings of stress, without trying to make others take responsibility for it.	Talking with a close friend about the difficulties you are having with speaking in front of class.
Humor	Positive	Finding the humor or irony of a situation. Differs from sarcasm, which is an anger response.	At the end of a day filled with conflict, finding humor in the ridiculous odds that "all those things" could happen in the same day.
Denial	Negative	Pretending a stressor is minor or does not exist.	Failing to recognize the possibility one has an alcohol problem after receiving a third DUI citation.
Rationalization	Negative	Defending or justifying personal actions and feelings others find unacceptable.	"I only smoke when I drink, so I'm not really a smoker."
Splitting	Negative	Categorization of others in one's life; idolizing one group and disenfranchising the other.	After a major argument with all four roommates, ignoring and shutting out those who disagreed with you, while spending all your time with those who did agree.
Repression	Negative	Blocking disturbing thoughts or experiences from the conscious mind.	Often used by those having experienced physical, emotional, or sexual abuse as children so the upsetting thoughts are not always present.

Source: Adapted from Levo L.M. Understanding defense mechanisms. *Lukenotes,* Saint Luke Institute, 2003, 7(4).

Defense Mechanisms

Defense mechanisms can be both positive and negative means of coping with stress. Sometimes we are aware that we are using a defense mechanism, and other times we may not be aware. **Table 10.1** describes some of the more common defenses.

Additional Ways to Manage Stress

Music

Listening to and creating music has a soothing effect. For most people, music is a popular way to relax. Individual tastes vary greatly regarding music. However, certain factors associated with music as a relaxation technique include the following:

- The music should be instrumental with a slow tempo. The music should be enjoyable rather than agitating.
- Minimize or eliminate all interruptions.
- Sit or recline in a comfortable position with eyes closed to minimize distractions.
- Make your own music by humming, singing, whistling a song, or playing an instrument.

Time-outs

Take time-outs to get away from the things that are bothering you. This will decrease your stress level.

Time-outs include power naps, meditation, daydreaming, a social conversation, a short walk, a refreshment break, or listening to music.

You have cycles throughout the day, peaks of energy and concentration interspersed with low energy and inefficiency. Watch for periods of low energy and take breaks when they occur.

A mid-morning break, lunch, a mid-afternoon break, and the evening meal divide a day into roughly 2-hour segments.

Relaxation Exercises

An effective relaxation technique is anything that helps reduce sensory overload by redirecting positive sensations through the five senses. However, just like throwing a football, building with wood, or sewing, it is a skill and must be practiced for an individual to be good at it (see **Figure 10.5** and **Lab 10-3**).

Meditation

Herbert Benson in his book *The Relaxation Response* describes a useful form of meditation. The components include the following (see Lab 10-3, Activity 3):

- Quiet room with minimal distractions.
- A comfortable sitting position with most of the body weight supported to avoid muscular tension or falling asleep.
- A focus word or phrase used to replace all other thoughts. It can be a repetition of a mantra (e.g., the word *one* or *peace*). Such a word can seem monotonous, but it will clear your mind of mental chatter.

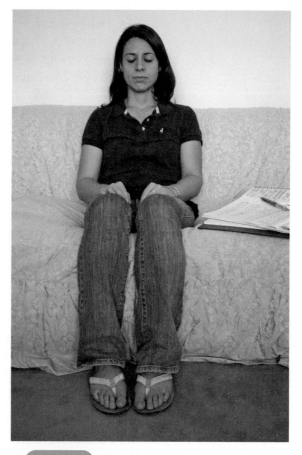

Figure 10.5

The relaxation response.

What's the word...

relaxation response
Reversal of stress symptoms.

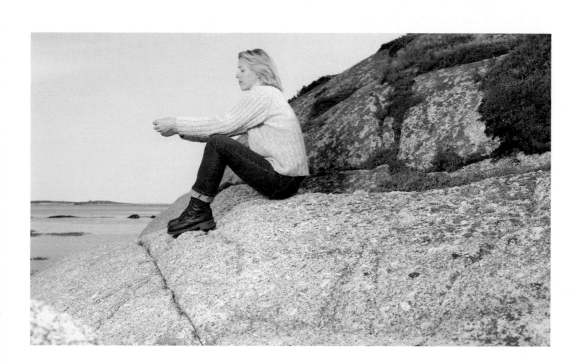

- Passive attitude. Disregard distracting thoughts or concerns. Any time your attention drifts, simply say, "no" or "Oh, well" to yourself and return to silently repeating your focus word or phrase.
- Proper breathing. As you breathe in through your nose, you should feel your lungs fill completely and your belly expand fully. As you exhale either through your nose or mouth, your belly will fall.

A session involves keeping your eyes closed and slowly inhaling and exhaling. At the end of each exhalation, mentally say the mantra (e.g., the word *one* or *peace*).

When you first start, go for 10 minutes. Gradually add time until a session is about 20 minutes daily, preferably at a specific time each day.

Progressive Muscle Relaxation

Muscle tension is the most common symptom of stress, but where each of us feels it varies. One woman might have a tight neck and shoulders, while another feels an iron band digging into her forehead. It is not always easy to locate and relax the muscles responsible.

Progressive muscle relaxation (PMR) teaches you to isolate specific sets of muscles, tense them briefly, and then relax them (see Lab 10-3, Activity 1). This exercise is especially helpful if your mind is racing, making it hard to settle down to other techniques.

It takes only about 10 minutes to exercise all the major body areas. There are several sequences. You can start with the hand muscles, progressing to others; begin at the top, moving from head to toe; or reverse the direction, going from bottom to top as explained here:

PMR Procedure

Find a comfortable position. Perform the steps while either sitting or lying down, preferably in a quiet, soothing environment.

Breathe deeply, allowing your stomach to rise as you inhale and fall as you exhale. Breathe this way for a few minutes before starting.

For each of the body areas, perform three contractions:

- First contraction: 100% intensity for 5 to 10 seconds
  - Release and relax (exhale)
  - Compare relaxation to contraction
- Second contraction: 50% intensity for 5 to 10 seconds
  - Release and relax (exhale)
  - Compare relaxation to contraction
- Third contraction: 5% to 10% intensity for 5 to 10 seconds
  - Release and relax (exhale)
  - Compare relaxation to contraction

Take your time, slowly working through each of these body areas:

1. Curl toes tightly.
2. Flex the feet.
3. Tighten the calves.
4. Tense the thighs.
5. Tighten the buttocks.
6. Tighten the lower back.
7. Tighten the abdomen.
8. Tense the upper chest.
9. Tense the upper back muscles.
10. Clench the fists.
11. Extend the fingers and flex the wrists.
12. Tighten the forearms.

What's the word. . .

progressive muscular relaxation Systematically tensing and relaxing the body's muscles from the feet to the head.

13. Tighten the upper arms.
14. Lift the shoulders gently toward the ears.
15. Wrinkle the forehead.
16. Squeeze your eyes shut.
17. Drop your chin, letting your mouth open wide.

Prayer

Prayer is one of the oldest and most commonly used methods of coping with life problems. If you are religious, prayer can promote mental and physical health.

A prayer commonly associated with stress seeks divine guidance or divine intervention. Such prayers are used when you need help yourself or when you pray for help to be given to others.

Mental Imagery

Imagination can produce feelings of relaxation. For example, visualize yourself feeling warm, calm, and relaxed. Picture a tranquil setting that appeals to you and create a mental picture of the details (see Figure 10.6 and Lab 10-3, Activity 2).

- Mental imagery is generating images that have a calming, healing effect.
- Visualization is mental imagery consciously directed by yourself.
- In guided mental imagery, images are suggested by another person, either live or on tape.

Mental imagery can be used in a stressful situation (e.g., before making a public speech, at the start of an exam, while waiting in line, while sitting in a dentist's chair, during a meeting).

The technique can also be used to change your habits or improve your performance in various activities. Visualize, or imagine, yourself doing something differently or performing successfully.

Exercise

Yoga

Based on Indian philosophy, yoga is an excellent way to invigorate the body and calm the mind. The many different types of yoga share certain basic elements: pranayamas (rhythmic breathing), meditation, and asanas (stretching postures). One of the most commonly practiced forms is hatha yoga, which has relatively gentle movements that can be tailored to your ability. Like tai chi and Qi Gong, yoga increases flexibility and coordination, releases muscle tension, and enhances tranquility.

Tai Chi

Tai chi, a series of slow, fluid, circular motions, originated as a martial art. Its low-intensity movements produce declines in blood pressure similar to those achieved with moderate-intensity aerobics.

Qi Gong

Qi Gong melds breathing, meditation, gentle exercise, and flowing movements. When practiced regularly, it can lower blood pressure, pulse, and demand for oxygen.

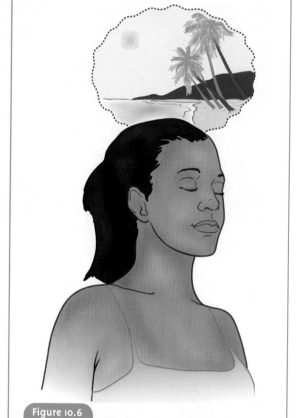

Figure 10.6

Visualize tranquil mental images to relax you when you are stressed.

What's the word. . .

asanas Various postures used in doing yoga exercises.

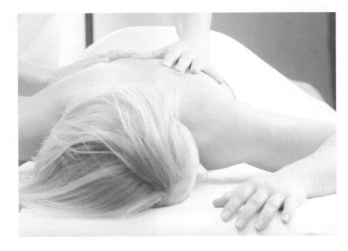

Rhythmic, Repetitive Activities

Rhythmic exercises, such as walking, jogging, swimming, or bicycling, can be calming and relaxing. Use a passive attitude and when disruptive thoughts intrude, gently turn your mind away from them and focus on moving and breathing rhythmically.

Massage

Research indicates that human touch is vital for well-being. For example, infants require human touch to thrive. People of all ages need it as well.

All forms of massage tend to be both relaxing and invigorating. Massage requires the assistance of someone else to achieve full benefit.

Hydrotherapy (e.g., baths, hot tubs, jacuzzis, saunas) is another form of muscle massage.

Pets

Animals can offer more than just friendship; they can decrease stress levels as well. You will often find that hospitals and dentists have aquariums—yes, even fish are capable of lowering our stress levels. The benefits of pet ownership have been studied a great deal. Numerous studies have confirmed that pets have beneficial effects on their owner's physical and emotional health.

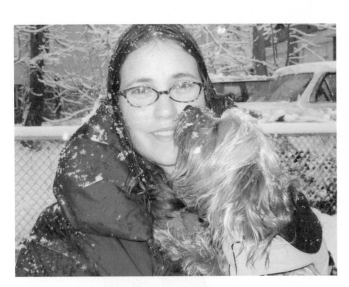

Sense of Humor

Humor may be the ultimate stress reliever. Studies show that humor promotes mental, emotional, physical, and spiritual well-being.

The author Norman Cousins, suffering from a connective tissue disease, credits his recovery to deliberate efforts to apply humor to his situation.

When you try to find the humorous side of life, you can inoculate yourself against the hazards of stressful perceptions.

The average American laughs 15 times per day. Under stress, laughter drops to zero.

Think of some ways in which you can experience humor to lift your spirits (e.g., listening to a humorous radio program, sharing funny stories, reading cartoons).

Hobbies

Hobbies promote clear thinking. They can help to take your mind off a problem and divert your attention to something else. When you return to the problem, you will be better able to deal with it. Many people find that time spent pursuing hobbies helps generate solutions to life problems.

Hobbies provide pleasure and involve creativity. A hobby can boost self-esteem, which transfers to other areas of life.

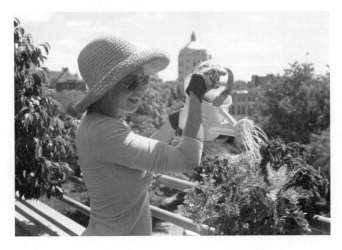

Tipping Point

101 Ways to Cope with Stress

Get up 15 minutes earlier
Prepare for the morning the night before
Avoid tight-fitting clothes
Avoid relying on chemical aids
Set appointments ahead
Don't rely on your memory . . . write it down
Practice preventive maintenance
Make duplicate keys
Say "no" more often
Set priorities in your life
Avoid negative people
Use time wisely
Simplify mealtimes
Always make copies of important papers
Anticipate your needs
Repair anything that doesn't work properly
Ask for help with the jobs you dislike
Break large tasks into bite-size portions
Look at problems as challenges
Look at challenges differently
Unclutter your life
Smile
Be prepared for rain
Tickle a baby
Pet a friendly dog/cat
Don't know all the answers
Look for a silver lining
Say something nice to someone
Teach a kid to fly a kite
Walk in the rain
Schedule play time into every day
Take a bubble bath
Be aware of the decisions you make
Believe in yourself
Stop saying negative things to yourself
Visualize yourself winning
Develop your sense of humor
Stop thinking tomorrow will be a better today
Have goals for yourself
Dance a jig
Say "hello" to a stranger
Ask a friend for a hug
Look up at the stars
Practice breathing slowly
Learn to whistle a tune
Read a poem
Listen to a symphony
Watch a ballet
Read a story curled up in bed
Do a brand new thing
Stop a bad habit
Buy yourself a flower
Take time to smell the flowers
Find support from others
Ask someone to be your "vent-partner"

Do it today
Work at being cheerful and optimistic
Put safety first
Do everything in moderation
Pay attention to your appearance
Strive for excellence *not* perfection
Stretch your limits a little each day
Look at a work of art
Hum a jingle
Maintain your weight
Plant a tree
Feed the birds
Practice grace under pressure
Stand up and stretch
Always have a plan "B"
Learn a new doodle
Memorize a joke
Be responsible for your feelings
Learn to meet your own needs
Become a better listener
Know your limitations and let others know them, too
Tell someone to have a good day in pig Latin
Throw a paper airplane
Exercise every day
Learn the words to a new song
Get to work early
Clean out one closet
Play patty cake with a toddler
Go on a picnic
Take a different route to work
Leave work early (with permission)
Put air freshener in your car
Watch a movie and eat popcorn
Write a note to a faraway friend
Go to a ballgame and scream
Cook a meal and eat it by candlelight
Recognize the importance of unconditional love
Remember that stress is an attitude
Keep a journal
Practice a monster smile
Remember you always have options
Have a support network of people, places, and things
Quit trying to fix other people
Get enough sleep
Talk less and listen more
Freely praise other people

Bonus: Relax, take each day at a time . . . you have the rest of your life to live!

Source: Courtesy of the Tripler Army Medical Center, Honolulu, Hawaii.

Reflect >>>> Reinforce >>>> Reinvigorate

Knowledge Check

Answers in Appendix D

1. Good stress is called:

    A. Eustress
    B. Distress
    C. Stressful
    D. No stress

2. Which categories are manifest signs of stress?

    A. Physical (e.g., aches, stomach problems)
    B. Emotional (e.g., anxiety, boredom)
    C. Mental (e.g., indecisiveness, confusion)
    D. Behavioral (e.g., drinking, yelling, swearing)
    E. All of the above

3. What are the three stages of the general adaptation syndrome?

    A. Flight, fright, sleep
    B. Confusion, hallucination, procrastination
    C. Alarm, resistance, exhaustion
    D. Anger, criticism, guilt

4. Dave was planning to go on a rafting trip next month but has just been told that his trip is cancelled. A travel agent recommended by a friend had arranged the trip. An appropriate way for Dave to reduce his stress would be to:

    A. Plan another vacation for the same time period
    B. Spend his vacation at home and read a book about river rafting
    C. Complain to his friend about his recommendation
    D. None of the above

5. Maria has four final exams and only 2 days left to study for them. An appropriate way for Maria to reduce her stress would be to:

    A. Take her mind off her own tests by helping a friend study
    B. Pick the hardest course and spend most of her time studying for that exam
    C. Set up a schedule so that she has some time to study for each test
    D. None of the above

6. Greg lives across from an all-night service station and is disturbed by the traffic noise. An appropriate way for Greg to reduce his stress would be to:

    A. Turn up his music to block out the noise
    B. Take a sleeping pill to help get to sleep
    C. Stay up later so that he can fall asleep more easily
    D. None of the above

7. Joyce must speak to a large group of people. She is well prepared to give the speech. However, she keeps remembering another time when she gave a speech and forgot what she was supposed to say. An appropriate way for Joyce to reduce her stress would be to:

    A. Set aside some time to sit quietly before the speech
    B. Look directly at the audience while she gives her speech
    C. Keep her hands busy while she gives the speech
    D. None of the above

8. A personality characterized by perfectionism, competitiveness, and a constant sense of urgency is a:

    A. Type-A personality
    B. Type-B personality
    C. Type-C personality
    D. Mental illness, not a personality type

9. Secretions from the brain designed to relieve pain are called:

    A. Glands
    B. Adrenaline
    C. Endorphins
    D. Homeostasis

10. A type of stress that raises your awareness and excitement level without causing negative responses is called:

    A. Distress
    B. Eustress
    C. Stressor
    D. Allostatic load

Modern Modifications

- Take 5 minutes each morning to visualize yourself being successful.
- Go for a brisk walk when you feel yourself becoming stressed during the day.
- Compile a CD with soothing music to listen to when you need to relax.
- Take a yoga class or rent a how-to video.
- Keep track of how many times you laugh in a day. If you are not laughing 15 times by the time you go to bed, try finding more humor in your life!

Critical Thinking

James is 1 year away from completing his degree. His advisors in the business department tell him his GPA is good, but not great, and that he will have to do an excellent job of selling himself to employers during his senior year. James finds that his sleeping patterns have changed, and he's not as rested as he would like to be. His friends, who are also getting close to graduation, go out often, and James usually accompanies them. Lately, James has been feeling down and has had more colds than normal.

Assess James's stress situation. Develop a list of the stressors he is most likely facing. Are his sources of stress positive or negative? What forms of coping is James using? How can he get himself back on track? If you were James, how would you handle the situation?

Going Above and Beyond

Websites

American Institute of Stress
http://www.stress.org

American Psychological Association
http://www.apa.org http://www.apa.org/helpcenter/index.aspx

The Humor Project
http://www.humorproject.com

National Institute for Occupational Safety and Health (NIOSH)
http://www.cdc.gov/niosh/stresshp.html

National Institute of Mental Health
http://www.nimh.nih.gov

National Sleep Foundation
http://www.sleepfoundation.org

References and Suggested Readings

Benson H. *The Relaxation Response.* New York: Avon/Wholecare, 2000.

Boscarino J. S. Diseases among men 20 years after exposure to severe stress: Implications for clinical research and medical care. *Psychosomatic Medicine* 1997; 59:605–614.

Clements K. and Turpin G. Life event exposure, physiological reactivity, and psychological strain. *Journal of Behavioral Medicine* 2000; 23:73–94.

Friedman M. and Ulmer D. *Treating Type A Behavior and Your Heart.* New York: Knopf, 1984.

Laitinen J. E., et al. Stress-related eating and drinking behavior and body-mass index and predictors of this behavior. *Preventive Medicine* 2002; 34:29–39.

McKinney C. H., et al. Effects of guided imagery and music (GIM) therapy on mood and cortisol in healthy adults. *Health Psychology* 1997; 16:390–400.

Miller M. A. and Rahe R. H. Life changes scaling for the 1990s. *Journal of Psychosomatic Research* 1997; 43:279–292.

Pashkow F. J. Is stress linked to heart disease? The evidence grows stronger. *Cleveland Clinic Journal of Medicine* 1999; 66:75–77.

Ross S., Niebling B., and Heckert T. Sources of stress among college students. *College Student Journal* 1999.

Scheufele P. M. Effects of progressive relaxation and classical music on measurements of attention, relaxation, and stress responses. *Journal of Behavioral Medicine* 2000; 23:207–228.

Seaward B. L. *Managing Stress: Principles and Strategies for Health and Wellness,* 5th ed. Sudbury, MA: Jones and Bartlett, 2006.

Selye H. *The Stress of Life,* rev. ed. New York: McGraw-Hill, 1978.

Stephens T. Physical activity and mental health in the United States and Canada: Evidence from four population surveys. *Preventive Medicine* 1988; 17:35–47.

Steptoe A. M. and Joekes K. Task demands and the pressures of everyday life: Associations between cardiovascular reactivity and work blood pressure and heart rate. *Healthy Psychology* 2000; 19:46–54.

Williams R. and Williams V. *Anger Kills.* New York: HarperCollins, 1993.

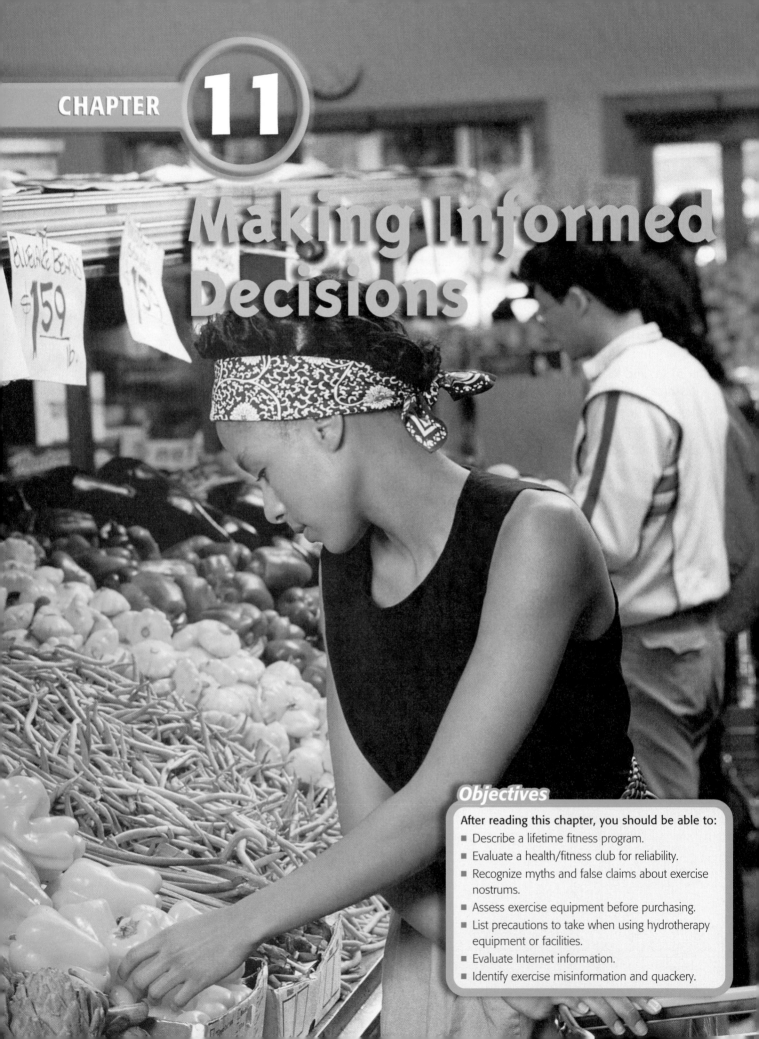

CHAPTER 11

Making Informed Decisions

Objectives

After reading this chapter, you should be able to:

- Describe a lifetime fitness program.
- Evaluate a health/fitness club for reliability.
- Recognize myths and false claims about exercise nostrums.
- Assess exercise equipment before purchasing.
- List precautions to take when using hydrotherapy equipment or facilities.
- Evaluate Internet information.
- Identify exercise misinformation and quackery.

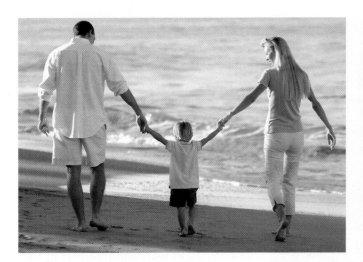

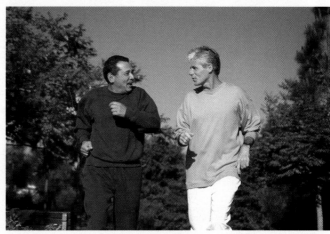

Childhood to Old Age

If you expect to become a parent, bear this in mind: A physically active life begins in childhood. You will do your children no favors if you allow them to watch television or play computer games most of the time. Encourage children to balance those activities with sports, games, or other physical activity that they enjoy. Also, remember that as a parent you are a model for your child. Take time to do activities with your children to encourage them to spend time exercising.

Continue to exercise as you age. You'll have a healthier heart and fitter body. Exercise can reduce blood pressure, make your joints more flexible, and increase muscular strength and endurance. Not only your body benefits: You will improve your mood and your cognitive functions as well.

Keeping your balance as you age is a major issue. Falls that a young person bounces back from can incapacitate or be fatal for older people. Falls in old age are usually the result of poor balance, and keeping fit improves balance.

Even if you did not start early, you can start late. Light to moderate exercise will improve your health at any age—for example, mall-walking, dancing, t'ai chi, or fitness classes designed for older people.

What's the word...

endurance Ability to work out for a period of time without fatigue.

mall-walking Walking a circuit around the lobby floors of an enclosed shopping mall in the morning, often before the stores open.

t'ai chi Thirteenth-century Chinese exercise routine involving graceful dance-like movements.

College Students

Now is the time to make exercise a permanent part of your life. Most colleges try to make it convenient for you. Did you know the following?

- Your college or university probably offers a variety of fitness and sports courses and intramural athletic programs.
- College gyms and athletic fields usually have times designated for recreational student use and have some of the best trainers and equipment.

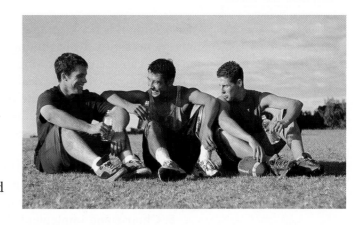

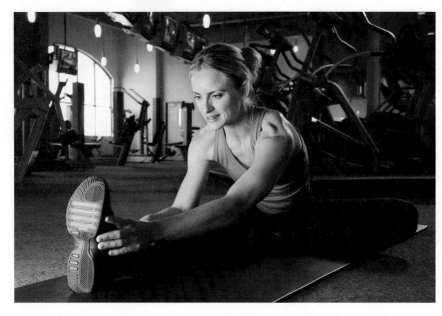

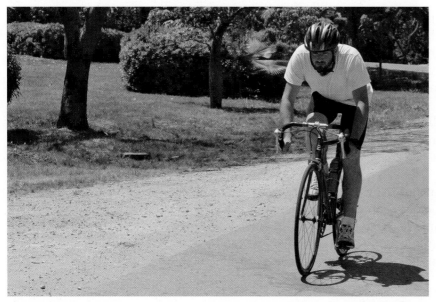

After College

It may take a bit more initiative, especially if your job is desk-bound, but you will be healthier if you create a personal program of physical activity and exercise after college.

Choose activities you like; you are more likely to stick with them throughout your life.

There are some simple ways to make a difference in your daily physical activity:

- Walk to work, at least part of the way.
- Use the stairs, not the elevator.
- Walk during lunchtime.
- Ride a bicycle.

To be more serious about it, you can exercise at home, join a fitness club, or use the exercise facilities in your office building.

If you like to exercise at home, you can buy barbells and hand weights for resistance training, and for aerobic exercise, use a rowing machine, stationary bike, treadmill, stair climber, or cross-country ski machine. A great way to decide whether these are the best pieces of equipment to purchase for home use is to try them out at a fitness club before buying them.

If you like the social aspects of belonging to a fitness club or find it more motivating, by all means join one, but look before you leap.

What's the word...

resistance training
Building muscle by working against the resistance of weights.

Steps in Decision Making

After reading this book, and especially this chapter, you should realize that many decisions are necessary for beginning and maintaining a healthy lifestyle. To make good decisions, you can use the following procedures. These procedures apply to any of life's decisions, not merely those dealing with a healthy lifestyle (**Lab 11-1 and 11-2**):

1. **Identify and clarify the problem.** You must recognize that a problem exists. Some may simply be annoyances, while others are big issues.
2. **Gather information.** Learn more about the problem situation. Look for possible causes and solutions.
3. **Evaluate the evidence.** How accurate is the information? Is it fact or opinion?
4. **Consider alternatives and implications.** Draw conclusions, then weigh the advantages and disadvantages of each alternative.
5. **Choose and implement the best alternative.**

Tipping Point

Selecting a Fitness Professional Who Is Right for You

• Is the fitness professional's workspace convenient to your workplace or home, or is training available in your home?

• Are new clients provided with a pre-exercise screening for health risk factors, and is a fitness program designed specifically for their needs?

• Does the fitness professional offer the expertise, programs, and services you need to achieve your fitness goals?

How to Choose a Fitness Facility

Gyms offer a great number of resources and allow you access to expensive equipment and a variety of fitness classes. But be wary of a high-pressure sales pitch. Once you walk into a gym with one of its promotional fliers, the sales staff will do everything in their power to persuade you to join that day. Take some steps to find out if this is the best gym for you and then take some time to assess whether you can afford the membership (Lab 11-3).

■ Find out how much it costs: Can you afford it? Never join a gym the first time you go. Ask to try out the club for a period of time before signing up. Then you can assess whether you will make the effort to go before making the financial investment. Membership frequently requires a year-long commitment.

■ Check equipment quality and general cleanliness. Check out the changing rooms and showers.

■ Interview the club's trainers. Ask for their credentials and names of clients you can call.

■ Ask them to describe a plan they might recommend for you.

■ Ask how long the club has been in business.

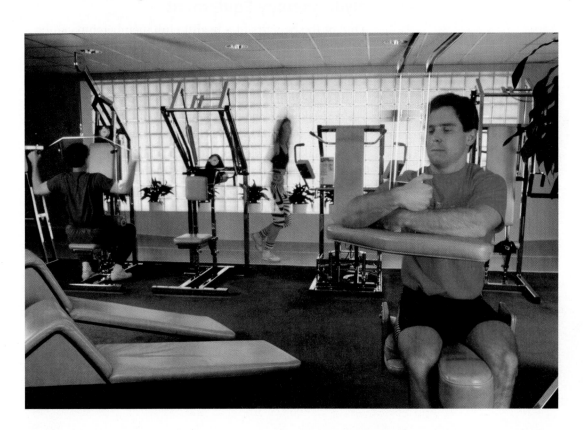

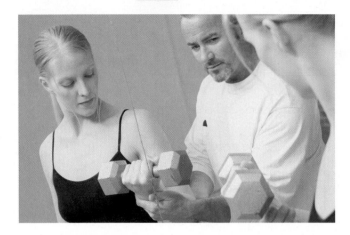

- Check references. Talk to current clients, the Better Business Bureau, and the consumer protection department of the local district attorney's office to see if there are any complaints against the club.
- Again, do not sign a contract on the spot. Double-check what the monthly fees are and ask what the initial joining fee is. Ask if fees exist for special programs, pool time, or court time.
- How do you end membership at the gym? Do you need to show proof of moving from the area? Do you have to pay a penalty for leaving before the contract ends?
- Check with your health insurance company. Often many insurance companies reimburse some or all of the cost of a gym membership.
- How far is the gym from your house and work? If it is too far out of the way, will you go often enough to make joining the gym a cost-effective decision?
- Does the fitness professional have CPR certification, the appropriate educational background, and fitness certification from nationally recognized organizations? Is the fitness professional accredited?
- Does the fitness professional abide by recognized regulations, standards, or guidelines accepted for personalized training in the fitness industry, and if so, what are they?

What's the word...

CPR (cardiopulmonary resuscitation) Clearing air passages to the lungs, giving mouth-to-mouth respiration, and massaging the heart to restore normal breathing after cardiac arrest.

pH Condition of a solution represented by a number on a scale of acidity to alkalinity.

Precautions When Using Hydrotherapy Equipment

One of the benefits of a health club membership can be using the sauna, steam bath, whirlpool, or hot tub. They do not do anything to make you more fit, but they can make you feel better. However, there are some precautions to keep in mind:

- Make sure the equipment is kept clean, and that a hot tub/whirlpool is chlorinated and has the right pH.
- Make sure the temperature is not hotter than 100°F for a whirlpool/hot tub, 120°F for a steam bath, or 190°F for a sauna.
- Shower with soap before and after using the facilities.
- Don't stay in longer than 10 to 15 minutes.
- Stay hydrated: Drink water before or during use.
- Be careful about overheating yourself:
  - Wait an hour after eating.
  - Cool down after exercising.
  - Don't drink alcohol beforehand.
  - Don't exercise while you are in the hot tub or sauna.
  - Get out immediately if you get a headache or feel dizzy, hot, chilled, or nauseated.

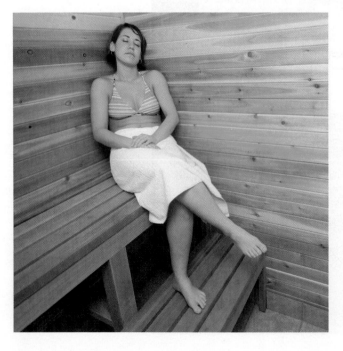

- Don't wear make-up, skin lotion, or jewelry.
- Don't go in by yourself.
- If you have any health problems or are on medication, check first with your doctor.
- Do not submerse you entire body if you have a heart condition or may be pregnant. The hot temperature may be harmful to the fetus.

Purchasing Exercise Equipment

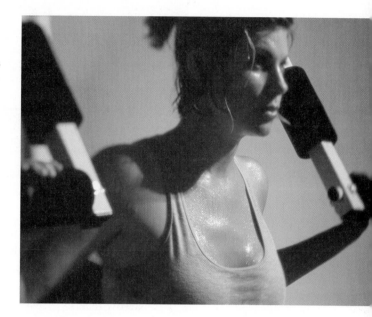

After checking the advertised claims for exercise equipment, consider these questions before buying (Lab 11-4):

- Most important, will the equipment help you achieve your desired goal—build strength, improve endurance, and so on?
- Will you use the equipment? Most home exercise equipment goes unused.
- Do you have room for it?
- Will you have to disassemble the equipment to store it?
- Is it so noisy it will bother your neighbors?
- Check out consumer and fitness magazines that rate exercise equipment.
- Test equipment at a local gym or retailer to find one that feels comfortable to you.
- What's the best deal? Shop around.
- Get details on warranties, guarantees, and return policies. Try to buy from a seller who offers a 30-day money-back guarantee.
- Check out the seller's customer service and support.

You may get a great deal from a secondhand store, consignment shop, yard sale, or the classified ads, but be aware:

- Items bought secondhand usually cannot be returned and don't carry the warranties of new equipment.
- Ask about total costs before buying. The ad may quote a low price, but not include shipping and handling fees, sales tax, and delivery and set-up fees.

Exercise Myths or Misconceptions

Misconceptions exist about what is exercise fact and what is exercise fiction. Here are some common exercise-related fallacies:

- Passive muscle stimulators expend energy from the electrical outlet in the wall, not from your cells. The energy expended to bring about fat loss must be from within your body.
- Taking a pill to bring about instant changes in fitness is an illusion. Fitness takes time and effort. The body systems (muscular, cardiovascular, and skeletal) become stronger in response to regular physical activity.
- Cellulite is not something a health gadget or cream can eliminate. Rapid gain or loss of body fat causes the dimpled look associated with the term *cellulite*.
- Shake, rattle, or roll your fat—it won't disappear. The *only* way to reduce body fat is to use more energy than you consume in calories.

What's the word. . .

cellulite Adipose tissue surrounded by stretched connective tissue.

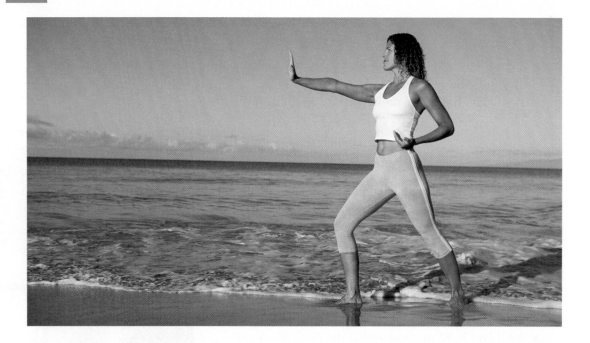

- Wearing rubberized suits, extra layers of clothing, or working out in a hot environment loses water, not fat. It takes a great deal of heat to melt fat. Such heat would melt the rest of you as well.
- If spot reduction worked, everyone who chewed gum or talked a lot would have a narrow face.
- Exercise does not turn fat cells into muscle cells, nor does inactivity turn muscle cells into fat. They are different types of cells. Eat too much and be inactive, and you will enlarge (hypertrophy) the fat cells in your body and shrink (atrophy) the muscle cells. Eat right and exercise to do the reverse.
- Rubbing lotions on the skin to lose fat, firm up muscles, or remove lactic acid does not work. Resistance training firms up muscles.
- Eating extra protein to build stronger muscles doesn't work. Eat more protein than your body uses and the extra will be stored by your body as fat. Increased muscle size comes through resistance training.
- Losing inches is not necessarily loss of fat. It can also be loss of water or lean muscle tissue.
- Exercise is only tiring momentarily. It then makes you feel more energetic as you become more fit.
- In women, resistance training mainly increases muscle strength, not size.
- Drinking liquids during exercise does not cause cramping. Cool water or other appropriate drinks (not soda) should be consumed before, during, and after exercising to replace lost fluids.

What's the word...

hypertrophy Enlargement of fat or muscle.

atrophy Shrinkage of fat or muscle.

cramping Muscular tightness and abdominal or limb pain from dehydration and high body temperature.

Evaluating the Quality of Internet Information Sources

You can find information on just about everything on the Internet. Of course, not all Internet sites are created equal. Some present research and information, some are trying to sell a product, and some are flat-out misinformation. Here are some suggestions on how to decide whether the information you find is quality and reputable:

1. **Check for the creator of the site.** It is important to be able to identify whom the authors or creators of the site are. The author should include his or her credentials

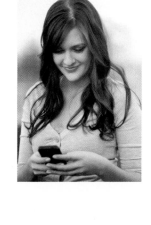

to demonstrate his or her training and expertise in the subject matter. If this information is missing, be cautious.

2. **Check the URL.** Website addresses that end with .edu are material from an educational or research institution. Those ending in .gov are government sources. Those ending with .com or .biz are commercial sites generally intended to sell a product. Because the content of websites is not monitored for accuracy, you may be reading inaccurate, biased, misleading, partial, or false information. This is much more likely to occur on commercial sites than on any other type of website. In addition, if the URL includes a personal name, the site may simply be an individual creating a forum for his or her personal opinion.

3. **Check for advertising.** Websites often accept advertising to help pay the cost of maintaining the site. If the products being advertised are the same as or related to the nature of the information you seek, be cautious. You'd hate to rely on information that has been biased so as not to offend or upset an advertiser. When that happens, you can be certain the information you are viewing is misleading.

4. **Look for accuracy.** Be on the lookout for sites that integrate personal opinions, testimonials, or leading statements about the material you are searching for. Do not assume the first site you visit has accurate information. Gather information from several sites on the same topic and look for common themes. Sites that go into greater depth with their information (as opposed to stating one "fact" and then presenting opinion afterward) are more likely to be accurate. Always back up data from Internet sources with other forms of information to make your data gathering more comprehensive and, in turn, more accurate.

5. **Look for timeliness.** Websites should always contain "updated on" dates to indicate when the information was created. If these dates are missing, you should find additional sources to support the materials' timeliness. Some websites are created but then never updated, and there is no systematic removal of old sites from the Internet. In addition, many sites contain links to other websites or other information. If many of the links are no longer available or contain outdated material, exercise caution regarding what you find. Make certain you find supporting materials from other sources.

Identifying Fitness Misinformation and Quackery

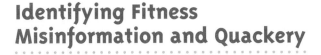

Some advertisers claim—without evidence—that their fitness products offer a quick, easy way to shape up, keep fit, and lose weight. There is no such thing as a no-work, no-sweat way to a healthy, fit body. To get the benefit, you have to do the work. Watch for these and other warning signs:

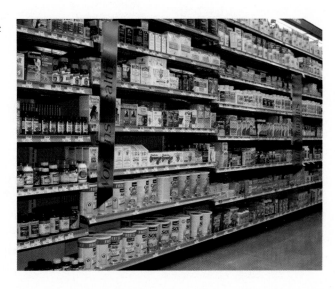

- If the claim sounds too good to be true, it probably is.
- If a product really worked, you would see it in headlines, not just in ads.
- The ads claim the product treats a wide range of ailments.
- The information given is unclear, vague, and highly emotional.
- Changes are promised to be quick, dramatic, or miraculous.
- Results are promised to be easy, effortless, guaranteed, or permanent.

11

- The ads claim relief from conditions for which there are few treatments and no cures.
- The promoter blames problems on a build up of toxins in the body.
- Ads declare the medical community to be against the discovery.
- The ads rely on a guru, testimonials, case histories, and before-and-after photos.
- Products are sold door-to-door, in fliers, through pop-up ads, or by mail order and television advertisements.
- The promoter uses high-pressure sales tactics, one-time-only deals, recruitment for a pyramid sales organization, or demands for large advance payments or long-term contracts.

Choosing Supplements

The next time you watch a TV commercial or see a flyer for a quick weight-loss program, take a moment to consider it. What is being said to you? Who is saying it? In today's day and age we find that to be healthy consumers we need to be educated consumers. The next time you see one of these ads, take a minute to answer the following questions:

- What claim is being made on behalf of this product?
- Who is making this claim? Is it an outside source or the company that makes the product?
- Is everything a testimony about how miraculous the product is?
- Does the ad list any studies that have been done to demonstrate the product's effectiveness?
- If yes, is this a credible source?
- Does it seem like a miracle cure or solution?
- How does it make you feel that ineffective or dangerous products may be marketed without any sound research?

Reflect >>>> Reinforce >>>> Reinvigorate

Knowledge Check

Answers in Appendix D

1. If you don't begin exercising when you are young, you will never get any benefit from it.
   A. True
   B. False
2. Perhaps the most important question to ask yourself when purchasing a piece of exercise equipment is:
   A. Do I have room for it?
   B. Will I use the equipment?
   C. Will the equipment help me achieve my goals (e.g., build strength)?

This statement has value claims that are not supported with scientific evidence.

No treatment contains everything each person needs to improve his or her health.

"Clinical proof" is a red flag. The medical experts and medical schools where their research has been conducted are not identified. Objective testing could show the product is neither safe nor effective. The ad should cite the specific effects of the product, including negative ones.

"Chemical-free" is a red flag; all matter, including herbs and other plants, is comprised of chemicals. Furthermore, scientific studies should be cited to provide evidence for these value claims.

A testimonial from an individual is not scientific evidence. This student's G.P.A. my have risen for a variety of reasons. Studies conducted to show that a treatment is useful should contain at least 30 subjects.

"Potency" is a vague and undefined red-flag term. Again, this testimonial is a value claim that is unsupported by scientific evidence.

This is irrelevant information. Where the product is sold has nothing to do with its quality or characteristics. The authors of the ad are simply trying to make their product look superior to other similar products.

This statement gives the impression that consumers have no time to investigate the product thoroughly. It is intended to make consumers think that the product will sell out if they wait, and they will miss out on a good thing. Again, this information is irrelevant.

This suggests that American scientists do not understand that medicines can be derived from plant sources, when, in fact, American researchers often rely on plants as sources of chemicals that have medicinal uses. No scientific evidence is cited to show that the herbs in Panacea have the touted properties. These two sentences, then, contain only value claims; thus, the information may be unreliable.

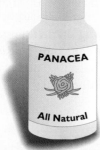

For centuries, doctors in the Orient have known about the wonders of herbal medicines— nature's botanical cures for human ailments.

PANACEA

All Natural

Finally, American scientists are recognizing the healthful benefits of these herbs.

A PANACEA PILL A DAY KEEPS THE EXPENSIVE DOCTORS AWAY!

* These statements have not been evaluated by the FDA.

SwayCon Pharmaceuticals has developed a capsule that contains everything you need to reduce suffering, enhance health, and regain youthful vigor.

A team of medical experts from three major medical schools in the United States have clinical proof that the ingredients of Panacea are effective! Panacea contains a chemical-free mixture of natural enzymes and exotic herbs that

- relieve up to 80% more arthritis pain than aspirin;
- lower blood pressure by up to 20%;
- lower cholesterol by up to 45%;
- reduce lung cancer risk by as much as 50%, even in smokers;
- and reduce the risk of heart attack by 75%.*

Other remarkable findings

Taking Panacea for a few months can improve intelligence. R.P., a college student at a large East Coast university, reports, "At the beginning of the fall semester, I started taking three capsules of Panacea a day. My G.P.A. went from a 1.8 to a 3.4! Panacea has helped me get all A's!"

Reports are coming into our offices that Panacea acts as a sexual stimulant, increasing potency. S.D., a computer programmer in St. Louis, writes, "Thanks for saving my marriage. Before taking Panacea, my husband complained about my lack of interest in sex. One of my friends told me that Panacea can help. Just a few days after taking the capsules, our marriage turned into a perpetual honeymoon."

Panacea is only available in fine health food stores. Order a three-month supply now, while supplies last

No scientific evidence is cited that a daily Panacea pill prevents serious illness. Additionally, this statement attacks conventional medical practitioners by implying that they are interested only in making money, which suggests that physicians can't be trusted.

Disclaimer

This ad is merely a collection of value claims that are not supported by scientific research. The ad further attempts to encourage the reader to purchase the product by suggesting that it is better (and less expensive) than conventional therapies. It claims to relieve a wide range of health conditions. The red-flag phrases and testimonials rather than scientific evidence, the lack of details concerning the medical experts' credentials, and the lack of caution about the hazards of using the product all suggest the ad is an unreliable source of health-related information.

3. What should you look for in using a hot tub?

   A. Its cleanliness

   B. It has 12, not 6, jets

   C. The bubbler signals you when to get out

4. Phil is a 55-year-old overweight salesman with high blood pressure. What course of action do you recommend to help him reach his 56th birthday?

   A. He should immediately join a gym and start vigorous daily workouts.

   B. He should check with his doctor about starting a program of gradually increasing daily physical activity coupled with a better diet.

   C. He should cut down a bit on the martinis at lunch.

   D. He doesn't need to change anything so long as he feels okay.

5. Sales of health and fitness club memberships are at an all-time high. What should you do in selecting a health/fitness club for your workouts?

A. Ask questions (e.g., What are the trainers' credentials?).

B. Check out the social amenities the club offers.

C. Look around to see if everyone in the club looks fit.

D. You should do all of the above.

6. Your mother has Alzheimer's disease. You want to help her in every way possible. In a magazine you read this advertisement: "Cure Alzheimer's Disease!!! My husband has Alzheimer's. On September 2, 1998, he began taking one teaspoon a day of Emu's Liver Oil. Now (in just 22 days) he mows the grass, cleans out the garage, weeds the flower beds, and we take our morning walk again. It hasn't helped his memory much yet, but he is more like himself!!!" What sends a warning signal that this product and its claims may not be valid?

A. The ad appeared in a magazine.

B. An unsupported testimonial is used to sell the product.

C. Emus do not develop Alzheimer's disease.

7. Which of the following is not a criterion for evaluating websites?

A. Sites should show the date they were last updated.

B. Site authors should explain their credentials.

C. Sites should have several links to related products.

D. Sites should be cross-referenced with other materials.

8. Which of the following product statements would support a product's safety?

A. "These statements have not been evaluated by the FDA."

B. "A 7-year study conducted at State University shows the product's effectiveness."

C. "Our product is 'chemical free'."

D. "This product was the best thing I've ever done for my health!"

Modern Modifications

- Look through your local community education or college intramurals programs for a new activity or sport class that you would like to try.
- Aerobic classes or sports not your style? Learn a new type of dance instead.
- Take a walk during your lunch break.
- Ride a bike or walk to work or class if you live a reasonable distance away.
- Check any supplements or home exercise equipment that you have at home using the guidelines provided in this chapter.

Critical Thinking

Identify three websites addressing the same health issue (e.g., Alzheimer's disease, colon cancer). Using the criteria set out in this chapter, discuss the quality of each site, specifically citing the items that make each a strong or weak example of a website.

Going Above and Beyond

Websites

American Dietetics Association
http://www.eatright.org

American Medical Association, Health Insight
http://www.ama-assn.org

Center for Science in the Public Interest
http://www.cspinet.org

Food and Drug Administration
http://www.fda.gov

Healthfinder
http://www.healthfinder.gov

Mayo Clinic
http://www.mayoclinic.com/

National Council Against Health Fraud
http://www.ncahf.org

Office of Dietary Supplements
http://ods.od.nih.gov/

Quackwatch
http://quackwatch.com

References and Suggested Readings

Angell M. and Kassirer J. P. Alternative medicine: The risks of untested and unregulated remedies. *New England Journal of Medicine* 1998; 339:839.

Armsey T. D. and Gree G. A. Nutrition supplements: Science vs. hype. *Physician and Sports Medicine* 1997; 25:76.

Kuntzleman C. T. and Wilkerson R. A primer to recommending home aerobic equipment. *American College of Sports Medicine Health and Fitness Journal* 1997; 1:24.

The mainstreaming of alternative medicine. *Consumer Reports* 2000; 65:17–25.

Stamford B. Choosing and using exercise equipment. *Physician and Sports Medicine* 1997; 25:107–108.

Injury Care and Prevention

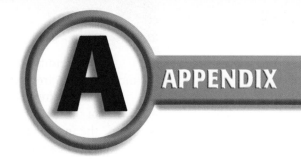

APPENDIX

Exercise-Related Injuries

Most exercise-related injuries do not threaten life, nor are they severe. However, exercise-related injuries demand that you make a decision about the proper care for an injury.

This section helps in such decision making with its decision table (If…, then…) format. Decision tables not only help identify what may be wrong (the "If" column) but also help determine what action to take (the "Then" column).

This appendix does not cover life-threatening conditions requiring rescue breathing and CPR, nor many other injuries and conditions that a quality first-aid course may cover. For a quality first-aid course, go to the American Academy of Orthopaedic Surgeons/American College of Emergency Physicians Emergency Care and Safety Institute website—http://www.ECSInstitute.org—to locate a training center near you. Many colleges and universities use the AAOS/ACEP first-aid, CPR, and AED (automated external defibrillator) program.

How to Examine for an Injury

See **Table A.1**.

Signs of an exercise-related injury may include:

- Loss of use. "Guarding" occurs when movement produces pain; the person refuses to use the injured part.
- A grating sensation (crepitus) can be felt, and sometimes even heard, when the ends of a broken bone rub together.

Table A.1	How to Examine for an Injury
What to Do	**How to Do It**
Determine the location of the problem.	Ask yourself or the injured person "What's wrong?" or "Where do you hurt?"
Find out if an injury exists.	Look and feel the area for one or more of the following signs of injury: deformity, open wounds, tenderness, and swelling. The mnemonic "D-O-T-S" helps in remembering the signs of an injury: • **D**eformities occur when bones are broken, causing an abnormal shape. Deformity might not be obvious. Compare the injured part with the uninjured part on the other side of the body. • **O**pen wounds break the skin and there is bleeding. • **T**enderness (pain) means sensitive when touched or pressed. It is commonly found only at the injury site. The person usually will be able to point to the site of the pain. • **S**welling is the body's response to injury that makes the area larger than usual. It appears later and is due to fluid from inflammation and/or bleeding.

For extremity (arms and legs) injuries, check blood flow and nerves. Use the mnemonic CSM (circulation, sensation, movement) as a way of remembering what to do.

- **Circulation:** For an arm injury, feel for the radial pulse (located on the thumb side of the wrist). For a leg injury, feel for the posterior tibial pulse (located between the inside ankle bone and the Achilles tendon). An arm or leg without a pulse requires immediate surgical care.
- **Sensation:** Lightly touch or squeeze one of the victim's fingers or toes and ask the victim what he or she feels. Loss of sensation is an early sign of nerve damage.
- **Movement:** Inability to move develops later. Check for nerve damage by asking the victim to wiggle his or her fingers or toes. If the fingers or toes are injured, do not have the victim try to move them.

A quick nerve and circulatory check is very important. The tissues of the arms and legs cannot survive for more than 3 hours without a continuous blood supply. If you note any disruption in the nerve and blood supply, seek immediate medical care.

RICE Procedures

RICE is the acronym—rest, ice, compression, and elevation—for the treatment of all bone, joint, and muscle injuries. The steps taken in the first 48 to 72 hours after such an injury can help to relieve, and even prevent, aches and pains.

Treat all extremity bone, joint, and muscle injuries with the RICE procedures. In addition to RICE, fractures and dislocations should be stabilized against movement.

R: Rest

Injuries heal faster if rested. Rest means to stay off the injured part and avoid moving it. Using any part of the body increases the blood circulation to that area, which can cause more swelling of an injured part.

I: Ice

An ice pack should be applied to the injured area for 20 to 30 minutes every 2 or 3 hours during the first 24 to 48 hours. Skin treated with cold passes through four stages: cold, burning, aching, and numbness. When the skin becomes numb, usually in 20 to 30 minutes, remove the ice pack. After removing the ice pack, compress the injured part with an elastic bandage and keep it elevated (the "C" and "E" of RICE).

Cold constricts the blood vessels to and in the injured area, which helps reduce the swelling and inflammation. Cold should be applied as soon as possible after the injury—healing time often is directly related to the amount of swelling that occurs. Heat has the opposite effect when applied to fresh injuries: It increases circulation to the area and greatly increases both the swelling and the pain.

Put crushed ice (or cubes) into a double plastic bag or commercial ice bag. Place the ice pack directly on the skin and then use an elastic bandage to hold the ice pack in place. Ice bags can conform to the body's contours.

C: Compression

Compressing the injured area may squeeze some fluid and debris out of the injury site. Compression limits the ability of the skin and of other tissues to expand and reduces internal bleeding. Apply an elastic bandage to the injured area, especially the foot, ankle, knee, thigh, hand, or elbow. Fill the hollow areas with padding, such as a sock or washcloth, before applying the elastic bandage.

Start the elastic bandage several inches below the injury and wrap in an upward, overlapping spiral with an even, slightly tight pressure. Pale skin, pain, numbness, and tingling are signs that the bandage is too tight. If any of these appear, immediately remove the elastic bandage. Rewrap later when the symptoms disappear.

For a bruise or strain, place a pad between the injury and the elastic bandage.

E: Elevation

Elevating the injured area, in combination with ice and compression, limits circulation to an area, helps limit internal bleeding, and minimizes swelling.

Returning to Physical Activity After an Injury

Returning to physical activity is generally permissible once an injury is fully healed. Fully healed means:

- No pain
- No swelling
- No limping, favoring, or instability

Full rehabilitation means:

- Return of full range of motion and flexibility
- Muscle strength and endurance in the affected extremity (arm or leg) equal to that of the unaffected extremity
- Resumption of pre-injury endurance levels
- Good balance and coordination

Sometimes, clearance to return to exercising should come from a physician (e.g., after surgery).

Definitions

- **Contusions:** Bruising of tissue.
- **Strains:** Muscles are stretched or torn.
- **Sprains:** Tearing or stretching of the joints that causes mild to severe damage to the ligaments and joint capsules.
- **Dislocations:** Bones are displaced from their normal joint alignment, out of their sockets, or out of their normal positions.
- **Tendinitis:** Inflammation of a tendon from overuse.

Specific Injuries

Foot

Foot injuries are common among exercisers because of the foot's role in bearing weight. Careless treatment can have consequences that may include lifelong disability Table A.2 .

Ankle

Most ankle injuries are sprains. About 85% of sprains involve the ankle's outside (lateral) ligaments and are caused by having the foot turned or twisted inward. If not treated properly, a sprained ankle becomes chronically susceptible for future injuries. See Table A.3 for symptoms and treatment.

Lower Leg

The two bones of the lower leg are the tibia ("shin bone") and fibula. Most shin injuries are "shin splints," which are strains from overuse. Occasionally, a bone is fractured from overuse. See Table A.4 .

A

Table A.2   Determining and Treating Foot Injuries

If...	Then...
Pain is at top of the heel (over Achilles tendon) Pain is aggravated by activity—worse at beginning of activity and improved with warm-up	Suspect **Achilles tendinitis**: • Apply ice to decrease inflammation and pain. • Reduce or stop activity until no more pain occurs while either walking or resting. • Elevate heel with a heel cup or pads in the shoe. • Calf muscles should be stretched after warm-up and cool-down.
Pain is at back of the heel Injury resembles Achilles tendinitis	Suspect **retrocalcaneal bursitis**: Treat the same as for Achilles tendinitis.
Pain, often disabling, is at bottom of the heel	Suspect **plantar fasciitis**: • Apply ice for 20–30 minutes after activity and 3–4 times daily. • Use a heel cup in the shoe and shoes with good support. • Reduce or stop activity and avoid going barefoot.
Pain is in fifth metatarsal bone, possibly with swelling	Suspect **fracture** (Jones fracture): • Apply ice. • Stop activity. • Seek medical care.
Pain is on ball of foot between second and third toes or sometimes between second and third toes	Suspect **Morton's neuroma**: • Wear wider, more supportive, softer shoes. • If there is no improvement, surgery may be required.
Pain is on ball of foot at the big toe	Suspect **sesamoiditis or a stress fracture**: • Apply ice for 20–30 minutes, 3–4 times daily. • Rest. • If pain persists, seek medical care.
Area on skin has a "hot spot" (not very painful, red area) from rubbing	Suspect a **blister**: • Cool the hot spot with an ice pack. AND/OR • Tape several layers of moleskin, which are cut into a "doughnut shape" to fit around the blister. OR • Apply duct tape over the painful area.
Blister is broken and fluid is seeping out	• Leave the "roof" on for protection. • Clean with soap and water. • Tape several layers of moleskin, cut into a "doughnut shape" to fit around the blister. • Apply an antibiotic ointment in the hole over the blister. • Cover with an uncut gauze pad and tape in place.
Blister on foot is very painful, affects walking, and is not broken	• Drain the blister by puncturing the roof with several holes. • Leave the "roof" on for protection. • Clean with soap and water. • Tape several layers of moleskin, cut into a "doughnut shape" to fit around the blister. • Apply an antibiotic ointment in the hole over the blister. • Place gauze pad over the moleskin and tape in place.

Table A.3	Determining and Treating Ankle Injuries (Ottawa Ankle Rules)
If...	**Then...**
Ankle is able to bear weight He/she is able to take four steps immediately after the injury and an hour later No tenderness or pain is felt when you push on the ankle knob bone	Suspect **ankle sprain:** • Use RICE procedures. • For the compression part of RICE, apply an elastic bandage over any soft pliable material (e.g., sock or T-shirt) placed in a "U" shape around the ankle knob with the curved part down. • If pain and swelling do not decrease within 48 hours, seek medical care.
Ankle is unable to bear weight He/she is unable to take four steps immediately after the injury and an hour later Tenderness and pain is felt when you push on the ankle knob bone	Suspect **ankle fracture:** • Use RICE procedures. • For the compression part of RICE, apply an elastic bandage over any soft pliable material (e.g., sock or T-shirt) placed in a "U" shape around the ankle knob with the curved part down. • Stabilize ankle against movement. • Seek medical care.

Table A.4	Determining and Treating Lower Leg Injuries
If...	**Then...**
Shin aches during activity, but: • Ache subsides significantly after activity stops • Ache is result of increase in workout routine (e.g., running longer, jogging on hills) • Shin is tender when pressed	Suspect **shin splints** (medial tibial stress syndrome): • Apply ice before activity and for 30 minutes after activity. • Stop activity until pain free. • Stretch calves several times daily.
Leg receives direct hit that produces: deformity, open wound, tenderness, and/or swelling	Suspect **fracture or bruise:** • Use RICE procedures. • Control any bleeding. If fracture is suspected: • Stabilize leg against movement. • Seek medical care.
He/she feels a pop or sudden, sharp, burning pain in calf muscle while running or jumping	Suspect a **muscle strain** (tear, pull): • Use RICE procedures.
He/she feels a pop while running or jumping causing pain just above the heel Leg is tender when pressed He/she is unable to bear weight on injured leg He/she has difficulty with controlling foot (flops around)	Suspect a **torn Achilles tendon:** • Use RICE procedures. • Seek medical care.
A muscle (most often the calf muscle) goes into an uncontrolled spasm and contraction, resulting in severe pain and restriction or loss of movement	Suspect a **muscle cramp:** • Gently stretch the affected muscle, or • Relax the muscle by applying pressure to it. • Apply ice to the muscle. • Drink lightly salted cool water (dissolve ¼ teaspoon salt in a quart of water). Do not give salt tablets.

Knee

Knee injuries are among the most serious joint injuries ⬤ Table A.5 ⬤. Their severity is difficult to determine; thus you should seek medical care.

Thigh

The thigh consists of a single bone, the femur, which is surrounded and protected by heavy muscle. The muscle group on the front of the thigh is the "quadriceps." Most thigh injuries are from direct hits. As with other leg muscles, a quadriceps strain can happen. See ⬤ Table A.6 ⬤.

Table A.5	Determining and Treating Knee Injuries
If...	**Then...**
Immediate swelling occurs after injury Knee locks Knee gives way Pain occurs below kneecap Pain occurs under the kneecap when climbing stairs	Suspect **knee injury** (acute and/or chronic): • Use RICE procedures. • Stabilize knee against movement. • Seek medical care.
Examining for an acute injury (not overuse type of injury): **Pittsburgh Knee Rules:** Any blunt trauma or fall-type injury and one of the following present: • Age younger than 12 years or over 50 years • Inability to walk four weight-bearing steps OR **Ottawa Knee Rules:** • Age over 55 years • Tenderness at the patella (kneecap) • Tenderness at head of fibula (bony knob on outside of knee) • Inability to flex knee to 90° angle • Inability to bear weight and take four steps immediately after injury and later	Suspect serious **knee injury:** • Use RICE procedures. • Stabilize knee against movement. • Seek medical care.
Deformity obvious, with the kneecap (patella) usually on the outside (lateral side) of the knee. Compare it with the other kneecap.	Suspect a **dislocated kneecap:** • Apply ice. • Stabilize against movement. • Seek medical care.

Table A.6	Determining and Treating Thigh Injuries
If...	**Then...**
Pain at front of thigh	Suspect a **bruise:** • Use RICE procedures.
Pain at back of thigh	Suspect a **muscle strain** (pulled hamstring): • Use RICE procedures.

Hip

See **Table A.7** for information on how to determine and treat hip injuries.

Finger

Most finger injuries are not severe. In rare cases a finger can dislocate, producing a grotesque deformity that requires immediate medical care. See **Table A.8**.

Elbow

More often than not, elbow injuries are nagging nuisances. Occasionally an elbow will be more seriously injured. Rarely will an elbow dislocate. See **Table A.9**.

Shoulder

Shoulder injuries can range from mild to those that pose medical emergencies **Table A.10**. A dislocated shoulder usually occurs during contact sports and requires immediate medical care. A shoulder dislocation can be confused with a shoulder separation. The key difference is that in separation the shoulder joint and upper arm remain mobile. In dislocation, the mobility is lost.

Table A.7	Determining and Treating Hip Injuries
If...	**Then...**
Pain is in groin	Suspect **muscle strain:** • Use RICE procedures.
Pain is on upper hip	Suspect **hip pointer:** • Use RICE procedures.
Pain is on outer thigh to knee	Suspect **muscle strain or bursitis:** • Use RICE procedures.

Table A.8	Determining and Treating Finger Injuries
If...	**Then...**

Deformed
Tender/painful
Swollen
	Suspect a possible **fracture and/or dislocation:**
	• Test for a finger fracture:
	  – If possible, straighten the fingers and place them flat on a hard surface.
	  – Tap the tip of the injured finger toward the hand. Pain lower down in the finger or into the hand can indicate a fracture.
	• Do **not** try to realign a dislocation.
	• Apply ice.
	• Stabilize finger against movement by "buddy" taping for support.
	Or
	• Keeping hand and fingers in cupping shape as though holding a baseball with extra padding in the palm, secure the hand, fingers, and arm to a rigid board or folded newspapers.
	• Seek medical care.

Table A.9	Determining and Treating Elbow Injuries
If...	**Then...**
Severe elbow pain after fall on arm	Suspect **dislocation or fracture:** • Apply ice. • Stabilize against movement. • Seek medical care.
Elbow pain on inside (medial)	Suspect **"little league, golf, or racquetball" elbow:** • Use RICE procedures. • Gently stretch by placing palms together in front of face, and slowly lowering. • Seek medical care if pain persists.
Elbow pain on outside (lateral)	Suspect **"tennis" elbow:** • Use RICE procedures. • Seek medical care if pain persists.
Elbow with: • Tenderness/pain • Swelling	Suspect a **bruise:** • Use RICE procedures. • Seek medical care if tingling and/or weakness continue for 24 hours (can be serious because of possible nerve injury).

Table A.10	Determining and Treating Shoulder Injuries
If...	**Then...**
Pain is on top of shoulder after a fall or being hit	Suspect a **separation:** • Apply ice. • Seek medical care.
Extreme pain is at front of shoulder after a fall Victim holds upper arm away from the body, supported by the uninjured arm Arm cannot be brought across the chest to touch the opposite shoulder Victim describes a history of previous dislocations	Suspect a **dislocation:** • Apply ice. • Stabilize shoulder against movement and immediately seek medical care.
Burning pain is felt down arm after twisting neck	Suspect a **"stinger":** • Apply ice. • Seek medical care.
Arm goes limp	Suspect a **subluxation:** • Apply ice. • Seek medical care.
Pain is felt when raising arm	Suspect a **rotator cuff injury:** • Apply ice. • Seek medical care.

Muscle

See **Table A.11** for information on how to determine and treat muscle injuries.

Chest

See **Table A.12** for symptoms and treatment of chest injuries.

Breathing Difficulty

See **Table A.13** for information on how to determine and treat breathing difficulty.

Table A.11	Determining and Treating Muscle Injuries
If...	**Then...**
Muscle pain occurs 12 to 72+ hours after physical activity	Suspect **delayed-onset muscle soreness:** • Apply ice (some experts suggest heat). • Perform gentle active motion of the area. • Gently stretch the muscle. • Do not use nonsteroidal medications (e.g., ibuprofen, aspirin).

Table A.12	Determining and Treating Chest Injuries
If...	**Then...**
Sudden, severe central chest pain: • Can occur at rest • Worse when exerting • Pain is crushing, vice-like • May radiate up to the jaws or down the left arm Nausea Breathlessness Sweating Blueness of lips	Suspect a **heart attack:** 1. Give one aspirin to chew (not any other analgesic, only aspirin). 2. Seek medical care immediately—usually by calling 9-1-1. 3. Monitor for possible cardiac arrest requiring CPR. 4. Help victim into least painful position—usually sitting with legs bent at the knees. 5. Ask if he or she is taking a medication known as nitroglycerin; if so, help person take it.
No chest pain, but: • Sudden general tiredness • Breathlessness as a new symptom • Sudden worsening of existing breathlessness	Suspect a **silent heart attack:** • Treat as you would a heart attack.

Table A.13	Determining and Treating Breathing Difficulty
If...	**Then...**

Coughing
Wheezing, especially when breathing out
Chest feels "tight"
Sweating, breathless, rapid pulse
Neck muscles strain in an attempt to increase breathing
As attack worsens, blue lips, tiredness, drowsiness
Confusion, coma
Poor response to usual medication
	Suspect **asthma** (asthma can be induced during exercise):
	1. Place victim in a comfortable, upright position to help breathing.
	2. Help victim use medicines (inhaler and/or pills).
	3. Give plenty of fluids.
	4. Seek medical care if:
	  • No improvement within 2 hours after using medications.
	  • There are repeated attacks.
	  • Attack is severe and prolonged.

A

How Heat Affects the Body

Human bodies dissipate heat by varying the rate and depth of blood circulation, by losing water through the skin and sweat glands, and—when blood is heated above 98.6°F—by panting. The heart begins to pump more blood, blood vessels dilate to accommodate the increased flow, and the bundles of tiny capillaries threading through the upper layers of skin are put into operation. The body's blood is circulated closer to the skin's surface, and excess heat drains off into the cooler atmosphere. At the same time, water diffuses through the skin as perspiration. The skin handles about 90% of the body's heat dissipating function.

Sweating, on its own, does nothing to cool the body, unless the water is removed by evaporation—and high relative humidity retards evaporation. The evaporation process works this way: The heat energy required to evaporate sweat is extracted from the body, thereby cooling it. Under conditions of high temperature (above 90°F) and high relative humidity, the body is doing everything it can to maintain an internal temperature of 98.6°F. The heart is pumping a torrent of blood through dilated circulatory vessels; the sweat glands are pouring liquid—including essential dissolved chemicals, like sodium and chloride—onto the surface of the skin.

Too Much Heat

Heat disorders generally occur from a reduction or collapse of the body's ability to shed heat by circulatory changes and sweating, or a chemical (salt) imbalance caused by too much sweating. When heat gain exceeds the level the body can remove, or when the body cannot compensate for fluids and salt lost through perspiration, the temperature of the body's inner core begins to rise and heat-related illness may develop.

Heat illnesses include a range of disorders (**Table A.14**). Some of them are common, but only heatstroke is life threatening. Untreated heatstroke victims always die.

Ranging in severity, heat disorders share one common feature: The individual has been overexposed or has overexercised for his or her age and physical condition in the existing thermal environment.

Studies indicate that, other factors being equal, the severity of heat disorders tends to increase with age—heat cramps in a 17-year-old may be heat exhaustion in a 40-year-old, and heatstroke in a person over age 60.

Acclimatization concerns adjusting the sweat–salt concentration, among other things. The idea is to lose enough water to regulate body temperature, with the least possible chemical disturbance.

The heat index (or apparent temperature) is how the heat and humidity in the air combine to make us feel (**Figure A.1**). Higher humidity plus higher temperatures often combine to make us feel a perceived temperature that is higher than the actual air temperature. The old saying, "It's not the heat, it's the humidity," holds true.

The National Weather Service is using a new "mean heat index" to alert people to the dangers of heat waves. The index, which went into use in May 2002, measures how hot a person will feel over a full day.

The idea is the same as the traditional heat index, which shows how hot a particular combination of heat and humidity feels. This index has usually been used to show the danger during the hottest part of the day.

The mean heat index averages the heat index from the hottest and coolest parts of a day.

Table A.14   Determining and Treating Heat-Related Illnesses

If...	Then...

Skin is extremely hot when touched—usually dry, but may be moist
Altered mental status, ranging from slight confusion, agitation, and disorientation to unresponsiveness
	Suspect **heatstroke:**
	Heatstroke is life threatening and must be treated immediately.
	1. Move victim to a cool place. Monitor breathing.
	2. Remove clothing down to victim's underwear.
	3. Keep victim's head and shoulders slightly raised.
	4. Quickly cool the victim:
	  • Spray the victim with water and vigorously fan. This method does not work well in high humidity.
	  • If ice is available, place ice packs into the armpits, sides of the neck, and groin.
	5. Stop cooling when mental status improves or if shivering occurs.
	6. Evacuate to medical care ASAP. Continue cooling during evacuation.

Sweating Thirsty Fatigued Flu-like symptoms—headache, nausea Shortness of breath Rapid pulse Differences from heatstroke: • No altered mental status • Skin is not hot, but clammy	Suspect **heat exhaustion:** Uncontrolled heat exhaustion can evolve into heatstroke. 1. Move victim to a cool place. 2. Have the victim remove excess clothing. 3. Have the victim drink cool fluids. 4. For more severe cases, give lightly salted cool water (dissolve ¼ teaspoon salt in a quart of water). Do not give salt tablets. 5. Raise victim's legs 8 to 12 inches (keep legs straight). 6. Cool the victim, but not as aggressively as for heatstroke. 7. If no improvement is seen within 30 minutes, seek medical care.
Painful muscle spasms that happen suddenly Affects muscle in the back of the leg or abdominal muscles Occurs during or after physical exertion	Suspect **heat cramp:** Relief may take several hours. 1. Have victim rest in a cool area. 2. Have victim drink lightly salted cool water (dissolve ¼ teaspoon salt in 1 quart of water) or a commercial sports drink. Do not give salt tablets. 3. Have victim stretch the cramped calf muscle or try acupressure method of pinching the upper lip just below the nose.
Victim is dizzy or faints	Suspect **heat syncope:** 1. If victim is unresponsive, check for breathing. Person usually recovers quickly. 2. If victim fell, check for injuries. 3. Have victim rest and lie down with legs raised in cool area. 4. Wet skin by splashing water on face. 5. If not nauseated, have victim drink lightly salted cool water (dissolve ¼ teaspoon salt in 1 quart of water) or a commercial sports drink. Do not give salt tablets.
Ankles and feet swell Occurs during first few days in a hot environment	Suspect **heat edema:** 1. Have victim wear support stockings. 2. Elevate legs.
Itchy rash on skin wet from sweating	Suspect **prickly heat:** 1. Dry and cool skin. 2. Limit heat exposure.

Relative Humidity (%)

°F (Air Temperature)	40	45	50	55	60	65	70	75	80	85	90	95	100
110	136												
108	130	137											
106	124	130	137										
104	119	124	131	137									
102	114	119	124	130	137								
100	109	114	118	124	139	136							
98	106	109	113	117	123	128	134						
96	101	104	108	112	116	121	126	132					
94	97	100	101	106	110	114	118	124	129	135			
92	94	96	99	101	105	108	112	116	121	125	131		
90	91	93	95	97	100	103	106	109	113	117	122	127	132
88	88	89	91	93	95	98	100	100	106	110	113	114	121
86	85	87	88	89	91	93	95	97	100	102	105	108	112
84	83	84	85	86	88	89	90	92	94	96	98	100	103
82	81	82	83	84	84	85	86	88	89	90	91	93	95
80	80	80	81	81	82	82	83	84	84	85	86	86	87

Heat Index (Apparent Temperature)

With Prolonged Exposure and/or Physical Activity
Extreme Danger
Heatstroke or sunstroke highly likely
Danger
Sunstroke, muscle cramps, and/or heat exhaustion likely
Extreme Caution
Sunstroke, muscle cramps, and/or heat exhaustion possible
Caution
Fatigue possible

Figure A.1

The heat index (or apparent temperature) shows how heat and humidity affect the human body. (*Source:* Courtesy of the National Weather Service.)

Sunburn

Sunburn, with its ultraviolet radiation burns, can significantly retard the skin's ability to shed excess heat.

See Table A.15 for information on how to determine and treat sunburns.

Table A.15 Determining and Treating Sunburns

If...	Then...
Skin that has been exposed to the sun later becomes: • Red • Mildly swollen • Tender and painful	Suspect **first-degree (superficial) sunburn:** 1. Immerse burned area in cold water or apply a wet, cold cloth until pain free, both in and out of the water (usually 10–45 minutes). If cold water is unavailable, use any cold liquid available. 2. Give ibuprofen (for children, give acetaminophen). 3. Have victim drink water. 4. Keep burned arm or leg raised. 5. After burn has been cooled, apply aloe vera gel or inexpensive moisturizer. First-degree burns do **not** have to be covered.
Skin that has been exposed to the sun later becomes: • Blistered • Swollen • Weeping of fluids • Severely painful	Suspect **second-degree (partial-thickness) sunburn:** • If skin affected is less than 20% of the body surface (victim's palm, not including fingers and thumb, equals 1% of body surface area): 1. Follow same procedures (steps 1–4) as for a first-degree burn, with these additions: a. After burn has been cooled, apply thin layer of antibacterial ointment (e.g., bacitracin, Neosporin). b. Cover burn with a dry, nonsticking, sterile dressing or clean cloth. • If skin has a large second-degree burn over more than 20% of the body surface area: 1. Follow steps 2–4 of first-degree burn care. 2. Seek medical care. Do **not** apply cold because it may cause hypothermia.

Cold-Related Injuries

Hypothermia

Hypothermia happens when the body's temperature (98.6°F, 37°C) drops more than 2 degrees (Table A.16). Hypothermia does not require subfreezing temperatures. Severe hypothermia is life threatening. Check also for possible frostbite.

Table A.16	Determining and Treating Hypothermia
If...	**Then...**

Shivering uncontrollably
Has the "umbles"—grumbles, mumbles, fumbles, and stumbles
Has cool abdomen when felt with a warm hand
	Suspect **mild hypothermia**:
	1. Stop heat loss:
	  • Get victim out of the cold.
	  • Handle victim gently.
	  • Replace wet clothing with dry clothing.
	  • Add insulation (e.g., blankets, towels, pillows, sleeping bags) beneath and around victim. Cover victim's head (50%–80% of body's heat loss is through the head).
	2. Keep in flat (horizontal) position.
	3. Allow the victim to shiver—do not stop the shivering by adding heat. Shivering, which generates heat, will rewarm mildly hypothermic victims. DO NOT use the following procedures because they stop shivering:
	  • Warm water immersion
	  • Body-to-body contact
	  • Chemical heat pads
	Warm drinks are unable to rewarm sufficiently. However, warm sugary liquids can provide calories for shivering to continue and may provide a psychological boost.
	DO NOT give alcohol to drink.

Muscles are rigid and stiff No shivering Skin feels ice cold and appears blue Altered mental status Slow pulse Slow breathing Victim appears to be dead	Suspect **severe hypothermia**: 1. Follow steps 1 and 2 from mild hypothermia for all hypothermic victims. 2. Check for breathing and give CPR as necessary. Gently evacuate victim to medical help for rewarming. Rewarming in a remote location is difficult and rarely effective. However, when the victim is far from medical care, the victim must be warmed by any available external heat source (e.g., body-to-body contact, warm water immersion).

Frostbite and Frostnip

Frostbite happens only in below-freezing temperatures (less than 32°F) **Figure A.2**. Mainly the feet, hands, ears, and nose are affected. The most severe results are gangrene requiring surgical amputation. See **Table A.17** for symptoms and treatment. Check for hypothermia, because it may also be present.

Frostnip is caused when water on the skin's surface freezes **Table A.18**.

Wind Chill Chart

Wind (mph)

Calm	5	10	15	20	25	30	35	40	45	50	55	60
40	36	34	32	30	29	28	28	27	26	26	25	25
35	31	27	25	24	23	22	21	20	19	19	18	17
30	25	21	19	17	16	15	14	13	12	12	11	10
25	19	15	13	11	9	8	7	6	5	4	4	3
20	13	9	6	4	3	1	0	−1	−2	−3	−3	−4
15	7	3	0	−2	−4	−5	−7	−8	−9	−10	−11	−11
10	1	−4	−7	−9	−11	−12	−14	−15	−16	−17	−18	−19
5	−5	−10	−13	−15	−17	−19	−21	−22	−23	−24	−25	−26
0	−11	−16	−19	−22	−24	−26	−27	−29	−30	−31	−32	−33
−5	−16	−22	−26	−29	−31	−33	−34	−36	−37	−38	−39	−40
−10	−22	−28	−32	−35	−37	−39	−41	−43	−44	−45	−46	−48
−15	−28	−35	−39	−42	−44	−46	−48	−50	−51	−52	−54	−55
−20	−34	−41	−45	−48	−51	−53	−55	−57	−58	−60	−61	−62
−25	−40	−47	−51	−55	−58	−60	−62	−64	−65	−67	−68	−69
−30	−46	−53	−58	−61	−64	−67	−69	−71	−72	−74	−75	−76
−35	−52	−59	−64	−68	−71	−73	−76	−78	−79	−81	−82	−84
−40	−57	−66	−71	−74	−78	−80	−82	−84	−86	−88	−89	−91
−45	−63	−72	−77	−81	−84	−87	−89	−91	−93	−95	−97	−98

Temperature (°F)

Note: Frostbite occurs in 15 minutes or less.

$$\text{Wind Chill (°F)} = 35.74 + 0.6215T - 35.75(V^{0.16}) + 0.4275T(V^{0.16})$$

Where T = Air Temperature (°F)

V = Wind Speed (mph)

Figure A.2

Wind chill chart. (*Source:* Courtesy of the National Weather Service.)

Table A.17 — Determining and Treating Frostbite

If...	Then...	
Skin color is white, waxy, or grayish-yellow Affected part is cold and numb Tingling, stinging, or aching sensation is felt Skin surface feels stiff or crusty, and underlying tissue feels soft when depressed gently	Suspect **superficial frostbite**	All frostbite injuries require the same first-aid treatment: 1. Get victim to a warm area. 2. Replace wet clothing or constricting items that could impair blood circulation (e.g., rings). 3. Do not rub or massage the area. 4. For deep frostbite, seek medical care. 5. When more than 1 hour from medical facility, place part in warm water (test by pouring some over the inside of your arm to test that it is warm, not hot). For ear or face, it is best but may be difficult to apply warm moist cloths, changing them frequently. May have to cover with warm hands. Give pain medication (preferably aspirin or ibuprofen). Rewarming may take 20 to 40 minutes or when parts become soft. **DO NOT:** • Rub or massage part. • Rewarm with stove, vehicle's tailpipe exhaust, or over a fire. • Break blisters.
Affected part feels cold, hard, and solid, and cannot be depressed—feels like a piece of wood or frozen meat Affected part is pale, and skin may appear waxy A painfully cold part suddenly stops hurting Blisters appear after rewarming	Suspect **deep frostbite**	• Allow victim to smoke or drink alcohol. • Rewarm if there is any possibility of refreezing. • Allow thawed part to refreeze. After thawing: • Place dry, sterile gauze between toes and fingers to prevent sticking. • Elevate part to reduce pain and swelling. • Give aspirin or ibuprofen for pain and inflammation. Do not give to children. • Apply thin layer of aloe vera on area. • Seek medical care.

Table A.18 — Determining and Treating Frostnip

If...	Then...
Skin appears red and sometimes swollen Painful	Suspect **frostnip** (it is difficult to tell the difference between frostnip and frostbite): 1. Gently warm area against a warm body part (e.g., armpit, stomach, bare hands) or by blowing warm air on the area. 2. Do not rub area.

Dietary Reference Intakes (DRIs)

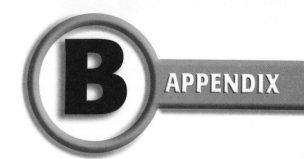

Dietary Reference Intakes (DRIs): Recommended Dietary Allowances and Adequate Intakes, Vitamins
Food and Nutrition Board, Institute of Medicine, National Academies

Life Stage Group	Vitamin A (µg/d)[a]	Vitamin C (mg/d)	Vitamin D (µg/d)[b,c]	Vitamin E (mg/d)[d]	Vitamin E (mg/d)[d]	Thiamin (mg/d)	Riboflavin (mg/d)	Niacin (mg/d)[e]	Vitamin B6 (mg/d)	Folate (µg/d)[f]	Vitamin B12 (µg/d)	Pantothenic Acid (mg/d)	Biotin (µg/d)	Choline (mg/d)[g]
Infants														
0–6 mo	400*	40*	10	4*	2.0*	0.2*	0.3*	2*	0.1*	65*	0.4*	1.7*	5*	125*
6–12 mo	500*	50*	10	5*	2.5*	0.3*	0.4*	4*	0.3*	80*	0.5*	1.8*	6*	150*
Children														
1–3 y	300	15	15	6	30*	0.5	0.5	6	0.5	150	0.9	2*	8*	200*
4–8 y	400	25	15	7	55*	0.6	0.6	8	0.6	200	1.2	3*	12*	250*
Males														
9–13 y	600	45	15	11	60*	0.9	0.9	12	1.0	300	1.8	4*	20*	375*
14–18 y	900	75	15	15	75*	1.2	1.3	16	1.3	400	2.4	5*	25*	550*
19–30 y	900	90	15	15	120*	1.2	1.3	16	1.3	400	2.4	5*	30*	550*
31–50 y	900	90	15	15	120*	1.2	1.3	16	1.3	400	2.4	5*	30*	550*
51–70 y	900	90	15	15	120*	1.2	1.3	16	1.7	400	2.4[h]	5*	30*	550*
>70 y	900	90	20	15	120*	1.2	1.3	16	1.7	400	2.4[h]	5*	30*	550*
Females														
9–13 y	600	45	15	11	60*	0.9	0.9	12	1.0	300	1.8	4*	20*	375*
14–18 y	700	65	15	15	75*	1.0	1.0	14	1.2	400[i]	2.4	5*	25*	400*
19–30 y	700	75	15	15	90*	1.1	1.1	14	1.3	400[i]	2.4	5*	30*	425*
31–50 y	700	75	15	15	90*	1.1	1.1	14	1.3	400[i]	2.4	5*	30*	425*
51–70 y	700	75	15	15	90*	1.1	1.1	14	1.5	400	2.4[h]	5*	30*	425*
>70 y	700	75	20	15	90*	1.1	1.1	14	1.5	400	2.4[h]	5*	30*	425*
Pregnancy														
14–18 y	750	80	15	15	75*	1.4	1.4	18	1.9	600[j]	2.6	6*	30*	450*
19–30 y	770	85	15	15	90*	1.4	1.4	18	1.9	600[j]	2.6	6*	30*	450*
31–50 y	770	85	15	15	90*	1.4	1.4	18	1.9	600[j]	2.6	6*	30*	450*

continues

B

Dietary Reference Intakes (DRIs): Recommended Dietary Allowances and Adequate Intakes, Vitamins, *continued*
Food and Nutrition Board, Institute of Medicine, National Academies

Life Stage Group	Vitamin A (μg/d)[a]	Vitamin C (mg/d)	Vitamin D (μg/d)[b,c]	Vitamin E (mg/d)[d]	Vitamin E (mg/d)[d]	Thiamin (mg/d)	Riboflavin (mg/d)	Niacin (mg/d)[e]	Vitamin B6 (mg/d)	Folate (μg/d)[f]	Vitamin B12 (μg/d)	Pantothenic Acid (mg/d)	Biotin (μg/d)	Choline (mg/d)[g]
Lactation
14–18 y	1,200	115	15	19	75*	1.4	1.6	17	2.0	500	2.8	7*	35*	550*
19–30 y	1,300	120	15	19	90*	1.4	1.6	17	2.0	500	2.8	7*	35*	550*
31–50 y	1,300	120	15	19	90*	1.4	1.6	17	2.0	500	2.8	7*	35*	550*

NOTE: This table (taken from the DRI reports, see www.nap.edu) presents Recommended Dietary Allowances (RDAs) in **bold type** and Adequate Intakes (AIs) in ordinary type followed by an asterisk (*). An RDA is the average daily dietary intake level; sufficient to meet the nutrient requirements of nearly all (97–98 percent) healthy individuals in a group. It is calculated from an Estimated Average Requirement (EAR). If sufficient scientific evidence is not available to establish an EAR, and thus calculate an RDA, an AI is usually developed. For healthy breastfed infants, an AI is the mean intake. The AI for other life stage and gender groups is believed to cover the needs of all healthy individuals in the groups, but lack of data or uncertainty in the data prevent being able to specify with confidence the percentage of individuals covered by this intake.

[a]As retinol activity equivalents (RAEs). 1 RAE = 1 μg retinol, 12 μg β-carotene, 24 μg α-carotene, or 24 μg β-cryptoxanthin. The RAE for dietary provitamin A carotenoids is two-fold greater than retinol equivalents (RE), whereas the RAE for preformed vitamin A is the same as RE.

[b]As cholecalciferol. 1 μg cholecalciferol = 40 IU vitamin D.

[c]Under the assumption of minimal sunlight.

[d]As α-tocopherol. α-Tocopherol includes *RRR*-α-tocopherol, the only form of α-tocopherol that occurs naturally in foods, and the *2R*-stereoisomeric forms of α-tocopherol (*RRR*-, *RSR*-, *RRS*-, and *RSS*-α-tocopherol) that occur in fortified foods and supplements. It does not include the *2S*-stereoisomeric forms of α-tocopherol (*SRR*-, *SSR*-, *SRS*-, and *SSS*- α-tocopherol), also found in fortified foods and supplements.

[e]As niacin equivalents (NE). 1 mg of niacin = 60 mg of tryptophan; 0–6 months = preformed niacin (not NE).

[f]As dietary folate equivalents (DFE). 1 DFE = 1 μg food folate = 0.6 μg of folic acid from fortified food or as a supplement consumed with food = 0.5 μg of a supplement taken on an empty stomach.

[g]Although AIs have been set for choline, there are few data to assess whether a dietary supply of choline is needed at all stages of the life cycle, and it may be that the choline requirement can be met by endogenous synthesis at some of these stages.

[h]Because 10 to 30 percent of older people may malabsorb food-bound B12, it is advisable for those older than 50 years to meet their RDA mainly by consuming foods fortified with B12 or a supplement containing B12.

[i]In view of evidence linking folate intake with neural tube defects in the fetus, it is recommended that all women capable of becoming pregnant consume 400 μg from supplements or fortified foods in addition to intake of food folate from a varied diet.

[j]It is assumed that women will continue consuming 400 μg from supplements or fortified food until their pregnancy is confirmed and they enter prenatal care, which ordinarily occurs after the end of the periconceptional period—the critical time for formation of the neural tube.

SOURCE: Reprinted with permission from Dietary Reference Intakes, 2011 by the National Academy of Sciences. Courtesy of the National Academies Press.

Dietary Reference Intakes (DRIs): Recommended Dietary Allowances and Adequate Intakes, Elements

Food and Nutrition Board, Institute of Medicine, National Academies

Life Stage Group	Calcium (mg/d)	Chromium (µg/d)	Copper (µg/d)	Fluoride (mg/d)	Iodine (µg/d)	Iron (mg/d)	Magnesium (mg/d)	Manganese (mg/d)	Molybdenum (µg/d)	Phosphorus (mg/d)	Selenium (µg/d)	Zinc (mg/d)	Potassium (g/d)	Sodium (g/d)	Chloride (g/d)
Infants															
0–6 mo	200*	0.2*	200*	0.01*	110*	0.27*	30*	0.003*	2*	100*	15*	2*	0.4*	0.12*	0.18*
6–12 mo	260*	5.5*	220*	0.5*	130*	11	75*	0.6*	3*	275*	20*	3	0.7*	0.37*	0.57*
Children															
1–3 y	**700**	11*	**340**	0.7*	**90**	**7**	**80**	1.2*	**17**	**460**	**20**	**3**	3.0*	1.0*	1.5*
4–8 y	**1,000**	15*	**440**	1*	**90**	**10**	**130**	1.5*	**22**	**500**	**30**	**5**	3.8*	1.2*	1.9*
Males															
9–13 y	**1,300**	25*	**700**	2*	**120**	**8**	**240**	1.9*	**34**	**1,250**	**40**	**8**	4.5*	1.5*	2.3*
14–18 y	**1,300**	35*	**890**	3*	**150**	**11**	**410**	2.2*	**43**	**1,250**	**55**	**11**	4.7*	1.5*	2.3*
19–30 y	**1,000**	35*	**900**	4*	**150**	**8**	**400**	2.3*	**45**	**700**	**55**	**11**	4.7*	1.5*	2.3*
31–50 y	**1,000**	35*	**900**	4*	**150**	**8**	**420**	2.3*	**45**	**700**	**55**	**11**	4.7*	1.5*	2.3*
51–70 y	**1,000**	30*	**900**	4*	**150**	**8**	**420**	2.3*	**45**	**700**	**55**	**11**	4.7*	1.3*	2.0*
>70 y	**1,200**	30*	**900**	4*	**150**	**8**	**420**	2.3*	**45**	**700**	**55**	**11**	4.7*	1.2*	1.8*
Females															
9–13 y	**1,300**	21*	**700**	2*	**120**	**8**	**240**	1.6*	**34**	**1,250**	**40**	**8**	4.5*	1.5*	2.3*
14–18 y	**1,300**	24*	**890**	3*	**150**	**15**	**360**	1.6*	**43**	**1,250**	**55**	**9**	4.7*	1.5*	2.3*
19–30 y	**1,000**	25*	**900**	3*	**150**	**8**	**310**	1.8*	**45**	**700**	**55**	**8**	4.7*	1.5*	2.3*
31–50 y	**1,000**	25*	**900**	3*	**150**	**18**	**320**	1.8*	**45**	**700**	**55**	**8**	4.7*	1.5*	2.3*
51–70 y	**1,200**	20*	**900**	3*	**150**	**8**	**320**	1.8*	**45**	**700**	**55**	**8**	4.7*	1.3*	2.0*
>70 y	**1,200**	20*	**900**	3*	**150**	**8**	**320**	1.8*	**45**	**700**	**55**	**8**	4.7*	1.2*	1.8*
Pregnancy															
14–18 y	**1,300**	29*	**1,000**	3*	**220**	**27**	**400**	2.0*	**50**	**1,250**	**60**	**12**	4.7*	1.5*	2.3*
19–30 y	**1,000**	30*	**1,000**	3*	**220**	**27**	**350**	2.0*	**50**	**700**	**60**	**11**	4.7*	1.5*	2.3*
31–50 y	**1,000**	30*	**1,000**	3*	**220**	**27**	**360**	2.0*	**50**	**700**	**60**	**11**	4.7*	1.5*	2.3*
Lactation															
14–18 y	**1,300**	44*	**1,300**	3*	**290**	**10**	**360**	2.6*	**50**	**1,250**	**70**	**13**	5.1*	1.5*	2.3*
19–30 y	**1,000**	45*	**1,300**	3*	**290**	**9**	**310**	2.6*	**50**	**700**	**70**	**12**	5.1*	1.5*	2.3*
31–50 y	**1,000**	45*	**1,300**	3*	**290**	**9**	**320**	2.6*	**50**	**700**	**70**	**12**	5.1*	1.5*	2.3*

NOTE: This table (taken from the DRI reports, see www.nap.edu) presents Recommended Dietary Allowances (RDAs) in **bold type** and Adequate Intakes (AIs) in ordinary type followed by an asterisk (*). An RDA is the average daily dietary intake level; sufficient to meet the nutrient requirements of nearly all (97–98 percent) healthy individuals in a group. It is calculated from an Estimated Average Requirement (EAR). If sufficient scientific evidence is not available to establish an EAR, and thus calculate an RDA, an AI is usually developed. For healthy breastfed infants, an AI is the mean intake. The AI for other life stage and gender groups is believed to cover the needs of all healthy individuals in the groups, but lack of data or uncertainty in the data prevent being able to specify with confidence the percentage of individuals covered by this intake.

SOURCE: Reprinted with permission from Dietary Reference Intakes, 2011 by the National Academy of Sciences. Courtesy of the National Academies Press.

B

Dietary Reference Intakes (DRIs): Tolerable Upper Intake Levels, Vitamins
Food and Nutrition Board, Institute of Medicine, National Academies

Life Stage Group	Vitamin A (µg/d)[a]	Vitamin C (mg/d)	Vitamin D (µg/d)	Vitamin E (mg/d)[b,c]	Vitamin K	Thiamin	Riboflavin	Niacin (mg/d)[c]	Vitamin B$_6$ (mg/d)	Folate (µg/d)[c]	Vitamin B$_{12}$	Pantothenic Acid	Biotin	Choline (g/d)	Carotenoids[d]
Infants															
0–6 mo	600	ND[e]	25	ND	ND	ND	ND	ND	ND	ND	ND	ND	ND	ND	ND
6–12 mo	600	ND	38	ND	ND	ND	ND	ND	ND	ND	ND	ND	ND	ND	ND
Children															
1–3 y	600	400	63	200	ND	ND	ND	10	30	300	ND	ND	ND	1.0	ND
4–8 y	900	650	75	300	ND	ND	ND	15	40	400	ND	ND	ND	1.0	ND
Males															
9–13 y	1,700	1,200	100	600	ND	ND	ND	20	60	600	ND	ND	ND	2.0	ND
14–18 y	2,800	1,800	100	800	ND	ND	ND	30	80	800	ND	ND	ND	3.0	ND
19–30 y	3,000	2,000	100	1,000	ND	ND	ND	35	100	1,000	ND	ND	ND	3.5	ND
31–50 y	3,000	2,000	100	1,000	ND	ND	ND	35	100	1,000	ND	ND	ND	3.5	ND
51–70 y	3,000	2,000	100	1,000	ND	ND	ND	35	100	1,000	ND	ND	ND	3.5	ND
>70 y	3,000	2,000	100	1,000	ND	ND	ND	35	100	1,000	ND	ND	ND	3.5	ND
Females															
9–13 y	1,700	1,200	100	600	ND	ND	ND	20	60	600	ND	ND	ND	2.0	ND
14–18 y	2,800	1,800	100	800	ND	ND	ND	30	80	800	ND	ND	ND	3.0	ND
19–30 y	3,000	2,000	100	1,000	ND	ND	ND	35	100	1,000	ND	ND	ND	3.5	ND
31–50 y	3,000	2,000	100	1,000	ND	ND	ND	35	100	1,000	ND	ND	ND	3.5	ND
51–70 y	3,000	2,000	100	1,000	ND	ND	ND	35	100	1,000	ND	ND	ND	3.5	ND
>70 y	3,000	2,000	100	1,000	ND	ND	ND	35	100	1,000	ND	ND	ND	3.5	ND
Pregnancy															
14–18 y	2,800	1,800	100	800	ND	ND	ND	30	80	800	ND	ND	ND	3.0	ND
19–30 y	3,000	2,000	100	1,000	ND	ND	ND	35	100	1,000	ND	ND	ND	3.5	ND
31–50 y	3,000	2,000	100	1,000	ND	ND	ND	35	100	1,000	ND	ND	ND	3.5	ND
Lactation															
14–18 y	2,800	1,800	100	800	ND	ND	ND	30	80	800	ND	ND	ND	3.0	ND
19–30 y	3,000	2,000	100	1,000	ND	ND	ND	35	100	1,000	ND	ND	ND	3.5	ND
31–50 y	3,000	2,000	100	1,000	ND	ND	ND	35	100	1,000	ND	ND	ND	3.5	ND

NOTE: A Tolerable Upper Intake Level (UL) is the highest level of daily nutrient intake that is likely to pose no risk of adverse health effects to almost all individuals in the general population. Unless otherwise specified, the UL represents total intake from food, water, and supplements. Due to a lack of suitable data, ULs could not be established for vitamin K, thiamin, riboflavin, vitamin B$_{12}$, pantothenic acid, biotin, and carotenoids. In the absence of a UL, extra caution may be warranted in consuming levels above recommended intakes. Members of the general population should be advised not to routinely exceed the UL. The UL is not meant to apply to individuals who are treated with the nutrient under medical supervision or to individuals with predisposing conditions that modify their sensitivity to the nutrient.

[a]As preformed vitamin A only.
[b]As α-tocopherol; applies to any form of supplemental α-tocopherol.
[c]The ULs for vitamin E, niacin, and folate apply to synthetic forms obtained from supplements, fortified foods, or a combination of the two.
[d]β-carotene supplements are advised only to serve as a provitamin A source for individuals at risk of vitamin A deficiency.
[e]ND = Not determinable due to lack of data of adverse effects in this age group and concern with regard to lack of ability to handle excess amounts. Source of intake should be from food only to prevent high levels of intake.

SOURCE: Reprinted with permission from Dietary Reference Intakes, 2011 by the National Academy of Sciences. Courtesy of the National Academies Press.

Dietary Reference Intakes (DRIs): Tolerable Upper Intake Levels, Elements

Food and Nutrition Board, Institute of Medicine, National Academies

Life Stage Group	Arsenic[a]	Boron (mg/d)	Calcium (mg/d)	Chromium	Copper (µg/d)	Fluoride (mg/d)	Iodine (µg/d)	Iron (mg/d)	Magnesium (mg/d)[b]	Manganese (mg/d)	Molybdenum (µg/d)	Nickel (mg/d)	Phosphorus (g/d)	Selenium (µg/d)	Silicon[c]	Vanadium (mg/d)[d]	Zinc (mg/d)	Sodium (g/d)	Chloride (g/d)
Infants																			
0–6 mo	ND[e]	ND	1,000	ND	ND	0.7	ND	40	ND	ND	ND	ND	ND	45	ND	ND	4	ND	ND
6–12 mo	ND	ND	1,500	ND	ND	0.9	ND	40	ND	ND	ND	ND	ND	60	ND	ND	5	ND	ND
Children																			
1–3 y	ND	3	2,500	ND	1,000	1.3	200	40	65	2	300	0.2	3	90	ND	ND	7	1.5	2.3
4–8 y	ND	6	2,500	ND	3,000	2.2	300	40	110	3	600	0.3	3	150	ND	ND	12	1.9	2.9
Males																			
9–13 y	ND	11	3,000	ND	5,000	10	600	40	350	6	1,100	0.6	4	280	ND	ND	23	2.2	3.4
14–18 y	ND	17	3,000	ND	8,000	10	900	45	350	9	1,700	1.0	4	400	ND	ND	34	2.3	3.6
19–30 y	ND	20	2,500	ND	10,000	10	1,100	45	350	11	2,000	1.0	4	400	ND	1.8	40	2.3	3.6
31–50 y	ND	20	2,500	ND	10,000	10	1,100	45	350	11	2,000	1.0	4	400	ND	1.8	40	2.3	3.6
51–70 y	ND	20	2,000	ND	10,000	10	1,100	45	350	11	2,000	1.0	4	400	ND	1.8	40	2.3	3.6
>70 y	ND	20	2,000	ND	10,000	10	1,100	45	350	11	2,000	1.0	3	400	ND	1.8	40	2.3	3.6
Females																			
9–13 y	ND	11	3,000	ND	5,000	10	600	40	350	6	1,100	0.6	4	280	ND	ND	23	2.2	3.4
14–18 y	ND	17	3,000	ND	8,000	10	900	45	350	9	1,700	1.0	4	400	ND	ND	34	2.3	3.6
19–30 y	ND	20	2,500	ND	10,000	10	1,100	45	350	11	2,000	1.0	4	400	ND	1.8	40	2.3	3.6
31–50 y	ND	20	2,500	ND	10,000	10	1,100	45	350	11	2,000	1.0	4	400	ND	1.8	40	2.3	3.6
51–70 y	ND	20	2,000	ND	10,000	10	1,100	45	350	11	2,000	1.0	4	400	ND	1.8	40	2.3	3.6
>70 y	ND	20	2,000	ND	10,000	10	1,100	45	350	11	2,000	1.0	3	400	ND	1.8	40	2.3	3.6
Pregnancy																			
14–18 y	ND	17	3,000	ND	8,000	10	900	45	350	9	1,700	1.0	3.5	400	ND	ND	34	2.3	3.6
19–30 y	ND	20	2,500	ND	10,000	10	1,100	45	350	11	2,000	1.0	3.5	400	ND	ND	40	2.3	3.6
61–50 y	ND	20	2,500	ND	10,000	10	1,100	45	350	11	2,000	1.0	3.5	400	ND	ND	40	2.3	3.6

continues

Dietary Reference Intakes (DRIs): Tolerable Upper Intake Levels, Elements, *continued*
Food and Nutrition Board, Institute of Medicine, National Academies

Life Stage Group	Arsenic[a]	Boron (mg/d)	Calcium (mg/d)	Chromium	Copper (µg/d)	Fluoride (mg/d)	Iodine (µg/d)	Iron (mg/d)	Magnesium (mg/d)[b]	Manganese (mg/d)	Molybdenum (µg/d)	Nickel (mg/d)	Phosphorus (g/d)	Selenium (µg/d)	Silicon[c]	Vanadium (mg/d)[d]	Zinc (mg/d)	Sodium (g/d)	Chloride (g/d)
Lactation																			
14–18 y	ND	17	3,000	ND	8,000	10	900	45	350	9	1,700	1.0	4	400	ND	ND	34	2.3	3.6
19–30 y	ND	20	2,500	ND	10,000	10	1,100	45	350	11	2,000	1.0	4	400	ND	ND	40	2.3	3.6
31–50 y	ND	20	2,500	ND	10,000	10	1,100	45	350	11	2,000	1.0	4	400	ND	ND	40	2.3	3.6

NOTE: A Tolerable Upper Intake Level (UL) is the highest level of daily nutrient intake that is likely to pose no risk of adverse health effects to almost all individuals in the general population. Unless otherwise specified, the UL represents total intake from food, water, and supplements. Due to a lack of suitable data, ULs could not be established for vitamin K, thiamin, riboflavin, vitamin B_{12}, pantothenic acid, biotin, and carotenoids. In the absence of a UL, extra caution may be warranted in consuming levels above recommended intakes. Members of the general population should be advised not to routinely exceed the UL. The UL is not meant to apply to individuals who are treated with the nutrient under medical supervision or to individuals with predisposing conditions that modify their sensitivity to the nutrient.

[a]Although the UL was not determined for arsenic, there is no justification for adding arsenic to food or supplements.

[b]The ULs for magnesium represent intake from a pharmacological agent only and do not include intake from food and water.

[c]Although silicon has not been shown to cause adverse effects in humans, there is no justification for adding silicon to supplements.

[d]Although vanadium in food has not been shown to cause adverse effects in humans, there is no justification for adding vanadium to food and vanadium supplements should be used with caution. The UL is based on adverse effects in laboratory animals and this data could be used to set a UL for adults but not children and adolescents.

[e]ND = Not determinable due to lack of data of adverse effects in this age group and concern with regard to lack of ability to handle excess amounts. Source of intake should be from food only to prevent high levels of intake.

SOURCE: Reprinted with permission from Dietary Reference Intakes, 2011 by the National Academy of Sciences. Courtesy of the National Academies Press.

Physical Activity Guidelines for Americans

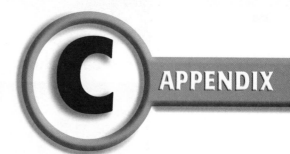

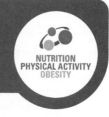

2008 Physical Activity Guidelines for Americans

Fact Sheet for Health Professionals on Physical Activity Guidelines for Adults

How much physical activity do adults need for health benefits?

Adults who are active are healthier, are less likely to develop many chronic diseases, and have better aerobic fitness than adults who are inactive. Adults need to do two types of physical activity each week to improve health – aerobic *and* muscle-strengthening activities.

Aerobic Activities

For **substantial health benefits**, adults need to do at least

- **2 hours and 30 minutes** (150 minutes) each week of **moderate-intensity*** aerobic activity,

OR

- **1 hour and 15 minutes** (75 minutes) each week of **vigorous-intensity*** aerobic activity,

OR

- An **equivalent mix of moderate- and vigorous-intensity** aerobic activity.

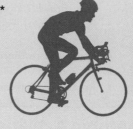

Aerobic activity should be performed for **at least 10 minutes at a time**, preferably, **spread throughout the week.**

*Intensity is the level of effort required to do an activity.
A person doing **moderate-intensity** aerobic activity can talk, but not sing, during the activity.
A person doing **vigorous-intensity** activity cannot say more than a few words without pausing for a breath.

Muscle Strengthening Activities

Muscle strengthening should be done **2 or more days a week.**
- All major muscle groups should be worked. These are the legs, hips, back, abdomen, chest, shoulders, and arms.
- Exercises for each muscle group should be **repeated 8 to 12** times per set. As exercises become easier, increase the weight or do another set.

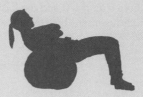

C

How can adults get additional health benefits?

> ### Aerobic Activities
>
> For **greater health benefits**, adults should do
> - **5 hours** (300 minutes) each week of **moderate-intensity** aerobic activity,
>
> OR
> - **2 hours and 30 minutes** (150 minutes) a week of **vigorous-intensity** aerobic activity,
>
> OR
> - An **equivalent mix of moderate- and vigorous-intensity** aerobic activity.

Health Benefits from Regular Physical Activity

Participating in regular physical activity provides many health benefits, as summarized below. Reducing risk of some of these conditions may require years of participation in regular physical activity. Other benefits, such as increased heart and lung—or cardiorespiratory—fitness, may require only a few weeks or months of participation.

> ### Strong Evidence for Health Benefits
>
> - **Lower risk of:**
>   - Early death
>   - Coronary heart disease
>   - Stroke
>   - High blood pressure
>   - High cholesterol or triglycerides
>   - Type 2 diabetes
>   - Metabolic syndrome
>   - Colon cancer
>   - Breast cancer
> - **Prevention of weight gain**
> - **Weight loss, particularly when combined with reduced calorie intake**
> - **Improved cardiorespiratory (aerobic) fitness and muscular strength**
> - **Prevention of falls**
> - **Reduced depression**

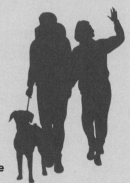

Aerobic Activities by Level of Intensity

There are different ways to classify intensity of exercise. **Absolute intensity** is the amount of energy expended per minute of activity. Moderate-intensity activities expend 3.0 to 5.9 times the amount of energy expended at rest. The energy expended in vigorous-intensity activities is 6.0 or more times the energy expended at rest.

Relative intensity is the effort required for an individual to do an activity. Relative intensity of aerobic activity is related to cardiorespiratory fitness. Less fit people generally require a higher level of effort than fitter people to do the same activity. Relative intensity can be estimated using a scale of 0 to 10, where sitting is 0 and the highest level of effort possible is 10. A moderate-intensity activity is a 5 or 6. A vigorous-intensity activity is a 7 or 8.

For most people, light daily activities such as shopping, cooking, or doing the laundry do not count toward the guidelines. Here are some examples of aerobic activities that require moderate-intensity and vigorous-intensity effort:

Level of Intensity	Type of Aerobic Activities
Moderate–Intensity A person doing **moderate-intensity** aerobic activity can talk, but not sing, during the activity.	• Brisk walking (3 miles-per-hour or faster, but not race walking) • Water aerobics • Bicycle riding slower than 10 miles per hour • Tennis (doubles) • Ballroom dancing • General gardening

Level of Intensity	Type of Aerobic Activities
Vigorous–Intensity A person doing **vigorous-intensity** activity cannot say more than a few words without pausing for a breath.	• Race walking, jogging, or running • Swimming laps • Tennis (singles) • Aerobic dancing • Bicycling 10 miles per hour or faster • Jumping rope • Heavy gardening (continuous digging or hoeing with heart rate increases) • Hiking uphill or with a heavy backpack

Muscle-Strengthening Activities

Adults also need to do muscle-strengthening activities **at least 2 days a week**, at a moderate to high level of intensity. These activities should **work all the major muscle groups**: the legs, hips, back, chest, abdomen, shoulders, and arms.

No specific amount of time is recommended for muscle strengthening, but exercises should be performed to the point at which it would be difficult to do another repetition. A **repetition** is one complete movement of an activity, like lifting a weight or doing a sit-up. Adults can do activities that strengthen muscles on the same or different days that they do aerobic activity, whichever works best. Muscle-strengthening activities do not count toward the aerobic activity total.

Below are some examples of muscle-strengthening physical activities for adults.

Types of Muscle-Strengthening Activity

• Lifting weights
• Working with resistance bands
• Doing exercises that use body weight for resistance (push-ups, sit-ups)

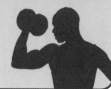

C

Ways for Adults to Get Physical Activity

To help adults understand the physical activity guidelines and to encourage them to add physical activity into their lives, the following materials are available at *www.cdc.gov/physicalactivity:*

- Tips on getting active

- Videos showing how to do muscle-strengthening activities and what counts as aerobic and muscle-strengthening activities

In addition, the following Health and Human Services (HHS) Web site has information and tools to help adults become and stay active: *www.health.gov/PAGuidelines.*

On this Web site you will find:

> *2008 Physical Activity Guidelines for Americans Toolkit* to assist organizations in promoting the physical activity guidelines.
> - Users' Guide – Promoting the Physical Activity Guidelines for Americans in Your Community: A Guide to Building Awareness and Participation
> - *Physical Activity Guidelines for Americans* booklet
> - *Be Active Your Way: A Guide for Adults*
> - Be Active Your Way: A Fact Sheet for Adults
> - At-A-Glance: A Fact Sheet for Professionals
> - Posters, event flyers, Frequently Asked Questions (FAQs)

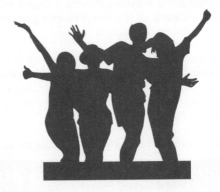

This appendix is reproduced from the 2008 Physical Activity Guidelines for Americans, Fact Sheet for Health Professionals on Physical Activity Guidelines for Children and Adolescents. Courtesy of the U.S. Department of Health and Human Services and the Centers for Disease Control and Prevention.

Knowledge Check Answers

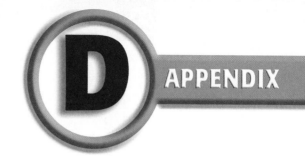

Chapter 1

1. C
2. D
3. B
4. C

5. B
6. D
7. C
8. D

Chapter 2

1. C
2. D
3. B
4. D

5. A
6. B
7. D
8. B

Chapter 3

1. B
2. D
3. D
4. B

5. C
6. B
7. D
8. C

Chapter 4

1. D
2. B
3. D
4. A
5. B

6. C
7. B
8. A
9. D
10. D

Chapter 5

1. A
2. B
3. B
4. A
5. C

6. B
7. B
8. B
9. B
10. B

Chapter 6

1. A
2. B
3. C
4. A
5. B

6. A
7. A
8. C
9. B
10. C

Chapter 7

1.	C	6.	A
2.	B	7.	C
3.	D	8.	C
4.	C	9.	A
5.	B	10.	C

Chapter 8

1.	A	6.	B
2.	A	7.	D
3.	A	8.	D
4.	C	9.	A
5.	D	10.	C

Chapter 9

1.	A	6.	C
2.	C	7.	C
3.	C	8.	A
4.	B	9.	C
5.	B	10.	B

Chapter 10

1.	A	6.	D
2.	E	7.	A
3.	C	8.	A
4.	A	9.	C
5.	C	10.	B

Chapter 11

1.	B	5.	A
2.	B	6.	B
3.	A	7.	C
4.	B	8.	B

Glossary

A

acute Rapid onset, severe symptoms, and short duration.

addiction Physiological and/or psychological need to perform a certain behavior.

adenosine triphosphate (ATP) The only form of energy used in the human body.

adrenaline A hormone that prepares the body to react during times of stress or in an emergency.

aerobic Using oxygen.

aerobic energy system System that provides energy for activities lasting longer than 2 minutes. This system requires oxygen.

aerobic exercise Exercise that depends on oxygen for energy production.

allostatic load The ongoing demand on the body from long-term exposure to stress hormones.

amenorrhea Absence of normal menstruation.

anabolic steroids Synthetic male hormones that increase muscle size and strength.

anaerobic Without using oxygen.

anaerobic energy system System that creates energy for activities that last less than 2 minutes or have frequent rest periods.

anemia A reduction in the number of red blood cells in the blood. Anemia is not a disease but rather a symptom of various diseases, including iron deficiency.

angina pectoris Chest pain caused by the early stages of cardiovascular disease.

angioplasty Technique used to open arteries blocked by plaque buildup.

anorexia nervosa Extreme restriction of food intake.

antioxidants A group of substances that can combine with or neutralize free radicals, thereby preventing oxidative damage to cells and tissues.

atherosclerosis Plaque buildup inside the arteries.

asanas Various postures used in doing yoga exercises.

atrophy Progressive loss (wasting) of muscle mass.

autonomic nervous system Part of the nervous system that controls automatic body functions, such as blood pressure, heart rate, and breathing. Subdivided into sympathetic and parasympathetic.

B

bacteria Microscopic organisms that cause disease.

ballistic stretching A form of stretching where repetitive bouncing occurs.

basal metabolic rate (BMR) Energy consumed (measured in calories) by the body at rest to keep vital functions going.

benzodiazepines Central nervous system depressants used to reduce anxiety and induce sleep.

binge eating Uncontrolled eating during a short time period.

bioelectrical impedance Measurement of the strength and speed of an electrical signal sent through the body.

blaming Placing the responsibility of an unmet goal on someone else.

blood clot Blockage that results from coagulation of blood.

body composition Proportion of fat, muscle, bone, and other tissues in the body.

body mass index (BMI) 1. Measure your height in inches (without shoes) and your weight in pounds (without clothing).

2. Multiply your weight by 703.

3. Divide that number by your height.

4. Divide again by your height.

botulism Poisoning by the toxin of the microorganism *Clostridium botulinum*.

bulimia Periodic bingeing followed by purging, or alternate days of bingeing and fasting.

C

calorie Unit of energy supplied by food; equals 1 kilocalorie (1 kcal), the amount if heated required to raise the temperature of 1 kilogram of water 1°C.

cancer A family of diseases characterized by rapid, uncontrolled growth of abnormal cells.

carbo loading Stuffing yourself with complex carbohydrates during the days before an endurance event.

carbohydrate Nutrient that is the body's main source of energy; consists of sugars and starches found in grains, vegetables, and fruits; two types are simple and complex.

carbon monoxide Most significant poisonous gas related to smoking.

cardiac catheterization Passage of a thin, flexible tube into the heart to provide treatment for heart disease.

cardiorespiratory endurance activity Exercise that contracts large muscle groups and increases breathing and heart rate.

cardiovascular disease Series of diseases affecting the heart and blood vessels.

cellulite Adipose tissue surrounded by stretched connective tissue.

cholesterol Wax-like substance made by the body's liver and found in animal and plant foods.

chronic Slow progression and long duration.

chronic disease Disease that takes many years to develop.

collars Devices used to secure weights to a barbell or dumbbell. Without collars the weights on one side of the bar will slip off.

complete protein A protein that contains all the essential amino acids.

compulsion An increase in the amount of time spent on an activity.

consistency The constant activity level needed to maintain fitness.

contusions Bruising of tissue.

cool-down The 5–10 minutes at the end of a workout involving light movement and stretching.

coronary bypass surgery Procedure used to reroute blood flow around a damaged or blocked artery.

CPR (cardiopulmonary resuscitation) Clearing air passages to the lungs, giving mouth-to-mouth respiration, and massaging the heart to restore normal breathing after cardiac arrest.

cramping Muscular tightness and abdominal or limb pain from dehydration and high body temperature.

creatine phosphate (CP) Chemical present in muscles that makes ATP rapidly for 30 seconds' worth of exercise. CP is produced in the body from the digestion of meat; it is also available as a supplement. Research is inconclusive as to its benefits or long-term risks.

cross-training Combining the components of fitness in a workout program, instead of focusing on only one area.

D

death rate Statistical representation of the significance of a disease or disorder in society.

diabetes Disease characterized by the body's inability to manage insulin.

diastolic pressure Lower blood pressure reading; measured when the heart relaxes between beats.

dietary fiber Nondigestible carbohydrates found in plants; two types are soluble and insoluble.

dislocations Bones are displaced from their normal joint alignment, out of their sockets, or out of their normal positions.

distress Harmful or bad response to a stressor.

drug Any nonfood substance that alters thought and/or behavior.

dynamic or active stretching Muscle is taken beyond its normal range of motion with help from a partner.

E

eating disorder A spectrum of abnormal eating patterns that eventually may endanger a person's health or increase the risk for other diseases. Generally, psychological factors play a key role.

endocrine system Consists of glands that produce hormones that control body functions.

endorphins Proteins produced in your brain that serve as your body's natural painkiller. Endorphins also reduce stress, depression, and anxiety.

endurance Ability to work out for a period of time without fatigue.

essential amino acids The nine protein amino acids that the body cannot make and, therefore, must come from foods you eat.

essential body fat Minimum amount of body fat needed for good health.

eustress Helpful or good response to a stressor.

exercise Planned, structured, and repetitive physical activity done to improve or maintain one or more components of physical fitness.

exercise log A record of your activity that includes the type, duration, and intensity of each exercise each day.

exercise machines Have a stack of weights that is lifted through an assortment of pulleys.

F

female athlete triad Combination of eating disorders, amenorrhea, and osteoporosis.

fitness The body's response to physical effort.

flexibility Ability to move a joint smoothly through a full range of motion.

free radicals Short-lived chemicals that can have detrimental effects on cells.

free weights Use barbells or hand weights.

frequency How often; the number of times an exercise or group of exercises is performed within a certain time frame.

G

general adaptation syndrome A series of body changes that result from stress. The syndrome occurs in three stages: alarm, resistance, and exhaustion.

genetic modification Manipulating the DNA of an organism to change some of its characteristics.

genetic testing Procedure used to investigate the pattern of human genes to determine the likelihood of disease development.

gland A group of cells that secretes hormones.

glucose Simple sugar circulating in the blood.

glycogen Complex carbohydrates stored primarily in the skeletal muscles and liver. When energy is needed, glycogen is converted to glucose.

H

health The World Health Organization's 1946 definition of health has been used as a foundation for the contemporary term of wellness: "Health is a state of complete physical, mental, and social well-being and not merely the absence of disease or infirmity."

heart attack Damage or death of all or part of the heart due to insufficient blood supply.

hemorrhagic stroke Disruption of blood flow to the brain caused by leaking of a blood vessel.

high-density lipoprotein (HDL) Carries cholesterol from the blood back to the liver, which processes the cholesterol for elimination from the body. It is often referred to as *good* cholesterol.

homeostasis Stability and consistency of a person's physiology.

hormone Chemical messenger released into the bloodstream that controls many body activities.

human immunodeficiency virus (HIV) The virus that causes AIDS.

hydrostatic (underwater) weighing Measuring a person's weight while he or she is suspended in water.

hypertension High blood pressure.

hypertrophy Increase in bulk or size by thickening of muscle fibers.

I

immediate energy system System using existing cellular ATP during first 10 seconds of activity.

incomplete protein A protein lacking one or more of the essential amino acids.

individual differences The variations in our physical ability.

insoluble fiber Does not dissolve in water.

insomnia Inability to sleep.

intensity How hard; the amount of energy exerted while performing an exercise.

irradiation Treatment with gamma rays, x-rays, or high-voltage electrons to kill pathogens and, in the case of food, to increase shelf life.

ischemic stroke Disruption of blood flow to the brain caused by blockage of an artery (clot).

isokinetic Muscle contraction where the maximum tension is generated in the muscle as it contracts at a constant speed over the full range of motion of the joint.

isometric Muscle contraction without movement at the joint.

isotonic Muscle contraction where tension is constant while length increases.

L

lactic acid Chemical formed when muscles must use stored glucose or blood-sugar to produce ATP.

lacto-ovo-vegetarian Person who includes milk, dairy products, and eggs in his or her diet.

lacto-vegetarian Person who includes some or all dairy products in his or her diet.

lipids Fats or fat-like substances characterized by their insolubility in water or solubility in fat.

lipoprotein Allows cholesterol to dissolve in the blood and carries it through the bloodstream to all parts of the body; two main types are high-density lipoprotein (HDL) and low-density lipoprotein (LDL).

locus of control The figurative place where a person locates the source of responsibility for the events in his or her life.

lordosis Excessive pelvic tilt.

low-density lipoprotein (LDL) Carries cholesterol from the liver to the rest of the body. When there is too much LDL cholesterol in the blood, it can be deposited on the walls of the coronary arteries. It is often referred to as *bad* cholesterol.

M

macrominerals Minerals needed by the body in amounts greater than 100 milligrams.

macronutrients Nutrients needed by your body in relatively large amounts.

mall-walking Walking a circuit around the lobby floors of an enclosed shopping mall in the morning before the stores open.

maximal oxygen uptake (VO_{2max}) How efficiently the cardiorespiratory system uses oxygen.

menopause The time when a woman's body stops producing ova and hormones related to fertility and menstruation.

metabolism The rate at which your body uses energy.

microminerals (trace minerals) Minerals needed by the body in amounts less than 100 milligrams.

micronutrients Nutrients needed by your body in relatively small amounts.

minerals Inorganic nutrients that regulate many chemical reactions in the body.

monounsaturated High concentrations of unsaturated fat in canola, peanut, and olive oils.

motivation The underlying drive behind making changes.

multiple-joint exercise An exercise in which two or more joints move together.

muscular endurance The ability of muscles to apply force repeatedly.

muscular strength The force muscles can exert against resistance.

myocardial infarction (MI) Heart attack.

N

nutrients Substances in food the body needs for normal function and good health.

O

obesity Excessive amounts of body fat.

osteoporosis Disease related to calcium deficiency in which bones become thin and brittle and fracture easily.

overload Placing a greater-than-normal amount of stress (within reason) on the body in an attempt to make it function at a higher capacity.

P

pH (powerHydrogen) Condition of a solution represented by a number on a scale of acidity to alkalinity.

physical activity Bodily movement produced by skeletal muscles that increases energy expenditure.

physical fitness Set of attributes that people have or achieve that relates to the ability to perform physical activity.

phytochemical Substance in plants (*phyto* = plant) that may have beneficial effects on the body.

plaque Artery-blocking deposits impeding blood flow.

plyometrics A form of training where muscles are subjected to rapid alternation of lengthening and shortening while resistance is continuously applied.

polyunsaturated High concentrations of unsaturated fat in sunflower, corn, soybean oils, and fish.

procrastination Pushing a task to a later point in time.

progression The gradual increase of the level and intensity of exercise.

progressive muscular relaxation Systematically tensing and relaxing the body's muscles from the feet to the head.

progressive overloading Increasing, from one session to another, the amount of weight you lift during a set.

protein Nutrient made up of amino acids that is needed for growth to build, repair, and maintain body tissues.

psychoneuroimmunology Study of nervous, endocrine, and immune system interaction.

pulmonary circulation Circulation between the heart and the lungs.

pulse The surge of blood that can be felt on certain points on the body each time the heart pumps blood into the arteries.

R

rate of perceived exertion (RPE) A person's own perception of the intensity of his or her exercise.

rationalization Making excuses for not carrying out a task.

reinforcement External support for a behavior.

relaxation response Reversal of stress symptoms.

repetition (rep) A single lifting and lowering of a weight.

repetition maximum (RM) The maximum weight you can lift successfully once while using proper form.

resistance training Building muscle by working against the resistance of weights.

rest A period of inactivity to allow your body to recover from strenuous exercise.

reversibility The principle that states that the results of physical fitness are not permanent.

S

safety Awareness of all aspects of your exercise routine to protect yourself from injury.

saturated fat Fat from meat, poultry, dairy products, and hardened vegetable fat.

sedatives Sleep and anxiety reduction drugs with small margin of safety.

sedentary Little or no physical activity.

semi- or partial vegetarian Person who eats no red meat, but may include chicken or fish, dairy products, and eggs in his or her diet.

set Number of reps performed without stopping to rest.

sexually transmitted infections (STIs) Infections and diseases transferred through intimate contact.

soluble fiber Partially dissolves in water.

specificity The type of physical changes you desire in your body relates directly to the type of exercise you choose.

spotter Another person who can help if the weight tilts or can help move a weight into position before or after a lift.

sprains Tearing or stretching of the joints that causes mild to severe damage to the ligaments and joint capsules.

ST2 Stress-related protein that may be a predictor of how well an individual will recover from heart attack.

static or passive stretching Muscle is stretched naturally without force being applied.

stent A mesh coil used to open blocked arteries.

stimulants Drugs used to increase activity in the central nervous system, causing increased energy and a sense of well-being.

storage fat Excess fat deposited in adipose tissue (fat cells) that protects organs and insulates the body.

strains Muscles are stretched or torn.

stress The physical and emotional tension that comes from situations the body perceives as threatening.

stress hormones (e.g., epinephrine) A hormone that prepares the body to react during times of stress or in an emergency.

stressor A source or cause of stress; may be physical, mental, social, or environmental.

stretch reflex An involuntary muscle contraction against a quick stretch.

stretching Primary method of improving flexibility.

sympathetic nervous system Subsystem of the autonomic system that triggers your body's response to stress—known as the fight-or-flight response.

systemic circulation Circulation between the heart and the rest of the body.

systolic pressure Higher blood pressure reading; measured when the heart contracts.

T

t'ai chi Thirteenth-century Chinese exercise routine involving graceful dance-like movements.

target heart rate range A range of heart rates used to maintain optimal effects during aerobic exercise.

tendonitis Inflammation of a tendon from overuse.

time How long; the duration an exercise or group of exercises takes to complete.

tolerance The condition where more of a drug or activity is required to reproduce the initial sensation.

trans fat Chemically derived fat present in hydrogenated foods; promotes plaque development and high cholesterol.

trans fatty acids Fats produced by heating liquid vegetable oils in the presence of hydrogen, a process called hydrogenation.

transgenic An organism into which hereditary (i.e., genetic) material from another organism has been introduced.

type The classification of exercise.

type 2 diabetes A disease that involves the inability to produce an adequate amount of insulin.

type A An individual exhibiting a sense of time urgency ("hurry sickness"), aggressiveness, and competitiveness, usually combined with hostility. Describes the majority of Americans.

type B An individual displaying no sense of time urgency, no hostility, noncompetitiveness, patience, and a secure sense of self-esteem.

U

underweight A BMI less than 19.

unsaturated fat Type of fat obtained from plant sources and fish; two types are mono-unsaturated and polyunsaturated.

V

vegan Person who eats only foods of plant origin.

vegetarian diet Diet in which vegetables are the foundation and meat products are restricted or eliminated.

vitamin Nutrient necessary for normal functioning of the body; two types are water soluble and fat soluble.

VO_{2max} Amount of oxygen the body uses when it reaches its maximum ability to supply oxygen during exercise.

W

warm-up The 5–10 minutes of low-intensity movement at the beginning of a workout that prepares the body for activity by increasing muscle temperature and metabolism.

wasting Occurs when the diet lacks protein; the body breaks down body tissue (e.g., muscle) and uses it as a protein source.

weight management The adoption of healthful and sustainable eating and exercise behaviors indicated for reduced disease risk and improved feelings of energy and well-being.

wellness An active process of becoming aware of and making choices toward a more successful existence.

Name _____ Section _____ Date _____

Date Due	Chapter	Assignment	Complete
_____	1	Lab 1-1: Healthstyle: A Self-Test	_____
_____	3	Lab 3-1: Determining Your Stage of Change	_____
_____	3	Lab 3-2: Personal Contract	_____
_____	4	Lab 4-1: PAR-Q & You: A Questionnaire for People Aged 15 to 69	_____
_____	4	Lab 4-2: Stages of Change: Continuous Measure	_____
_____	4	Lab 4-3: Barriers to Being Active	_____
_____	5	Lab 5-1: Activity 1: Measuring Your Heart Rate	_____
_____	5	Lab 5-1: Activity 2: Determining Your Target Heart Rate Range	_____
_____	5	Lab 5-2: Activity 1: Rockport Fitness Walking Test™	_____
_____	5	Lab 5-2: Activity 2: Cooper's 1.5-Mile Run/Walk Test	_____
_____	5	Lab 5-2: Activity 3: YMCA Step Test	_____
_____	5	Lab 5-3: Activity 1: Tracking Your Cardiorespiratory Endurance Ratings	_____
_____	5	Lab 5-3: Activity 2: Cardiorespiratory Training Log	_____
_____	6	Lab 6-1: Activity 1: Sit-and-Reach Test	_____
_____	6	Lab 6-1: Activity 2: Shoulder Flexibility Test	_____
_____	6	Lab 6-1: Activity 3: Other Flexibility Tests	_____
_____	6	Lab 6-2: Activity 1: Tracking Your Flexibility	_____
_____	6	Lab 6-2: Activity 2: Stretching Log	_____
_____	6	Lab 6-3: Posture Assessment	_____
_____	7	Lab 7-1: Activity 1: YMCA Bench-Press Test	_____
_____	7	Lab 7-1: Activity 2: Push-up Test for Muscular Endurance	_____
_____	7	Lab 7-1: Activity 3: YMCA Half Sit-up Test (Partial Curl-up Test)	_____
_____	7	Lab 7-2: Activity 1: One-Repetition Maximum Test (1 RM)	_____
_____	7	Lab 7-2: Activity 2: Hand Grip Strength Test	_____
_____	7	Lab 7-3: Activity 1: Tracking Your Muscular Endurance	_____
_____	7	Lab 7-3: Activity 2: Tracking Your Muscular Strength	_____
_____	7	Lab 7-3: Activity 3: Tracking Your Grip Strength	_____
_____	7	Lab 7-3: Activity 4: Resistance Training	_____

LAB MANUAL ASSIGNMENTS

Date Due	Chapter	Assignment	Complete
_____	8	Lab 8-1: On-Line Diet/Nutrition Analysis	_____
_____	8	Lab 8-2: Fast-Food Analysis	_____
_____	8	Lab 8-3: Food Labels	_____
_____	8	Lab 8-4: Grocery Store Scavenger Hunt	_____
_____	9	Lab 9-1: Activity 1: Calculate Your Waist Circumference	_____
_____	9	Lab 9-1: Activity 2: Calculate Your Waist-to-Hip Ratio	_____
_____	9	Lab 9-1: Activity 3: Calculate Your BMI	_____
_____	9	Lab 9-1: Activity 4: Calculate Your Waist-to-Height Ratio	_____
_____	9	Lab 9-1: Activity 5: Calculate Your Skinfold Measurements	_____
_____	9	Lab 9-2: Assess Your Total Daily Energy Needs	_____
_____	9	Lab 9-3: Tracking Your Body Composition	_____
_____	10	Lab 10-1: Activity 1: The College Life-Stress Scale	_____
_____	10	Lab 10-1: Activity 2: The Inventory of College Students' Recent Life Experiences	_____
_____	10	Lab 10-2: Activity 1: Ranking Tasks	_____
_____	10	Lab 10-2: Activity 2: Scheduling	_____
_____	10	Lab 10-3: Activity 1: Progressive Muscle Relaxation	_____
_____	10	Lab 10-3: Activity 2: Meditation	_____
_____	10	Lab 10-3: Activity 3: Track and Record Your Relaxation Technique	_____
_____	10	Lab 10-4: Activity 1: Scenarios	_____
_____	10	Lab 10-4: Activity 2: Problem-Solving Steps	_____
_____	11	Lab 11-1: Decision-Making: Paired Comparison Analysis	_____
_____	11	Lab 11-2: Health Food Store Visit	_____
_____	11	Lab 11-3: Fitness Club Visit	_____
_____	11	Lab 11-4: Shopping for Exercise Equipment	_____

Name _____ Section _____ Date _____

Healthstyle: A Self-Test

This self-test, which is a modified version of the one developed by the U.S. Public Health Service, assesses several health-related behaviors. Although these behaviors apply to most individuals, pregnant women and people with chronic health concerns should follow the advice of their physicians. Answer each of the following questions by circling the number of the response that applies best to you. Add the number of points under each health-related behavior category to obtain a score for that category. Use the scoring guide at the end of the test to determine the level of risk you are incurring by your health-related behavior.

Tobacco, Alcohol, and Other Drugs

If you have never used tobacco products, enter a score of 10 for this section, and skip questions 1 and 2.

	Almost always	Sometimes	Almost never
1. I avoid using tobacco products.	2	1	0
2. I smoke only low-tar cigarettes.	2	1	0
Smoking Score:			
3. I avoid drinking alcoholic beverages, or I drink no more than one or two drinks per day.	2	1	0
4. I avoid using alcohol or other drugs (especially illegal drugs) as a way of handling stressful situations or problems in my life.	2	1	0
5. I avoid driving while under the influence of alcohol and other drugs.	2	1	0
6. I am careful not to drink alcohol when taking certain pain medications or when pregnant.	2	1	0
7. I read and follow the label directions when using prescribed and over-the-counter drugs.	2	1	0
Alcohol and Other Drugs Score:			

Eating Habits

	Almost always	Sometimes	Almost never
8. I eat a variety of foods each day, including fruits and vegetables, whole-grain products, lean meats, low-fat dairy products, seeds, nuts, and dry beans.	3	1	0
9. I limit the amount of fat that I eat, especially animal fats such as cream, butter, cheese, and fatty meats.	3	1	0

Eating Habits, continued

	Almost always	Sometimes	Almost never
10. I limit the amount of salt that I eat, by avoiding salty foods and not using salt at the table.	2	1	0
11. I avoid eating too much sugar, by eating few sweet snacks and limiting sugary soft drinks.	2	1	0
Eating Habits Score:			

Exercise/Fitness

	Almost always	Sometimes	Almost never
12. I maintain a body weight that is reasonable for my height.	3	1	0
13. I do vigorous exercise (for example, running, swimming, or brisk walking) for at least 30 minutes at least three times per week.	3	1	0
14. I do exercises to enhance my muscle tone and flexibility (for example, yoga or calisthenics) for 15 to 30 minutes at least three times per week.	2	1	0
15. I use part of my leisure time participating in individual, family, or team activities that increase my level of physical fitness (for example, gardening, bowling, or golf).	2	1	0
Exercise/Fitness Score:			

Stress Management

	Almost always	Sometimes	Almost never
16. I take time every day to relax.	2	1	0
17. I find it easy to express my feelings.	2	1	0
18. I recognize and prepare for events or situations that are likely to be stressful.	2	1	0
19. I have close friends, relatives, or others I can talk to about personal matters and contact for help when needed.	2	1	0
20. I participate in hobbies that I enjoy or group activities such as religious or community organizations.	2	1	0
Stress Management Score:			

Safety

	Almost always	Sometimes	Almost never
21. I wear a seat belt while riding in a motor vehicle.	2	1	0

© 2013 Jones & Bartlett Learning, LLC

Safety, continued

	Almost always	Sometimes	Almost never
22. I obey traffic rules and speed limits while driving.	2	1	0
23. I have a working smoke detector in my home.	2	1	0
24. I am careful when using potentially harmful products or substances, such as household cleaners, poisons, and electrical devices.	2	1	0
25. I avoid smoking in bed.	2	1	0
Safety Score:			

What Your Scores Mean

Scores of 9 or 10 for each section: Excellent! Your responses show that you are aware of the importance of this area to your health, and that you are practicing good health-related habits. As long as you continue to do so, this area of health should not pose a risk.

Scores of 6 to 8 for each section: Your health practices in this area are good, but there is room for improvement. Look at the items that you answered with "Sometimes" or "Almost Never." What lifestyle changes can you make to improve your score and reduce your risk?

Scores of 3 to 5 for each section: Your health-related behaviors are risky. What lifestyle changes can you make to improve your score in this area of health and reduce your risk?

Scores of 0 to 2 for each section: You may be taking serious and unnecessary risks with your health and, possibly, the health of others. What lifestyle changes can you make to improve your score and reduce your risk?

Source: Healthstyle: A self-test. Hyattsville, MD: U.S. Public Health Service, 1981.

Name _____ Section _____ Date _____

Determining Your Stage of Change

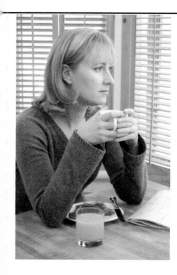

Throughout Chapter 3, we've asked you to think about your behavior—in particular, items you would like to change. Most people have a health behavior they would like to adopt or an unhealthy behavior they would like to eliminate. Follow the steps below to see how ready you are for a health-related behavior change.

Step 1: Identify a health behavior to change (write it on the line below and be specific):

_____

_____

Step 2: Find Your Current Stage of Change
Change the behavior from Step 1 to a question and write it on the line below. (e.g., Do I get 7 to 9 hours of sleep most nights of the week? Do I consistently limit fat in my diet? Do I exercise for at least 30 minutes on most days of the week?)

_____

_____

_____

Step 3: Read all of the possible answers to your question in Step 2 carefully. Choose the best response for your question.

_____ A. YES, I have been for MORE than 6 months.

_____ B. YES, I have been, but for LESS than 6 months.

_____ C. NO, but I intend to in the next 30 days.

_____ D. NO, but I intend to in the next 6 months.

_____ E. NO, and I do NOT intend to in the next 6 months.

Scoring:

Answer choice (A) — Maintenance Stage

Answer choice (B) — Action Stage

Answer choice (C) — Preparation Stage

Answer choice (D) — Contemplation Stage

Answer choice (E) — Precontemplation Stage

Which stage are you in with your current health behavior?

_____

Determining Your Stage of Change

Name _____ Section _____ Date _____

Personal Contract

Start Date: _____ Finish Date: _____

The Goal: _____

Motivation (benefits): _____

Identify current stage of change (use Lab 3-1): _____

Match your current stage of change and other stages you anticipate progressing through with the appropriate processes of change (see main text, Figure 3.3):

_____   _____

_____   _____

What specific techniques will you use for each of the processes identified above (see main text, Table 3.1)?

Processes	Specific techniques

Stage of change on the finish date: _____

I, _____, agree to work toward a healthier lifestyle, and in doing so shall comply with the terms and dates of this contract.

Signature: _____   Date: _____

Witness: _____   Date: _____

Name _____ Section _____ Date _____

PAR-Q & You: A Questionnaire for People Aged 15 to 69

Regular physical activity is fun and healthy, and increasingly more people are starting to become more active every day. Being more active is very safe for most people. However, some people should check with their doctor before they start becoming more physically active.

If you are planning to become much more physically active than you are now, start by answering the seven questions in the box below. If you are between the ages of 15 and 69, the PAR-Q will tell you whether you should check with your doctor before you start. If you are older than 69 years of age, and you are not used to being very active, check with your doctor.

Common sense is your best guide when you answer these questions. Please read the questions carefully and answer each one honestly. Check Yes or No.

Yes	No	
☐	☐	1. Has your doctor ever said that you have a heart condition *and* that you should only do physical activity recommended by a doctor?
☐	☐	2. Do you feel pain in your chest when you do physical activity?
☐	☐	3. In the past month, have you had chest pain when you were not doing physical activity?
☐	☐	4. Do you lose your balance because of dizziness or do you ever lose consciousness?
☐	☐	5. Do you have a bone or joint problem (for example, back, knee, or hip) that could be made worse by a change in your physical activity?
☐	☐	6. Is your doctor currently prescribing drugs (for example, water pills) for your blood pressure or heart condition?
☐	☐	7. Do you know of *any other reason* why you should not do physical activity?

If you answered YES to one or more questions

Talk with your doctor by phone or in person BEFORE you start becoming much more physically active or BEFORE you have a fitness appraisal. Tell your doctor about the PAR-Q and which questions you answered YES.

- You may be able to do any activity you want—as long as you start slowly and build up gradually. Or, you may need to restrict your activities to those that are safe for you. Talk with your doctor about the kinds of activities you wish to participate in and follow his or her advice.

- Find out which community programs are safe and helpful for you.

If you answered NO to all questions

If you answered NO honestly to *all* PAR-Q questions, you can be reasonably sure that you can:

- Start becoming much more physically active—begin slowly and build up gradually. This is the safest and easiest way to go.

- Take part in a fitness appraisal—this is an excellent way to determine your basic fitness so that you can plan the best way for you to live actively. It is also highly recommended that you have your blood pressure evaluated. If your reading is over 144/94, talk with your doctor before you start becoming much more physically active.

Delay Becoming Much More Active:

- If you are not feeling well because of a temporary illness such as a cold or a fever—wait until you feel better; or

- If you are or may be pregnant—talk to your doctor before you start becoming more active.

Please Note:

If your health changes so that you then answer YES to any of the preceding questions, tell your fitness or health professional.

Ask whether you should change your physical activity plan.

Informed Use of the PAR-Q: The Canadian Society for Exercise Physiology, Health Canada and their agents assume no liability for persons who undertake physical activity, and if in doubt after completing this questionnaire, consult your doctor prior to physical activity.

No changes permitted. You are encouraged to photocopy the PAR-Q but only if you use the entire form.

NOTE: If the PAR-Q is being given to a person before he or she participates in a physical activity program or a fitness appraisal, this section may be used for legal or administrative purposes.

"I have read, understood, and completed this questionnaire. Any questions I had were answered to my full satisfaction."

NAME _____

SIGNATURE _____ DATE _____

SIGNATURE OF PARENT _____ WITNESS _____

or GUARDIAN (for participants under the age of majority)

Note: This physical activity clearance is valid for a maximum of 12 months from the date it is completed and becomes invalid if your condition changes so that you would answer YES to any of the seven questions.

Source: Reproduced from Physical Activity Readiness Questionnaire (PAR-Q) © 2002. Used with permission from the Canadian Society for Exercise Physiology, www.cesp.ca.

Name _____ Section _____ Date _____

Stages of Change: Continuous Measure

Directions

Please use the following definition of exercise when answering these questions:
Regular exercise is any planned physical activity (brisk walking, aerobics, jogging, bicycling, swimming, rowing) performed to increase physical fitness. Such activity should be performed 3 to 5 times per week for 20 to 60 minutes per session. Exercise does not have to be painful to be effective but should be done at a level that increases your breathing rate and causes you to break a sweat.

Please check off all statements that apply to your lifestyle.

1. As far as I'm concerned, I don't need to exercise regularly. _____

2. I have been exercising regularly for a long time, and I plan to continue. _____

3. I don't exercise, and right now I don't care. _____

4. I am finally exercising regularly. _____

5. I have been successful at exercising regularly, and I plan to continue. _____

6. I am satisfied with being a sedentary person. _____

7. I have been thinking that I might want to start exercising regularly. _____

8. I have started exercising regularly within the last 6 months. _____

9. I could exercise regularly, but I don't plan to. _____

10. Recently, I have started to exercise regularly. _____

11. I don't have the time or energy to exercise regularly right now. _____

12. I have started to exercise regularly, and I plan to continue. _____

13. I have been thinking about whether I will be able to exercise regularly. _____

14. I have set up a day and a time to start exercising regularly within the next few weeks. _____

15. I have managed to keep exercising regularly through the last 6 months. _____

16. I have been thinking that I may want to begin exercising regularly. _____

17. I have arranged with a friend to start exercising regularly within the next few weeks. _____

18. I have completed 6 months of regular exercise. _____

19. I know that regular exercise is worthwhile, but I won't have time for it in the near future. _____

20. I have been calling friends to find someone to start exercising with in the next few weeks. _____

21. I think regular exercise is good, but I can't figure it into my schedule right now. _____

22. I really think I should work on getting started with a regular exercise program in the next 6 months. _____

23. I am preparing to start a regular exercise group in the next few weeks. _____

24. I am aware of the importance of regular exercise but I can't do it right now. _____

In the box below, circle the numbers that correspond with the numbers of the statements you checked off. For example, if you checked off statement number 17, find and circle 17 in the box below.

Stages of Change:
Precontemplation (nonbelievers in exercise) items: 1, 3, 6, 9
Precontemplation (believers in exercise) items: 11, 19, 21, 24
Contemplation items: 7, 13, 16, 22
Preparation items: 14, 17, 20, 23
Action items: 4, 8, 10, 12
Maintenance items: 2, 5, 15, 18

Source: Cancer Prevention Research Center (CPRC). *Measures. Exercise: Stages of change—Continuous measure.* http://www.uri.edu/ research/cprc/Measures/Exercise01.htm [October 14, 2008].

• What stage of change had the most numbers circled?

• Do you think this is an accurate measure of where you are in regard to increasing physical activity in your life?

Source: Courtesy of Dr. James O. Prochaska.

Name _____ Section _____ Date _____

Barriers to Being Active

What Keeps You from Being More Active?

Directions

Listed below are reasons that people give to describe why they do not get as much physical activity as they think they should. Please read each statement and indicate how likely you are to say it.

How likely are you to say?	Very likely	Somewhat likely	Somewhat unlikely	Very unlikely
1. My day is so busy now; I just don't think I can make the time to include physical activity in my regular schedule.	3	2	1	0
2. None of my family members or friends like to do anything active, so I don't have a chance to exercise.	3	2	1	0
3. I'm just too tired after work to get any exercise.	3	2	1	0
4. I've been thinking about getting more exercise, but I just can't seem to get started.	3	2	1	0
5. I'm getting older, so exercise can be risky.	3	2	1	0
6. I don't get enough exercise because I have never learned the skills for any sport.	3	2	1	0
7. I don't have access to jogging trails, swimming pools, bike paths, and so forth.	3	2	1	0
8. Physical activity takes too much time away from other commitments—work, family, and so on.	3	2	1	0
9. I'm embarrassed about how I will look when I exercise with others.	3	2	1	0
10. I don't get enough sleep as it is. I just couldn't get up early or stay up late to get some exercise.	3	2	1	0
11. It's easier for me to find excuses not to exercise than to go out and do something.	3	2	1	0

How likely are you to say?	Very likely	Somewhat likely	Somewhat unlikely	Very unlikely
12. I know of too many people who have hurt themselves by overdoing it with exercise.	3	2	1	0
13. I really can't see learning a new sport at my age.	3	2	1	0
14. It's just too expensive. You have to take a class or join a club or buy the right equipment.	3	2	1	0
15. My free times during the day are too short to include exercise.	3	2	1	0
16. My usual social activities with family or friends do not include physical activity.	3	2	1	0
17. I'm too tired during the week and I need the weekend to catch up on my rest.	3	2	1	0
18. I want to get more exercise, but I just can't seem to make myself stick to anything.	3	2	1	0
19. I'm afraid I might injure myself or have a heart attack.	3	2	1	0
20. I'm not good enough at any physical activity to make it fun.	3	2	1	0
21. If we had exercise facilities and showers at work, then I would be more likely to exercise.	3	2	1	0

Follow these instructions to score yourself:

• Enter the circled number in the spaces provided below, putting together the number for statement 1 on line 1, statement 2 on line 2, and so on.

• Add the three scores on each line. Your barriers to physical activity fall into one or more of seven categories: lack of time, social influences, lack of energy, lack of will-power, fear of injury, lack of skill, and lack of resources. A score of 5 or above in any category shows that this is an important barrier for you to overcome.

____ + ____ + ____ = _____
 1   8   15   Lack of time

____ + ____ + ____ = _____
 2   9   16   Social influence

____ + ____ + ____ = _____
 3   10   17   Lack of energy

____ + ____ + ____ = _____

  4   11   18   Lack of motivation

____ + ____ + ____ = _____

  5   12   19   Fear of injury

____ + ____ + ____ = _____

  6   13   20   Lack of skill

____ + ____ + ____ = _____

  7   14   21   Lack of resources

What To Do

For high-scoring barriers (5 or more scored), use the following strategies. Place a check mark next to the strategies attempted.

Suggestions for Overcoming Physical Activity Barriers

Lack of Time

_____ Identify available time slots. Monitor your daily activities for one week. Identify at least three 30-minute time slots you could use for physical activity.

_____ Add physical activity to your daily routine. For example, walk or ride your bike to work or shopping, organize school activities around physical activity, walk the dog, exercise while you watch TV, park farther away from your destination, and so forth.

_____ Make time for physical activity. For example, walk, jog, or swim during your lunch hour, or take fitness breaks instead of coffee breaks.

_____ Select activities requiring minimal time, such as walking, jogging, or stairclimbing.

Social Influence

_____ Explain your interest in physical activity to friends and family. Ask them to support your efforts.

_____ Invite friends and family members to exercise with you. Plan social activities involving exercise.

_____ Develop new friendships with physically active people. Join a group, such as the YMCA or a hiking club.

Lack of Energy

_____ Schedule physical activity for times in the day or week when you feel energetic.

_____ Convince yourself that if you give it a chance, physical activity will increase your energy level; then, try it.

Lack of Motivation

_____ Plan ahead. Make physical activity a regular part of your daily or weekly schedule and write it on your calendar.

_____ Invite a friend to exercise with you on a regular basis and write it on both your calendars.

_____ Join an exercise group or class.

Fear of Injury

_____ Learn how to warm up and cool down to prevent injury.

_____ Learn how to exercise appropriately considering your age, fitness level, skill level, and health status.

_____ Choose activities involving minimum risk.

Lack of Skill

_____ Select activities requiring no new skills, such as walking, climbing stairs, or jogging.

_____ Exercise with friends who are at the same skill level as you are.

_____ Find a friend who is willing to teach you some new skills.

_____ Take a class to develop new skills.

Lack of Resources

_____ Select activities that require minimal facilities or equipment, such as walking, jogging, jumping rope, or calisthenics.

_____ Identify inexpensive, convenient resources available in your community (community education programs, park and recreation programs, worksite programs, etc.).

Weather Conditions

_____ Develop a set of regular activities that are always available regardless of weather (indoor cycling, aerobic dance, indoor swimming, calisthenics, stair climbing, rope skipping, mall walking, dancing, gymnasium games, etc.).

_____ Look on outdoor activities that depend on weather conditions (cross-country skiing, outdoor swimming, outdoor tennis, etc.) as "bonuses"—extra activities possible when weather and circumstances permit.

Travel

_____ Put a jump rope in your suitcase and jump rope.

_____ Walk the halls and climb the stairs in hotels.

_____ Stay in places with swimming pools or exercise facilities.

_____ Join the YMCA or YWCA (ask about reciprocal membership agreement).

_____ Visit the local shopping mall and walk for half an hour or more.

_____ Bring a small tape recorder and your favorite aerobic exercise tape.

Family Obligations

_____ Trade babysitting time with a friend, neighbor, or family member who also has small children.

_____ Exercise with the kids—go for a walk together, play tag or other running games, get an aerobic dance or exercise tape for kids (there are several on the market) and exercise together. You can spend time together and still get your exercise.

_____ Hire a babysitter and look at the cost as a worthwhile investment in your physical and mental health.

_____ Jump rope, do calisthenics, ride a stationary bicycle, or use other home gymnasium equipment while the kids are busy playing or sleeping.

_____ Try to exercise when the kids are not around (e.g., during school hours or their nap time).

_____ Encourage exercise facilities to provide child care services.

Retirement Years

_____ Look upon your retirement as an opportunity to become more active instead of less. Spend more time gardening, walking the dog, and playing with your grandchildren. Children with short legs and grandparents with slower gaits are often great walking partners.

_____ Learn a new skill you have always been interested in, such as ballroom dancing, square dancing, or swimming.

_____ Now that you have the time, make regular physical activity a part of every day. Go for a walk every morning or every evening before dinner. Treat yourself to an exercycle and ride every day while reading a favorite book or magazine.

Content in the "Personal Barriers" section was taken from *Promoting Physical Activity: A Guide for Community Action* (USDHHS, 1999).

Source: CDC Division of Nutrition and Physical Activity (1999). *Promoting Physical Activity: A Guide for Community Action.* http://www.cdc.gov/physicalactivity/everyone/health/index.html

Name _____ Section _____ Date _____

Your Heart Rate

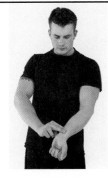

Activity 1: Measuring Your Heart Rate

1. Use your fingertips, not your thumb, to find your pulse at the radial artery (at your wrist, below your thumb).

2. Count the beats for 15 seconds.

3. Multiply this number by 4 to get your heart rate in beats per minute (bpm).

Note: Some prefer other methods, such as the following:

a. Count the beats for 10 seconds and multiply by 6 to get the heart rate.

b. Count the beats for 30 seconds and multiply by 2 to get the heart rate.

c. Count the beats for 6 seconds and multiply by 10 to get the heart rate.

Caution: Some prefer feeling the carotid artery in the neck. Your heart's rhythm may be affected if the carotid artery is felt, massaged, or rubbed.

For each of the methods, record your resting heart rate.

15 seconds × 4 = _____ _____

10 seconds × 6 = _____ _____

30 seconds × 2 = _____ _____

6 seconds × 10 = _____ _____

Which method is the least accurate? _____

Which method do you prefer? _____ Why? _____

_____

_____

_____

_____

_____

_____

_____

_____

Activity 2: Determining Your Target Heart Rate Range

Maximum Heart Rate (HRmax) Method

The heat rate provides a convenient way to monitor exercise intensity. Cardiorespiratory fitness will not increase unless the heart rate during exercise rises to at least a predetermined minimum level. This level is known as the target heart rate range and is about 60% to 80% of the maximum heart rate (maximum heart rate is the highest number of times your heart can beat in 1 minute). When you exercise, you should strive to keep your heart rate inside this range.

Use your findings in Lab 5-1, Activity 1 for determining your heart rate for 1 minute. Complete the chart below to derive your target heart rate range (low end and high end).

Most people have misinterpreted the target heart rate range, believing that exercise has to be very tense or it is useless. This is not true, but the belief discourages many from participating in, and benefiting from, exercise.

Example of a 25-year-old with resting heart rate of 70 at 60% to 80% training range:

Low end	High end
HRmax = 208 − (0.7 × age) HRmax = 208 − (0.7 × 25) = 190.5	HRmax = 208 − (0.7 × age) HRmax = 208 − (0.7 × 25) = 190.5
HRR = HRmax − HRrest HRR = 190.5 − 70 = 120.5	HRR = HRmax − HRrest HRR = 190.5 − 70 = 120.5

Low-end target range % = HRR ×
    intensity % + HRrest
60% intensity = 120.5 × 0.60 + 70 =
    142 bpm
	High-end target range % = HRR ×
	    intensity % + HRrest
	80% intensity = 120.5 × 0.80 + 70 =
	    166 bpm

Key to abbreviations:

HRmax = Maximum heart rate

HRR = Heart rate reserve

HRrest = Resting heart rate

bpm = beats per minute

Age = _____
Resting heart rate (HRrest) = _____
Low-end intensity level = _____
High-end intensity level = _____

Low end	High end
HRmax =	HRmax =
HRR =	HRR =
Low-end target range pulse per minute =	Low-end target range pulse per minute =

Name _____ Section _____ Date _____

Cardiorespiratory Assessments

Activity 1: Rockport Fitness Walking Test™

This activity assesses cardiorespiratory (aerobic) fitness. To perform the test, you need a watch with a second hand to record your time, and you need to wear good walking shoes and loose clothes. You should have your physician's consent before undertaking this exercise test.

Instructions

1. Find a measured track or measure 1 mile using your car's odometer on a level, uninterrupted road.

2. Warm up by walking slowly for 5 minutes.

3. Walk 1 mile as fast as you can, maintaining a steady pace. Note the time that you began walking.

4. When you complete the mile walk, record your time to the nearest second and keep walking at a slower pace. Count your pulse for 15 seconds and multiply by 4, then record this number. This gives your heart rate per minute after your test walk.

   Heart rate at the end of 1-mile walk: _____ beats per minute

   Time to walk the mile: _____ minutes

5. Remember to stretch once you have cooled down.

6. To find your cardiorespiratory fitness level, refer to the appropriate Rockport Fitness Walking Test™ charts (Figure 5.A1) based on your age and sex. These show established fitness norms from the American Heart Association.

   Using your fitness level chart from Figure 5.A1, find your time in minutes and your heart rate per minute. Follow these lines until they meet, and mark this point on your chart. This tells you how fit you are compared to other individuals of your sex and age category.

   These charts are based on weights of 170 lb for men and 125 lb for women. If you weigh substantially less, your cardiovascular fitness will be slightly underestimated. Conversely, if you weigh substantially more, your cardiovascular fitness will be slightly overestimated.

   How fit you are compared to others of the same age and gender: _____

   Level 5 = high
   Level 4 = above average
   Level 3 = average
   Level 2 = below average
   Level 1 = low

Figure 5.A1 Find your fitness level using the Rockport Fitness Walking Test™

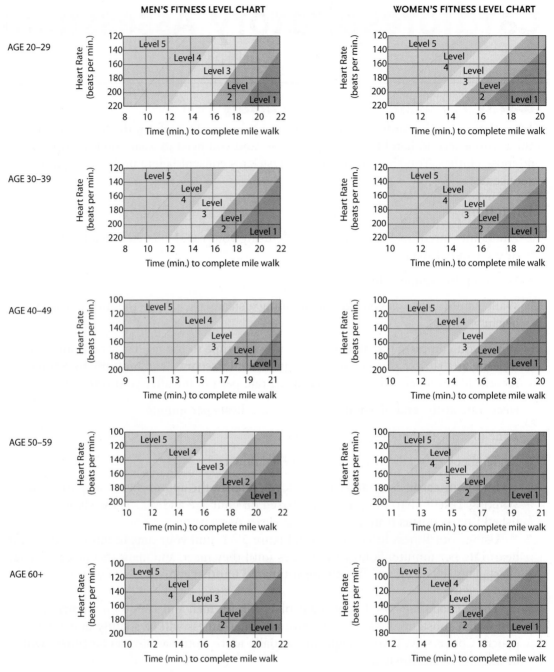

Source: Courtesy of the Rockport Company, Inc.

Cardiorespiratory Assessments

Activity 2: Cooper's 1.5-Mile Run/Walk Test

The 1.5-mile run/walk test is recommended for those who are motivated, experienced in running, and in good condition before taking the test. Do not take the test unless you can already jog nonstop for 15 minutes. It is not recommended for the following people:

- Those failing the PAR-Q questionnaire

- Sedentary people older than 30 years of age

- Severely deconditioned people

- Those with joint problems

- Obese individuals

Sedentary individuals (especially those older than 30 years of age) should participate in a walking/running program for 1 to 2 months before taking the test. For those in hot or cold environments, do not take this test unless you have been exercising in these conditions.

Preparation

You will need the following:

- Stopwatch, watch, or clock with a second hand

- Oval running track

- Appropriate running shoes and clothing

Warm up for 5 to 10 minutes before the test.

Procedure

1. Complete a 1.5-mile distance in the shortest possible time. If outdoors, the test should be conducted in favorable weather conditions. Physically fit individuals can cover the distance either by running or jogging. Less fit individuals can run and jog, but may need to walk some of the time.

2. Attempt to keep a steady pace throughout the test.

3. When completed, record the time (minutes and seconds) it took to complete the 1.5-mile distance.

    Time to finish the 1.5-mile distance: _____

4. See Table 5.A1 to find your fitness rating.

    Fitness rating: _____

Table 5.A1
Fitness Categories for Cooper's 1.5-Mile Run Test to Determine Cardiorespiratory Fitness

Fitness category	Age (years)					
	13–19	**20–29**	**30–39**	**40–49**	**50–59**	**60+**
Men						
Very poor	>15:30	>16:00	>16:30	>17:30	>19:00	>20:00
Poor	12:11–15:30	14:01–16:00	14:46–16:30	15:36–17:30	17:01–19:00	19:01–20:00
Average	10:49–12:10	12:01–14:00	12:31–14:45	13:01–15:35	14:31–17:00	16:16–19:00
Good	9:41–10:48	10:46–12:00	11:01–12:30	11:31–13:00	12:31–14:30	14:00–16:15
Excellent	8:37–9:40	9:45–10:45	10:00–11:00	10:30–11:30	11:00–12:30	11:15–13:59
Superior	<8:37	<9:45	<10:00	<10:30	<11:00	<11:15
Women						
Very poor	>18:30	>19:00	>19:30	>20:00	>20:30	>21:00
Poor	16:55–18:30	18:31–19:00	19:01–19:30	19:31–20:00	20:01–20:30	20:31–21:31
Average	14:31–16:54	15:55–18:30	16:31–19:00	17:31–19:30	19:01–20:00	19:31–20:30
Good	12:30–14:30	13:31–15:54	14:31–16:30	15:56–17:30	16:31–19:00	17:31–19:30
Excellent	11:50–12:29	12:30–13:30	13:00–14:30	13:45–15:55	14:30–16:30	16:30–18:00
Superior	<11:50	<12:30	<13:00	<13:45	<14:30	<16:30

Times are given in minutes and seconds (> = greater than, < = less than)

Source: Reprinted with permission from The Cooper Institute, Dallas, Texas. Available online at www.CooperInstitute.org.

Activity 3: YMCA Step Test

Complete the PAR-Q questionnaire. Do not take the test if you suffer joint problems in your ankles, knees, or hips, or if you are obese.

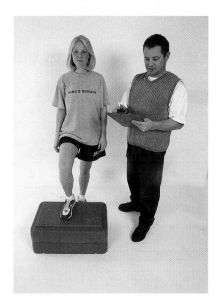

Preparation

You will need the following:

- 12-inch-high sturdy bench

- Metronome

- Stopwatch, watch, or clock with a second hand

Warm up for 5 minutes before taking the test. Practice before, but you should be well rested with no prior exercise of any kind for several hours before the test.

Procedure

1. Set the metronome at 96 beats per minute (four clicks of the metronome equals one step-cycle: up—1, 2; down—3, 4).

2. Step up and down on the 12-inch bench for 3 minutes.

3. After the 3 minutes of stepping, sit down and within 5 seconds count your radial pulse for 1 full minute.

4. See Table 5.A2 for your fitness rating.

Table 5.A2
YMCA 3-Minute Step Test:
Post-Exercise 1-Minute Heart Rate (beats/minute)

Age (years) Gender	18–25		26–35		36–45	
	Male	**Female**	**Male**	**Female**	**Male**	**Female**
Excellent	50–76	52–81	51–76	58–80	49–76	51–84
Good	79–84	85–93	79–85	85–92	80–88	89–96
Above average	88–93	96–102	88–94	95–101	92–98	100–104
Average	95–100	104–110	96–102	104–110	100–105	107–112
Below average	102–107	113–120	104–110	113–119	108–113	115–120
Poor	111–119	122–131	114–121	122–129	116–124	124–132
Very poor	124–157	135–169	126–161	134–171	130–163	137–169

Age (years) Gender	46–55		56–65		Over 65	
	Male	**Female**	**Male**	**Female**	**Male**	**Female**
Excellent	56–82	63–91	60–77	60–92	59–81	70–92
Good	87–93	95–101	86–94	97–103	87–92	96–101
Above average	95–101	104–110	97–100	106–111	94–102	104–111
Average	103–111	113–118	103–109	113–118	104–110	116–121
Below average	113–119	120–124	111–117	119–127	114–118	123–126
Poor	121–126	121–132	119–128	129–135	121–126	128–133
Very poor	131–159	137–171	131–154	141–174	130–151	135–155

Note: Pulse is to be counted for 1 full minute after 3 minutes of stepping at 24 steps per minute on a 12-inch bench.

Source: Adapted with permission from *YMCA Fitness Testing and Assessment Manual, 4th ed.* © 2000 by YMCA of the USA, Chicago. All rights reserved.

Name _____   Section _____   Date _____

Tracking Your Cardiorespiratory Endurance Progress

Activity 1: Tracking Your Cardiorespiratory Endurance Ratings

The following charts will help you to track your cardiorespiratory endurance ratings on different dates. Try to measure yourself at the same time and under the same conditions. These records can provide information as you pursue a physical activity program.

Choose one or more of the tests in Lab 5-2 to evaluate your cardiorespiratory endurance rating. You do not have to complete all of the fitness tests.

Test 1 Date _____

Test	Values	Fitness rating
1-mile walk test	Time: Pulse rate:	
1.5-mile run/walk test	Time:	
3-minute step test	Pulse rate:	

Test 2 Date _____

Test	Values	Fitness rating
1-mile walk test	Time: Pulse rate:	
1.5-mile run/walk test	Time:	
3-minute step test	Pulse rate:	

Test 3 Date _____

Test	Values	Fitness rating
1-mile walk test	Time: Pulse rate:	
1.5-mile run/walk test	Time:	
3-minute step test	Pulse rate:	

Test 4 Date _____

Test	Values	Fitness rating
1-mile walk test	Time: Pulse rate:	
1.5-mile run/walk test	Time:	
3-minute step test	Pulse rate:	

Activity 2: Cardiorespiratory Training Log

Track your workouts by recording the date, activity, intensity, and duration for each workout.

Cardiorespiratory Training Log

Date	Activity	Intensity (heart rate)	Duration (time)	Comments (e.g., rating of perceived exertion, pain, observations)
Sept. 15	Walk/jog	60% of HRR	30 min.	Great being outdoors

LAB 6-1

Muscular Endurance Assessments

Activity 1: YMCA Bench-Press Test

The YMCA developed a bench-press test for muscular endurance, using a standardized weight. This test offers several advantages, but it discriminates against lighter individuals.

Preparation

You will need the following:

• Barbell with weights and collars to hold them in place

• For the test, men use an 80-pound barbell and women use a 35-pound barbell

• Another person to "spot" for you

• Flat bench

• Metronome, set for 60 bpm

Warm-up should include doing a few bench presses with a small amount of weight to practice bench pressing. Give yourself a couple of minutes to recover after warm-up before beginning the test.

Procedure

• Lie on the flat bench with your feet on the floor.

• Your spotter hands the barbell to you. The down position is the starting position (elbows flexed, hands shoulder-width apart, palms facing up).

• Press the barbell upward to fully extend (straighten) the elbows. After each extension, the barbell is returned to the original down position with the bar touching the chest. Do not bounce the bar on your chest. Do not arch your back.

• Keep up with the rhythm of the metronome—lift the barbell on one beat and lower it on the next. Your spotter counts the number of bench presses you perform (each time the barbell is in the down position); each click represents a movement up or down for 30 lifts per minute.

• Perform as many reps as you can without stopping, and keep with the rhythm. Stop the test when any of these occur: (1) you are unable to reach full extension of the elbows, (2) you are unable to keep up with the rhythm of the metronome, or (3) you are unable to do any more bench presses.

• See Table 6.A1 for your fitness level.

Table 6.A1
YMCA Bench-Press Test Scoring

Your score is the number of completed bench presses. Refer to the appropriate portion of the table below for a rating of your upper body endurance. Record your rating below and in the chart at the end of this lab.

Rating: _____

Number of bench presses							
Men	**Very poor**	**Poor**	**Below average**	**Average**	**Above average**	**Good**	**Excellent**
Age: 18–25	Below 13	13–19	20–23	24–28	29–33	34–43	Above 43
26–35	Below 12	12–16	17–20	21–25	26–29	30–40	Above 40
36–45	Below 9	9–13	14–17	18–21	22–25	26–35	Above 35
46–55	Below 5	5–8	9–11	12–15	16–20	21–27	Above 27
56–65	Below 2	2–4	5–8	9–11	12–16	17–23	Above 23
Over 65	Below 2	2–3	4–6	7–9	10–11	12–19	Above 19
Women	**Very poor**	**Poor**	**Below average**	**Average**	**Above average**	**Good**	**Excellent**
Age: 18–25	Below 9	9–15	16–19	20–24	25–29	30–41	Above 41
26–35	Below 9	9–13	14–17	18–23	24–28	29–39	Above 39
36–45	Below 6	6–11	12–15	16–20	21–25	26–32	Above 32
46–55	Below 2	2–6	7–9	10–13	14–19	20–28	Above 28
56–65	Below 2	2–4	5–7	8–11	12–16	17–23	Above 23
Over 65	Below 1	1–2	3–4	5–7	8–11	12–17	Above 17

Source: Adapted with permission from *YMCA Fitness Testing and Assessment Manual*, 4th ed. © 2000 by YMCA of the USA, Chicago. All rights reserved.

Activity 2: Push-up Test for Muscular Endurance

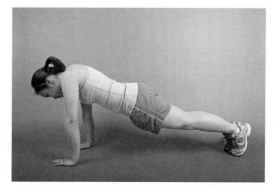

Preparation

- Use a large space on the floor, clear of obstructions.

- Warm up for 3 to 5 minutes before starting. Give yourself a couple of minutes to recover after warm-up before beginning the test.

Procedure

Men

- Assume the standard position for a push-up, with the body rigid and straight, toes tucked under, and hands about shoulder-width apart and straight under the shoulders.

- Lower the body until the elbows reach 90°. Some prefer to place an object such as a paper cup beneath to touch.

- Return to the starting position with the arms fully extended.

- The most common error is not keeping the back straight and rigid throughout the entire push-up.

- Perform as many push-ups as you can without stopping.

- See Table 6.A2 for your fitness level.

Table 6.A2
Ratings for the Push-up and Modified Push-up Tests

Number of push-ups						
Men	**Very poor**	**Poor**	**Fair**	**Good**	**Excellent**	**Superior**
Age: 18–29	Below 22	22–28	29–36	37–46	47–61	Above 61
30–39	Below 17	17–23	24–29	30–38	39–51	Above 51
40–49	Below 11	11–17	18–23	24–29	30–39	Above 39
50–59	Below 9	9–12	13–18	19–24	25–38	Above 38
60+	Below 6	6–9	10–17	18–22	23–27	Above 27

Number of modified push-ups						
Women	**Very poor**	**Poor**	**Fair**	**Good**	**Excellent**	**Superior**
Age: 18–29	Below 17	17–22	23–29	30–35	36–44	Above 44
30–39	Below 11	11–18	19–23	24–30	31–38	Above 38
40–49	Below 6	6–12	13–17	18–23	24–32	Above 32
50–59	Below 6	6–11	12–16	17–20	21–27	Above 27
60+	Below 2	2–4	5–11	12–14	15–19	Above 19

Source: Reprinted with permission from The Cooper Institute, Dallas, Texas from a book called *"Physical Fitness Assessments and Norms for Adults and Law Enforcement"*. Available online at www.CooperInstitute.org.

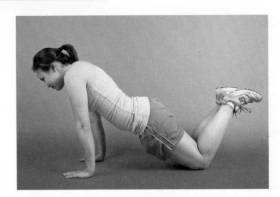

Women

Women tend to have less upper body strength and therefore should use the modified push-up position to assess their upper body endurance. The test is performed as follows:

- Directions are the same for women as for men, except that women should perform the test with the knees remaining on the floor. Make sure that your hands are slightly ahead of your shoulders in the up position so that when you are in the down position, your hands are directly under the shoulders.

- Keep the back straight and rigid throughout the entire push-up.

- Perform as many push-ups as you can without stopping.

- See Table 6.A2 for your fitness level.

Activity 3: YMCA Half Sit-up Test (Partial Curl-up Test)

Preparation

You will need the following:

- Ruler for measuring 3 inches

- Stopwatch, watch, or clock with a second hand

- Adhesive tape

- Metronome

Sit on a mat or carpet with your legs bent 90° (your feet must remain flat on the floor). Extend your arms so that both hands' longest fingertips touch a strip of tape placed on the floor perpendicular to the body. A second strip of tape is placed on the floor 3 inches toward the feet and parallel to the first. Alternatives to the two tape marks are a 3-inch-width piece of cardboard or two pieces of athletic tape (each is 1.5 inches and can be applied next to each other or a yardstick or similar piece of wood used for the mark nearest the feet).

- Warm-up should include a few sit-ups. Give yourself a couple of minutes to recover after warm-up before beginning the test.

- Set the metronome for 50 bpm.

Procedure

- While lying on the mat or carpet, the curl-up is done by raising your trunk (e.g., curling upward) with arms straight. Fingers slide along the floor until your longest fingertip of each hand touches the second strip of tape or object and then returns to the starting position. You then curl down so that your upper back touches the floor. Keep the 90° bend in your legs. Your feet should not be held down.

- Perform curl-ups to the rhythm of the metronome—curl up on one beat and down on the second beat.

- Perform as many curl-ups as you can without stopping and keep with the rhythm. Stop the test when either of these occurs: (1) You are unable to keep up with the rhythm of the metronome or (2) you are unable to do any more curl-ups. At the end of the test, check your fingertip position. If the fingertips do not touch the near side of the line, your score is not accurate.

- See Table 6.A3 for your fitness level.

Table 6.A3
Ratings for the Partial Curl-up Test

		Number of curl-ups				
Men	**Needs improvement**	**Fair**	**Good**	**Very good**	**Excellent**
Age: 15–19	Below 16	16–20	21–22	23–24	25
20–29	Below 13	13–20	21–22	23–24	25
30–39	Below 13	13–20	21–22	23–24	25
40–49	Below 11	11–15	16–21	22–24	25
50–59	Below 9	9–13	14–19	20–24	25
60–69	Below 4	4–9	10–15	16–24	25
Women					
Age: 15–19	Below 16	16–20	21–22	23–24	25
20–29	Below 13	13–18	19–22	23–24	25
30–39	Below 11	11–15	16–21	22–24	25
40–49	Below 6	6–12	13–20	21–24	25
50–59	Below 4	4–8	9–15	16–24	25
60–69	Below 2	2–5	6–10	11–17	18–25

Assessing Muscular Strength

The one-repetition maximum (1 RM) test for muscular strength is not recommended for older individuals and unconditioned individuals because of possible injury. The 1 RM test should be used only after several weeks of strength training. Muscular strength can be measured by the 1 RM test, which measures the maximum amount of weight that can be lifted one time.

Activity 1: One-Repetition Maximum Test (1 RM)

Preparation
You will need the following:

- Barbell and various weights with collars

- One or two spotters for safety

- The bench press, shoulder press (military press), and arm curl are the most common methods for assessing muscular strength. Warm up by performing the selected lift to be used several times.

Procedure

- For the selected muscle group to be tested, choose a starting weight that you can lift without a great deal of stress. Then, gradually add weight until you reach the maximum weight that you can lift one time. Rest 2 to 3 minutes between each trial or new attempt to lift the new weight.

- If you can lift the weight more than once, add more weight until you reach a level of resistance that can be performed only once.

- Compute your strength score by dividing your 1 RM weight (in pounds) by your body weight (in pounds) and then multiply by 100.

$$\frac{1 \text{ RM weight (lb)}}{\text{body weight (lb)}} \times 100 = \text{muscle strength score}$$

- See Table 6.A4 for your fitness rating for the bench press.

Table 6.A4
Strength Ratings for the Maximum Bench-Press Test

	Pounds lifted/body weight (lb)					
Men	**Very poor**	**Poor**	**Fair**	**Good**	**Excellent**	**Superior**
Age: Under 20	Below 0.89	0.89–1.05	1.06–1.18	1.19–1.33	1.34–1.75	Above 1.75
20–29	Below 0.88	0.88–0.98	0.99–1.13	1.14–1.31	1.32–1.62	Above 1.62
30–39	Below 0.78	0.78–0.87	0.88–0.97	0.98–1.11	1.12–1.34	Above 1.34
40–49	Below 0.72	0.72–0.79	0.80–0.87	0.88–0.99	1.00–1.19	Above 1.19
50–59	Below 0.63	0.63–0.70	0.71–0.78	0.79–0.89	0.90–1.04	Above 1.04
60 and over	Below 0.57	0.57–0.65	0.66–0.71	0.72–0.81	0.82–0.93	Above 0.93
Women	**Very poor**	**Poor**	**Fair**	**Good**	**Excellent**	**Superior**
Age: Under 20	Below 0.53	0.53–0.57	0.58–0.64	0.65–0.76	0.77–0.87	Above 0.87
20–29	Below 0.51	0.51–0.58	0.59–0.69	0.70–0.79	0.80–1.00	Above 1.00
30–39	Below 0.47	0.47–0.52	0.53–0.59	0.60–0.69	0.70–0.81	Above 0.81
40–49	Below 0.43	0.43–0.49	0.50–0.53	0.54–0.61	0.62–0.76	Above 0.76
50–59	Below 0.39	0.39–0.43	0.44–0.47	0.48–0.54	0.55–0.67	Above 0.67
60 and over	Below 0.38	0.38–0.42	0.43–0.46	0.47–0.53	0.54–0.71	Above 0.71

Source: Reprinted with permission from The Cooper Institute, Dallas, Texas from a book called *"Physical Fitness Assessments and Norms for Adults and Law Enforcement"*. Available online at www.CooperInstitute.org.

Activity 2: Hand Grip Strength Test

Preparation

You will need the following:

- Dynamometer

- Dry hands

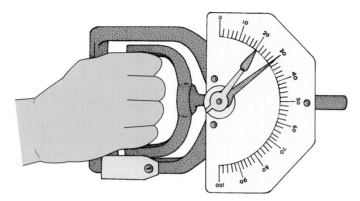

Figure 6.A1 Dynamometer.

Procedure

- Adjust and comfortably place the dynamometer in the hand to be tested. The second joint of the hand should fit snugly under the handle, which is gripped between the fingers and the palm at the base of the thumb (see Figure 6.A1).

- Bend forward slightly, with the hand to be tested out in front of your body. Neither the hand nor the arm should be touching the body or any other object. The arm can be slightly bent.

- During the test, an all-out effort should be given for between 2 and 3 seconds. No swinging or pumping of the arm is allowed. The dial can face you.

- The score comes from the sum of both hands, based on the best of two to four trials each.

- See Table 5.A1 for your fitness level.

Table 6.A5 Grip Strength for Males and Females of All Ages

Norms and percentiles by age groups and sex for combined right- and left-hand grip strength (kg)

Age Sex	15–19 M	15–19 F	20–29 M	20–29 F	30–39 M	30–39 F	40–49 M	40–49 F	50–59 M	50–59 F	60–69 M	60–69 F
Excellent	≥113	≥71	≥124	≥71	≥123	≥73	≥119	≥73	≥110	≥65	≥102	≥60
Above avg.	130–112	64–70	113–123	65–70	113–122	66–72	110–118	65–72	102–109	59–64	93–101	54–59
Average	95–102	59–63	106–112	61–64	105–112	61–65	102–109	59–64	96–101	55–58	86–92	51–53
Below avg.	84–94	54–58	97–105	55–60	97–104	56–60	94–101	55–58	87–95	51–54	79–85	48–50
Weak	≤83	≤53	≤96	≤54	≤96	≤55	≤93	≤54	≤86	≤50	≤78	≤47

Age Sex	15–19 M	15–19 F	20–29 M	20–29 F	30–39 M	30–39 F	40–49 M	40–49 F	50–59 M	50–59 F	60–69 M	60–69 F
Percentiles												
95	125	78	136	78	135	80	128	80	119	72	111	67
90	119	74	127	74	127	76	123	76	114	69	106	62
85	113	71	124	71	123	73	119	73	110	65	102	60
80	110	69	120	70	120	71	117	71	108	63	99	58
75	108	67	118	68	117	69	115	69	105	62	96	56
70	105	65	115	67	115	68	112	67	103	60	94	55
65	103	64	113	65	113	66	110	65	102	59	93	54
60	101	63	111	64	111	65	108	64	100	58	91	53
55	99	61	109	63	109	63	106	62	99	57	89	52
50	97	60	107	62	107	62	104	61	97	56	88	52
45	95	59	106	61	105	61	102	59	96	55	86	51
40	93	58	104	59	104	60	100	58	94	54	84	50
35	90	57	102	58	101	59	98	57	92	53	82	49
30	87	56	100	56	99	58	96	56	90	53	81	49
25	84	54	97	55	97	56	94	55	87	51	79	48
20	81	53	95	53	94	55	91	53	85	50	76	47
15	77	51	91	52	91	53	89	51	83	48	73	45
10	73	49	87	50	87	51	84	49	80	46	69	43
5	67	45	81	47	81	48	76	46	74	42	62	39

© 2013 Jones & Bartlett Learning, LLC

Name _____ Section _____ Date _____

Track and Record Your Muscular Strength and Endurance Progress

Activity 1: Tracking Your Muscular Endurance

The following charts will help you to track your muscular endurance on different dates. Try to measure yourself at the same time and under the same conditions. These records can provide information as you pursue a physical activity program. Perform the activities in Lab 6-1 to obtain values and classifications.

Test 1 Date: _____

Assessment technique	Value	Classification
YMCA bench-press test		
Push-up test		
YMCA half sit-up test		

Test 2 Date: _____

Assessment technique	Value	Classification
YMCA bench-press test		
Push-up test		
YMCA half sit-up test		

Test 3 Date: _____

Assessment technique	Value	Classification
YMCA bench-press test		
Push-up test		
YMCA half sit-up test		

Test 4 Date: _____

Assessment technique	Value	Classification
YMCA bench-press test		
Push-up test		
YMCA half sit-up test		

Activity 2: Tracking Your Muscular Strength

The following charts will help you to track your muscular strength on different dates. Try to measure yourself at the same time and under the same conditions. These records can provide information as you pursue a physical activity program. Perform the activities in Lab 6-2, Activity 1 to obtain values and classifications.

Test 1 Date: _____

Assessment technique	Value	Classification
Bench press		

Test 2 Date: _____

Assessment technique	Value	Classification
Bench press		

Test 3 Date: _____

Assessment technique	Value	Classification
Bench press		

Test 4 Date: _____

Assessment technique	Value	Classification
Bench press		

Activity 3: Tracking Your Grip Strength

The following charts will help you to track your grip strength on different dates. Try to measure yourself at the same time and under the same conditions. These records can provide information as you pursue a physical activity program. Perform the activities in Lab 6-2, Activity 2 to obtain values and classifications.

Test 1 Date: _____

Assessment technique	Value	Classification
Grip strength		

Test 2 Date: _____

Assessment technique	Value	Classification
Grip strength		

Test 3 Date: _____

Assessment technique	Value	Classification
Grip strength		

Test 4 Date: _____

Assessment technique	Value	Classification
Grip strength		

Activity 4: Resistance Training

Table 6.A6
Sample of Resistance Exercises

Muscle Group	Training with Weights (free weights or resistance machines)	Without Weights
Chest	Bench press	Push-ups; modified push-ups
Shoulder	Shoulder press	Pull-ups, chin-ups, modified dips
Arm (bicep)	Bicep curl	Arm curl, chin-ups
Arm (tricep)	Tricep curl	Pull-ups, modified dips
Hip/leg	Lunges	Lunges
Leg (thigh)	Half squat	
Leg (calf)	Heel raise	Heel raise

Monitor your workouts by recording the number of sets, repetitions, and the amount of weight.

Muscle group/ exercises	Date: _____ set × rep / wt	Date: _____ set × rep / wt	Date: _____ set × rep / wt	Date: _____ set × rep / wt	Date: _____ set × rep / wt
	× /	× /	× /	× /	× /
	× /	× /	× /	× /	× /
	× /	× /	× /	× /	× /
	× /	× /	× /	× /	× /
	× /	× /	× /	× /	× /
	× /	× /	× /	× /	× /
	× /	× /	× /	× /	× /
	× /	× /	× /	× /	× /
	× /	× /	× /	× /	× /
	× /	× /	× /	× /	× /

Muscle group/ exercises	Date: _____ set × rep / wt	Date: _____ set × rep / wt	Date: _____ set × rep / wt	Date: _____ set × rep / wt	Date: _____ set × rep / wt
	× /	× /	× /	× /	× /
	× /	× /	× /	× /	× /
	× /	× /	× /	× /	× /
	× /	× /	× /	× /	× /
	× /	× /	× /	× /	× /
	× /	× /	× /	× /	× /
	× /	× /	× /	× /	× /
	× /	× /	× /	× /	× /
	× /	× /	× /	× /	× /
	× /	× /	× /	× /	× /

Muscle group/ exercises	Date: _____ set × rep / wt	Date: _____ set × rep / wt	Date: _____ set × rep / wt	Date: _____ set × rep / wt	Date: _____ set × rep / wt
	× /	× /	× /	× /	× /
	× /	× /	× /	× /	× /
	× /	× /	× /	× /	× /
	× /	× /	× /	× /	× /
	× /	× /	× /	× /	× /
	× /	× /	× /	× /	× /
	× /	× /	× /	× /	× /
	× /	× /	× /	× /	× /
	× /	× /	× /	× /	× /
	× /	× /	× /	× /	× /

Muscle group/ exercises	Date: _____ set × rep / wt	Date: _____ set × rep / wt	Date: _____ set × rep / wt	Date: _____ set × rep / wt	Date: _____ set × rep / wt
	× /	× /	× /	× /	× /
	× /	× /	× /	× /	× /
	× /	× /	× /	× /	× /
	× /	× /	× /	× /	× /
	× /	× /	× /	× /	× /
	× /	× /	× /	× /	× /
	× /	× /	× /	× /	× /
	× /	× /	× /	× /	× /
	× /	× /	× /	× /	× /
	× /	× /	× /	× /	× /

Muscle group/ exercises	Date: _____ set × rep / wt	Date: _____ set × rep / wt	Date: _____ set × rep / wt	Date: _____ set × rep / wt	Date: _____ set × rep / wt
	× /	× /	× /	× /	× /
	× /	× /	× /	× /	× /
	× /	× /	× /	× /	× /
	× /	× /	× /	× /	× /
	× /	× /	× /	× /	× /
	× /	× /	× /	× /	× /
	× /	× /	× /	× /	× /
	× /	× /	× /	× /	× /
	× /	× /	× /	× /	× /
	× /	× /	× /	× /	× /

Track and Record Your Muscular Strength and Endurance Progress

Name _____ Section _____ Date _____

Flexibility Assessments

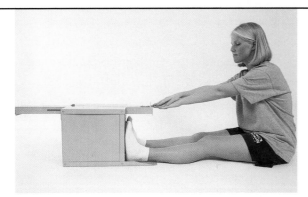

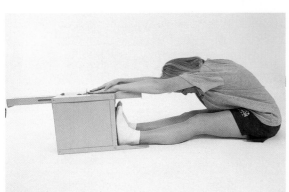

Activity 1: Sit-and-Reach Test

Precautions

1. Warm up.

2. Stop the test if pain occurs.

3. Do not be competitive. This is a test to help assess your spine/back flexibility, not a game. Do not perform fast, jerky movements.

4. If any of the following apply, seek medical advice before performing tests:

    A. You are presently suffering from acute back pain

    B. You are currently receiving treatment for back pain

    C. You have had a surgical operation on your back

    D. A health-care professional told you to never exercise your back

Procedure

Step 1: Sit on the floor with your legs straight, knees together, and toes pointing upward toward the ceiling.

Step 2: Place one hand over the other. The tips of your two middle fingers should be on top of each other.

Step 3: Slowly stretch forward without bouncing or jerking. Stop when tightness or discomfort occurs in the back or legs.

Step 4: Repeat this test two more times and record scores as follows:

- First attempt: _____ points

- Second attempt: _____ points

- Third attempt: _____ points

- Total points = _____ divided by 3 = _____ points, which is rated as _____.

How to score (average of 3 attempts)	
Reached well past toes	1 point; excellent
Reached just to toes	2 points; good
Up to 4 inches from toes	3 points; fair
More than 4 inches from toes	4 points; poor

Source: Data from Imrie D. *The Backpower Program*, 1st ed. Wiley Publishing, Inc., 1990.

Name _____ Section _____ Date _____

Activity 2: Shoulder Flexibility Test

Precautions

- Briefly warm up with a few minutes of stretching.
- Avoid rapid or jerky movements during the test.

Procedure

Step 1: Bring the right hand around to the back of the neck.

Step 2: Bring the left hand around to the small of the back.

Step 3: Try to touch the fingertips of both hands behind the back.

Step 4: Have someone measure the distance between the fingertips.

Step 5: Do the test the other way, left hand to the back of the neck, right hand to the small of the back.

Step 6: Try to touch the fingertips of both hands behind the back.

Step 7: Have someone measure the distance between the fingertips.

How to score	
Can clasp hands together	Very good flexibility
Fingertips almost touch	Good, but needs work
Not within an inch of touching fingertips together	Poor, needs a lot of work

Source: Adapted from Schlosberg S. *Fitness for Dummies*, 3rd ed. Wiley Publishing, Inc., 2005.

Name _____ Section _____ Date _____

Activity 3: Other Flexibility Tests

Perform the following tests to assess your flexibility.

Tests	What to Do	Your flexibility is good if . . .	Your flexibility needs work if . . .	Your flexibility needs a lot of work if . . .
Thigh (front) Precaution: Do not perform if you have had knee problems or knee surgery.	Lie on stomach with one leg straight and bend other knee so heel moves toward buttocks. Test both legs.	Heel easily touches buttocks	Heel comes close, but does not touch buttocks	Heel does not come within 6 inches of touching buttocks
Calf	Sit on floor with legs straight and feet flat against a wall. While keeping heels against wall, point toes and feet away from wall, back toward head, as far a possible.	Soles of feet move more than 4 inches from the wall	Soles of feet move several inches from the wall	Soles of feet barely move from the wall
Hamstring	Sit with one leg straight, one leg bent. Put the sole of foot next to the knee of straight leg. Gently curl upper body toward knee of straight leg.	Able to touch straight leg with upper body	Able to move more than half the distance toward straight leg	Able to move a few inches toward straight leg
Groin	Sit on floor with knees bent and heels of feet together 6 inches from buttocks. Push knees toward floor as far as possible with elbows.	Knees or calf muscles able to touch floor	Knees able to move about half the distance toward floor	Knees able to move only a few inches toward floor
Hip flexors	Lie on back with knees bent. Bring right leg toward chest by holding knee with both hands. Hold it there tightly. Gently straighten left leg out to the floor, but do not let right leg move away from chest.	Able to hold one leg firmly against chest with other leg flat against floor	Able to hold one leg against chest while other knee is bent 2 to 4 inches off floor	Unable to get one leg firmly against chest without causing pain or discomfort and other leg raises off floor 4 or more inches

Source: Reproduced from Schlosberg S. *Fitness for Dummies*, 3rd ed. Wiley Publishing, Inc., 2005, with permission of John Wiley & Sons, Inc.

Name _____ Section _____ Date _____

Track and Record Your Flexibility

Activity 1: Tracking Your Flexibility

Procedure

The following charts will help you to track your flexibility on different dates. Use the tests in Lab 7-1 to assess your flexibility. Try to measure yourself at the same time under the same conditions. These records can provide information as you pursue a physical activity.

Test 1 Date: _____

Assessment technique	Value	Classification
Sit-and-reach		
Shoulder	left arm right arm	
Thigh	left right	
Calf	left right	
Hamstring	left right	
Groin		
Hip flexors	left right	

Test 2 Date: _____

Assessment technique	Value	Classification
Sit-and-reach		
Shoulder	left arm right arm	
Thigh	left right	
Calf	left right	
Hamstring	left right	
Groin		
Hip flexors	left right	

Test 3 Date: _____

Assessment technique	Value	Classification
Sit-and-reach		
Shoulder	left arm right arm	
Thigh	left right	
Calf	left right	
Hamstring	left right	
Groin		
Hip flexors	left right	

Test 4 Date: _____

Assessment technique	Value	Classification
Sit-and-reach		
Shoulder	left arm	
	right arm	
Thigh	left	
	right	
Calf	left	
	right	
Hamstring	left	
	right	
Groin		
Hip flexors	left	
	right	

Test 5 Date: _____

Assessment technique	Value	Classification
Sit-and-reach		
Shoulder	left arm	
	right arm	
Thigh	left	
	right	
Calf	left	
	right	
Hamstring	left	
	right	
Groin		
Hip flexors	left	
	right	

Test 6 Date: _____

Assessment technique	Value	Classification
Sit-and-reach		
Shoulder	left arm	
	right arm	
Thigh	left	
	right	
Calf	left	
	right	
Hamstring	left	
	right	
Groin		
Hip flexors	left	
	right	

Name _____ Section _____ Date _____

Activity 2: Stretching Log

Step 1: Select stretching exercises and write them in the left column.

Step 2: Circle the days of each week you stretched.

Exercise	Week of _____	Week of _____	Week of _____
	S M T W Th F Sa	S M T W Th F Sa	S M T W Th F Sa
	S M T W Th F Sa	S M T W Th F Sa	S M T W Th F Sa
	S M T W Th F Sa	S M T W Th F Sa	S M T W Th F Sa
	S M T W Th F Sa	S M T W Th F Sa	S M T W Th F Sa
	S M T W Th F Sa	S M T W Th F Sa	S M T W Th F Sa
	S M T W Th F Sa	S M T W Th F Sa	S M T W Th F Sa
	S M T W Th F Sa	S M T W Th F Sa	S M T W Th F Sa
	S M T W Th F Sa	S M T W Th F Sa	S M T W Th F Sa
	S M T W Th F Sa	S M T W Th F Sa	S M T W Th F Sa
	S M T W Th F Sa	S M T W Th F Sa	S M T W Th F Sa
	S M T W Th F Sa	S M T W Th F Sa	S M T W Th F Sa
	S M T W Th F Sa	S M T W Th F Sa	S M T W Th F Sa

Exercise	Week of _____	Week of _____	Week of _____
	S M T W Th F Sa	S M T W Th F Sa	S M T W Th F Sa
	S M T W Th F Sa	S M T W Th F Sa	S M T W Th F Sa
	S M T W Th F Sa	S M T W Th F Sa	S M T W Th F Sa
	S M T W Th F Sa	S M T W Th F Sa	S M T W Th F Sa
	S M T W Th F Sa	S M T W Th F Sa	S M T W Th F Sa
	S M T W Th F Sa	S M T W Th F Sa	S M T W Th F Sa
	S M T W Th F Sa	S M T W Th F Sa	S M T W Th F Sa
	S M T W Th F Sa	S M T W Th F Sa	S M T W Th F Sa
	S M T W Th F Sa	S M T W Th F Sa	S M T W Th F Sa
	S M T W Th F Sa	S M T W Th F Sa	S M T W Th F Sa
	S M T W Th F Sa	S M T W Th F Sa	S M T W Th F Sa
	S M T W Th F Sa	S M T W Th F Sa	S M T W Th F Sa

Exercise	Week of _____	Week of _____	Week of _____
	S M T W Th F Sa	S M T W Th F Sa	S M T W Th F Sa
	S M T W Th F Sa	S M T W Th F Sa	S M T W Th F Sa
	S M T W Th F Sa	S M T W Th F Sa	S M T W Th F Sa
	S M T W Th F Sa	S M T W Th F Sa	S M T W Th F Sa
	S M T W Th F Sa	S M T W Th F Sa	S M T W Th F Sa
	S M T W Th F Sa	S M T W Th F Sa	S M T W Th F Sa
	S M T W Th F Sa	S M T W Th F Sa	S M T W Th F Sa
	S M T W Th F Sa	S M T W Th F Sa	S M T W Th F Sa
	S M T W Th F Sa	S M T W Th F Sa	S M T W Th F Sa
	S M T W Th F Sa	S M T W Th F Sa	S M T W Th F Sa
	S M T W Th F Sa	S M T W Th F Sa	S M T W Th F Sa
	S M T W Th F Sa	S M T W Th F Sa	S M T W Th F Sa

Exercise	Week of _____	Week of _____	Week of _____
	S M T W Th F Sa	S M T W Th F Sa	S M T W Th F Sa
	S M T W Th F Sa	S M T W Th F Sa	S M T W Th F Sa
	S M T W Th F Sa	S M T W Th F Sa	S M T W Th F Sa
	S M T W Th F Sa	S M T W Th F Sa	S M T W Th F Sa
	S M T W Th F Sa	S M T W Th F Sa	S M T W Th F Sa
	S M T W Th F Sa	S M T W Th F Sa	S M T W Th F Sa
	S M T W Th F Sa	S M T W Th F Sa	S M T W Th F Sa
	S M T W Th F Sa	S M T W Th F Sa	S M T W Th F Sa
	S M T W Th F Sa	S M T W Th F Sa	S M T W Th F Sa
	S M T W Th F Sa	S M T W Th F Sa	S M T W Th F Sa
	S M T W Th F Sa	S M T W Th F Sa	S M T W Th F Sa
	S M T W Th F Sa	S M T W Th F Sa	S M T W Th F Sa

Exercise	Week of _____	Week of _____	Week of _____
	S M T W Th F Sa	S M T W Th F Sa	S M T W Th F Sa
	S M T W Th F Sa	S M T W Th F Sa	S M T W Th F Sa
	S M T W Th F Sa	S M T W Th F Sa	S M T W Th F Sa
	S M T W Th F Sa	S M T W Th F Sa	S M T W Th F Sa
	S M T W Th F Sa	S M T W Th F Sa	S M T W Th F Sa
	S M T W Th F Sa	S M T W Th F Sa	S M T W Th F Sa
	S M T W Th F Sa	S M T W Th F Sa	S M T W Th F Sa
	S M T W Th F Sa	S M T W Th F Sa	S M T W Th F Sa
	S M T W Th F Sa	S M T W Th F Sa	S M T W Th F Sa
	S M T W Th F Sa	S M T W Th F Sa	S M T W Th F Sa
	S M T W Th F Sa	S M T W Th F Sa	S M T W Th F Sa
	S M T W Th F Sa	S M T W Th F Sa	S M T W Th F Sa

Track and Record Your Flexibility

Exercise	Week of _____	Week of _____	Week of _____
	S M T W Th F Sa	S M T W Th F Sa	S M T W Th F Sa
	S M T W Th F Sa	S M T W Th F Sa	S M T W Th F Sa
	S M T W Th F Sa	S M T W Th F Sa	S M T W Th F Sa
	S M T W Th F Sa	S M T W Th F Sa	S M T W Th F Sa
	S M T W Th F Sa	S M T W Th F Sa	S M T W Th F Sa
	S M T W Th F Sa	S M T W Th F Sa	S M T W Th F Sa
	S M T W Th F Sa	S M T W Th F Sa	S M T W Th F Sa
	S M T W Th F Sa	S M T W Th F Sa	S M T W Th F Sa
	S M T W Th F Sa	S M T W Th F Sa	S M T W Th F Sa
	S M T W Th F Sa	S M T W Th F Sa	S M T W Th F Sa
	S M T W Th F Sa	S M T W Th F Sa	S M T W Th F Sa
	S M T W Th F Sa	S M T W Th F Sa	S M T W Th F Sa

Exercise	Week of _____	Week of _____	Week of _____
	S M T W Th F Sa	S M T W Th F Sa	S M T W Th F Sa
	S M T W Th F Sa	S M T W Th F Sa	S M T W Th F Sa
	S M T W Th F Sa	S M T W Th F Sa	S M T W Th F Sa
	S M T W Th F Sa	S M T W Th F Sa	S M T W Th F Sa
	S M T W Th F Sa	S M T W Th F Sa	S M T W Th F Sa
	S M T W Th F Sa	S M T W Th F Sa	S M T W Th F Sa
	S M T W Th F Sa	S M T W Th F Sa	S M T W Th F Sa
	S M T W Th F Sa	S M T W Th F Sa	S M T W Th F Sa
	S M T W Th F Sa	S M T W Th F Sa	S M T W Th F Sa
	S M T W Th F Sa	S M T W Th F Sa	S M T W Th F Sa
	S M T W Th F Sa	S M T W Th F Sa	S M T W Th F Sa
	S M T W Th F Sa	S M T W Th F Sa	S M T W Th F Sa

Name _____ Section _____ Date _____

Posture Assessment

Purpose
Identify basic posture deviations.

Procedure
Ideal posture varies among individuals, but it is possible to identify certain basic posture flaws. One method featured in Figure 7.A2 requires two people and a plumb line (a string with an attached weight).

1. The evaluator suspends the plumb line about 3 feet in front of a blank wall.

2. The subject should stand between the wall and the line facing the wall.

3. The plumb line should pass down the middle of the subject's back.

4. The evaluator should stand about 10 feet directly behind the plumb line.

5. After the back view has been evaluated using the posture rating chart (Figure 7.A1), the person being examined makes a one-quarter turn to the left or right.

6. The plumb line should pass along the ankle bone.

7. The evaluator then judges the side view.

Use Figures 7.A1 and 7.A2 to evaluate and score the back and side views.

Results
1. Score 5 points for left column, 3 points for the middle column, or 1 point for the right column.

2. Add points from the 13 views.

3. Divide total points by 13 for an average score.

What are your total points? _____   5 = good

Your average is _____   3 = fair

Your rating is _____   1 = poor

Are there any deviations? Yes _____ No _____

List the deviations considered poor or fair (needing improvement).

_____

_____

_____

_____

Figure 7.A1 Posture rating chart.

Score:

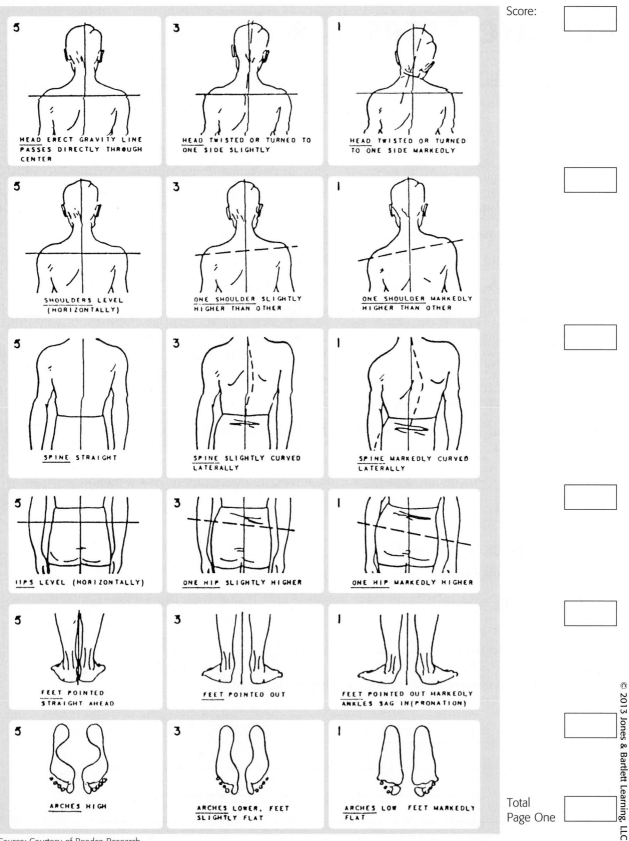

Total
Page One

Source: Courtesy of Reedco Research.

Score:

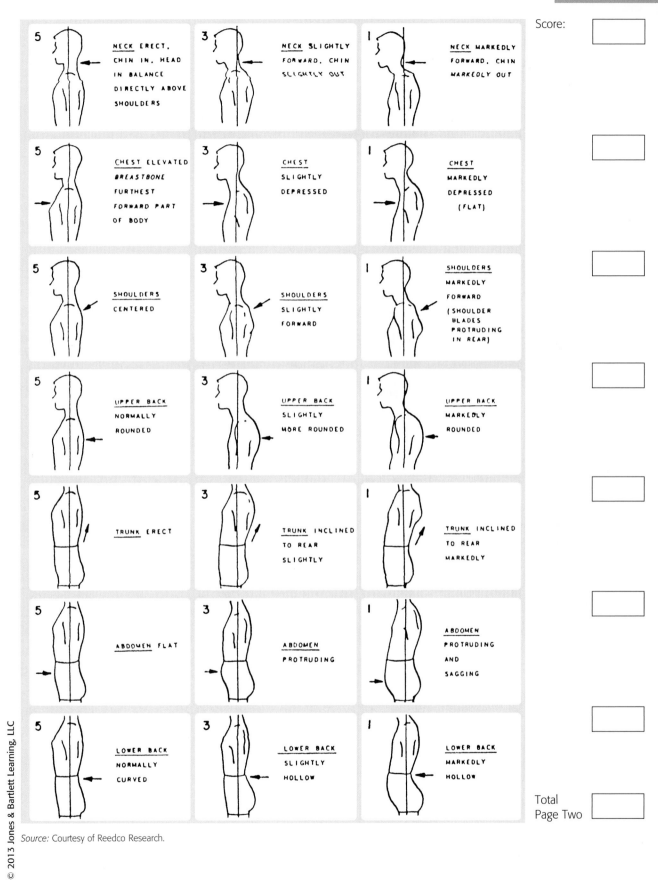

5   NECK ERECT, CHIN IN, HEAD IN BALANCE DIRECTLY ABOVE SHOULDERS

3   NECK SLIGHTLY FORWARD, CHIN SLIGHTLY OUT

1   NECK MARKEDLY FORWARD, CHIN MARKEDLY OUT

5   CHEST ELEVATED BREASTBONE FURTHEST FORWARD PART OF BODY

3   CHEST SLIGHTLY DEPRESSED

1   CHEST MARKEDLY DEPRESSED (FLAT)

5   SHOULDERS CENTERED

3   SHOULDERS SLIGHTLY FORWARD

1   SHOULDERS MARKEDLY FORWARD (SHOULDER BLADES PROTRUDING IN REAR)

5   UPPER BACK NORMALLY ROUNDED

3   UPPER BACK SLIGHTLY MORE ROUNDED

1   UPPER BACK MARKEDLY ROUNDED

5   TRUNK ERECT

3   TRUNK INCLINED TO REAR SLIGHTLY

1   TRUNK INCLINED TO REAR MARKEDLY

5   ABDOMEN FLAT

3   ABDOMEN PROTRUDING

1   ABDOMEN PROTRUDING AND SAGGING

5   LOWER BACK NORMALLY CURVED

3   LOWER BACK SLIGHTLY HOLLOW

1   LOWER BACK MARKEDLY HOLLOW

Total Page Two

Source: Courtesy of Reedco Research.

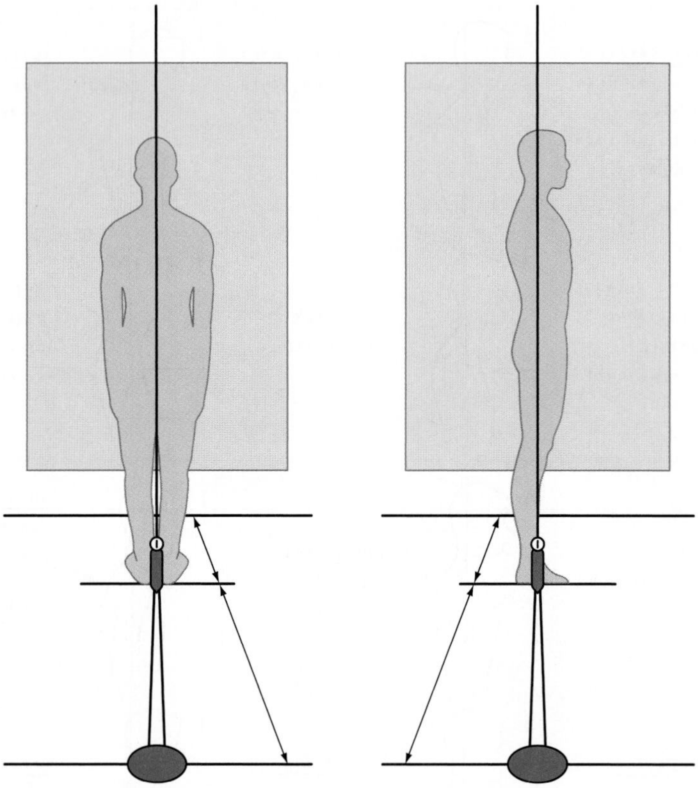

Figure 7.A2 Plumb-line posture assessment.

Name _____ Section _____ Date _____

On-Line Diet/Nutrition Analysis

A diet analysis is a valuable tool for understanding your diet. Although you may be able to recall the foods you have eaten generally, these recollections do not always provide adequate details on whether your diet is healthy or balanced. An analysis of your diet can identify areas that you need to address to improve it.

For 1 day, carry a small notebook or 3 × 5 index card with you to record each item you eat and drink and how much of it (e.g., cups, ounces, or tablespoons). It is easier to remember the foods you eat with each meal, but it is the snacks and foods you eat between meals that you do not always remember.

Go to ChooseMyPlate.gov at www.choosemyplate.gov and click on "Analyze my diet," and then click on "Assess Your Food Intake."

Follow the directions to register and enter your Personal Profile. Then click on "Proceed to Food Intake" and enter each food and quantity you ate for the day. Once you are done, you can click on "Save & Analyze." Then, click on "Calculate Nutrient Intakes from Foods" and later "Calculate MyPyramid Stats" to compare your food intake with what is recommended for you.

Print both analyses.

Self-analysis:

1. From the Calculate Nutrient Intakes page, how many of the nutrients were in the acceptable range? _____

2. How many of the nutrients were not in the acceptable range? _____

3. From the Comparison of Your Intake with MyPyramid, complete this table:

Categories	Your Intake	Recommended Intake	Percent of Recommendation
Milk			
Meat and Beans			
Vegetables			
Fruits			
Grains			

4. Was this day's food intake typical of other days? ___ Yes   ___ No

5. Identify one action you can take to improve your food choices.

Name _____ Section _____ Date _____

Fast-Food Analysis

Fast-foods have become popular, and it is prudent to know the nutrient content of the foods eaten.

    For nutritional information use one of these: (1) Fast Food Facts (www.foodfacts.info), (2) The Fast Food Explorer (www.fatcalories.com), (3) restaurant company's website (see below for some examples), or (4) visit fast-food restaurants in person for a printed brochure.

Arby's: www.arbysrestaurant.com

Burger King: www.burgerking.com

Domino's Pizza: www.dominos.com

Hardees: www.hardees.com

KFC: www.kfc.com

McDonald's: www.mcdonalds.com

Subway: www.subway.com

Taco Bell: www.tacobell.com

Wendy's: www.wendys.com

1. Choose one fast-food restaurant and access their nutritional information.

    Restaurant: _____

2. Select one fast-food item (e.g., hamburger, pizza, milkshake) from the selected restaurant and list the following information:

    Food selected: _____

    a. Total calories:

    b. Grams of protein:

    c. Total grams of fat:

    d. Total grams of saturated fat:

    e. mg of cholesterol:

    f. mg of salt:

    g. grams of fiber:

3. Give one reason for selecting this fast-food restaurant:

4. What did you learn from this assignment?

Name _____   Section _____   Date _____

Food Labels

Select a food with a food label.

Answer the following questions/calculations:

Name of product: _____

Serving size: _____

Servings per container: _____

Total calories per container: _____

Per serving: Fat calories _____, carbohydrate calories _____, and protein calories _____

Per serving: Percent of fat _____, carbohydrate _____, and protein _____

What does the percent of fat per serving in this food item tell you?

Percent of saturated fat per serving _____

What does the percent of saturated fat per serving in this food item tell you?

Can the manufacturers of this item make a claim of "high in," a "good source of," and/ or "healthy" regarding the product? Circle yes or no and **list all nutrients that make it possible or list the nutrients that prevent the claim.**

Healthy: Yes No   Why:

High in: Yes No   Why:

Good source of: Yes No   Why:

List all the "buzz" words on the label (low, organic, light/lite . . .). Are these buzz words nutritionally correct?

LAB 8-4

Name _____ Section _____ Date _____

Grocery Store Scavenger Hunt

1. Name of supermarket visited. _____

2. Location _____

3. Locate the following frozen desserts:

   • Well-known brand of chocolate ice cream

   • Store-brand chocolate ice cream

   • Fat-free frozen yogurt

   Which one do you think is the healthiest choice and why?

4. What percentage of fat calories is found in the following products
   (list the brand name you chose):

   • Any LEAN CUISINE dinner?

   • Any frozen pizza?

   • Any brand of chicken hot dogs?

5. Find a frozen dinner choice (different from the above) that contains less than 30 percent
   of its calories from fats. What is the product and what is the percentage?

6. Of all the cheese in the store that you can find, which one has the lowest percent of fat?

   Cheese _____ Percent fat _____

7. Locate any brand of chocolate chip cookie. Identify the brand name. List all types
   of sugars found in the ingredients. How many calories per cookie are there?

8. Find the lowest calorie cookie or sweet cracker you can. What is it and how many
   calories per cookie does it provide?

9. It is suggested that an individual limit sodium levels to 2400 mg per day.

   Find a "low-sodium" product. Product _____ Sodium mg _____

   Find a "high-sodium" product. Product _____ Sodium mg _____

10. Find three cereals that contain three grams or more of fiber per serving.

    Cereal Name   Amount of Fiber

    1. _____   _____

    2. _____   _____

    3. _____   _____

Summarize three of the most important things you learned from doing this assignment.

1.

2.

3.

Grocery Store Scavenger Hunt

Name _____   Section _____   Date _____

Assess Your Body Composition

Activity 1: Calculate Your Waist Circumference

Preparation
You will need a nonstretchable tape measure.

Procedure
How to measure waist circumference:

- Remove clothing to make sure the measuring tape is positioned correctly.

- Locate the upper hip bone and the top of the right iliac crest (see Figure 9.A1).

- Place a measuring tape in a horizontal plane around the abdomen at the level of the iliac crest. (Using a full-length mirror will help ensure that the tape is level all around the abdomen.)

Figure 9.A1 Measuring waist circumference.

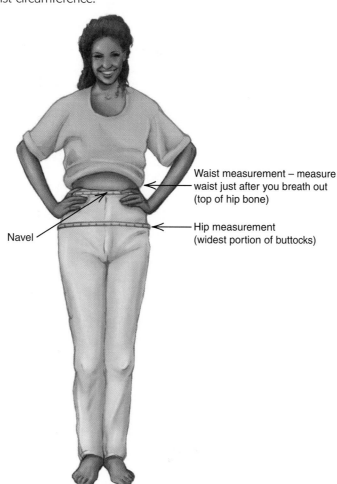

Waist measurement – measure waist just after you breath out (top of hip bone)

Hip measurement (widest portion of buttocks)

Navel

- Before reading the tape measure, ensure that the tape is snug but does not compress the skin, and is parallel to the floor.

- The measurement is made at the end of an exhalation (breathing out).

You are more likely to develop heart disease, high blood pressure, diabetes, and certain cancers when your waist circumference exceeds these measurements:

- Men: More than 40 inches (102 cm)

- Women: More than 35 inches (88 cm)

Activity 2: Calculate Your Waist-to-Hip Ratio

In addition to your waist circumference, it is helpful to know your waist-to-hip ratio (WHR). This ratio determines your pattern of fat distribution (e.g., where you store body fat).

$$\frac{\text{Waist circumference (inches)}}{\text{Hip circumference (inches)}} = \text{_____} \text{ Your WHR}$$

The appropriate ratios for men and women are listed in Table 9.A1. Ratios greater than these indicate a tendency toward central (torso) obesity. People who store excess fat centrally, as opposed to in their extremities, are at an increased risk for cardiorespiratory diseases and diabetes.

Table 9.A1 Standards for Waist-to-Hip Ratios

Men	<0.95 (known as "apples")
Women	<0.8 (known as "pears")

Activity 3: Calculate Your BMI

The body mass index (BMI) is commonly calculated to assess body composition. BMI is the ratio of body weight (in pounds) to body height (in inches). Calculate your BMI by dividing your weight in pounds by your height in inches; divide that answer by your height in inches; multiply that answer by 703.

A quick method for determining BMI is using Table 9.A3. You can interpret BMI values for adults with one fixed number, regardless of age or sex, using the guidelines in Table 9.A2.

Table 9.A2 Classification for BMI Ratios

Ratio	Classification
≤18.5	Underweight
18.6 to 24.9	Normal
25 to 29.9	Overweight
≥ 30	Obese

Table 9.A3 Body Mass Index

BMI	19	20	21	22	23	24	25	26	27	28	29	30	31	32	33	34	35	36	37	38	39	40	41	42	43	44	45	46	47	48	49	50	51	52	53	54
	Normal						Overweight					Obese										Extreme Obesity														
Height (inches)																						Body Weight (pounds)														
58	91	96	100	105	110	115	119	124	129	134	138	143	148	153	158	162	167	172	177	181	186	191	196	201	205	210	215	220	224	229	234	239	244	248	253	258
59	94	99	104	109	114	119	124	128	133	138	143	148	153	158	163	168	173	178	183	188	193	198	203	208	212	217	222	227	232	237	242	247	252	257	262	267
60	97	102	107	112	118	123	128	133	138	143	148	153	158	163	168	174	179	184	189	194	199	204	209	215	220	225	230	235	240	245	250	255	261	266	271	276
61	100	106	111	116	122	127	132	137	143	148	153	158	164	169	174	180	185	190	195	201	206	211	217	222	227	232	238	243	248	254	259	264	269	275	280	285
62	104	109	115	120	126	131	136	142	147	153	158	164	169	175	180	186	191	196	202	207	213	218	224	229	235	240	246	251	256	262	267	273	278	284	289	295
63	107	113	118	124	130	135	141	146	152	158	163	169	175	180	186	191	197	203	208	214	220	225	231	237	242	248	254	259	265	270	278	282	287	293	299	304
64	110	116	122	128	134	140	145	151	157	163	169	174	180	186	192	197	204	209	215	221	227	232	238	244	250	256	262	267	273	279	285	291	296	302	308	314
65	114	120	126	132	138	144	150	156	162	168	174	180	186	192	198	204	210	216	222	228	234	240	246	252	258	264	270	276	282	288	294	300	306	312	318	324
66	118	124	130	136	142	148	155	161	167	173	179	186	192	198	204	210	216	223	229	235	241	247	253	260	266	272	278	284	291	297	303	309	315	322	328	334
67	121	127	134	140	146	153	159	166	172	178	185	191	198	204	211	217	223	230	236	242	249	255	261	268	274	280	287	293	299	306	312	319	325	331	338	344
68	125	131	138	144	151	158	164	171	177	184	190	197	203	210	216	223	230	236	243	249	256	262	269	276	282	289	295	302	308	315	322	328	335	341	348	354
69	128	135	142	149	155	162	169	176	182	189	196	203	209	216	223	230	236	243	250	257	263	270	277	284	291	297	304	311	318	324	331	338	345	351	358	365
70	132	139	146	153	160	167	174	181	188	195	202	209	216	222	229	236	243	250	257	264	271	278	285	292	299	306	313	320	327	334	341	348	355	362	369	376
71	136	143	150	157	165	172	179	186	193	200	208	215	222	229	236	243	250	257	265	272	279	286	293	301	308	315	322	329	338	343	351	358	365	372	379	386
72	140	147	154	162	169	177	184	191	199	206	213	221	228	235	242	250	258	265	272	279	287	294	302	309	316	324	331	338	346	353	361	368	375	383	390	397
73	144	151	159	166	174	182	189	197	204	212	219	227	235	242	250	257	265	272	280	288	295	302	310	318	325	333	340	348	355	363	371	378	386	393	401	408
74	148	155	163	171	179	186	194	202	210	218	225	233	241	249	256	264	272	280	287	295	303	311	319	326	334	342	350	358	365	373	381	389	396	404	412	420
75	152	160	168	176	184	192	200	208	216	224	232	240	248	256	264	272	279	287	295	303	311	319	327	335	343	351	359	367	375	383	391	399	407	415	423	431
76	156	164	172	180	189	197	205	213	221	230	238	246	254	263	271	279	287	295	304	312	320	328	336	344	353	361	369	377	385	394	402	410	418	426	435	443

Source: Courtesy of the National Heart, Lung and Blood Institute.

Activity 4: Calculate Your Waist-to-Height Ratio (WHtR)

Recent research shows that the waist-to-height ratio (WHtR) is a much better measure than BMI, waist-to-hip ratio, and waist circumference for assessing obesity, cardiovascular risk, and other health risks associated with excess body fat.

The WHtR is calculated by dividing waist size by height, and takes gender into account.

The following chart helps determine if your WHtR falls in a healthy range (the ratios are percentages):

Women (the ratios are percentages)	
Ratio less than 35	Abnormally underweight to underweight
Ratio 35 to 42	Underweight
Ratio 42 to 46	Slightly underweight to healthy
Ratio 46 to 49	Healthy
Ratio 49 to 54	Overweight
Ratio 54 to 58	Seriously overweight
Ratio over 58	Highly obese

Men (the ratios are percentages)	
Ratio less than 35	Extremely underweight to underweight
Ratio 35 to 43	Underweight
Ratio 43 to 46	Slightly underweight to healthy
Ratio 46 to 53	Healthy
Ratio 53 to 58	Overweight
Ratio 58 to 63	Extremely overweight to obese
Ratio over 63	Highly obese

What is your WHtR? _____

Activity 5: Calculate Your Skinfold Measurements

There are three sites where skinfolds are most commonly measured (see Figures 9.A2 and 9.A3):

Men	
Chest	Measure halfway between the right shoulder crease and the nipple.
Abdomen	Measure about 1 inch to the right of the navel.
Thigh	Measure on the front of the right thigh, midway between the hip and the knee joint.

Figure 9.A2 Measuring skinfolds.

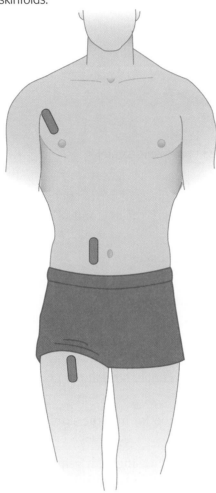

Women	
Triceps	Measure on the back of the right arm, half the distance between the tip of the shoulder and the tip of the elbow.
Suprailium	Measure at the top of the right iliac crest.
Thigh	Measure on the front of the right thigh, midway between the hip and the knee joint.

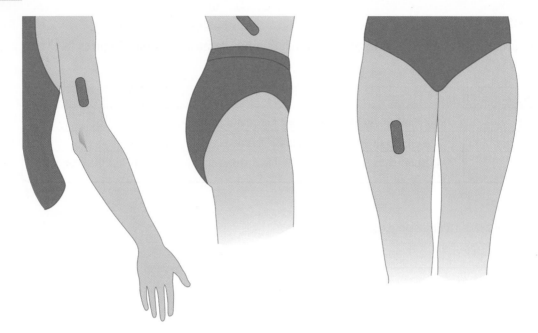

Figure 9.A3 Anatomical sites used to measure skinfolds.

Techniques for Taking Skinfolds

1. Before measuring, if you prefer, mark the anatomical site with a water-soluble felt-tip pen.

2. Take all measurements on the right side.

3. Grasp the skinfold firmly by the thumb and finger of your left hand and pull away from the body. This is usually easier on thin people. Do not pinch the skinfold too hard. The skinfolds are normally pinched in a vertical rather than a horizontal line.

4. With your right hand, hold the caliper perpendicular with the skinfold, keeping the skinfold dial up so that it can be read. The caliper should be a quarter- to a half-inch away from the thumb and the forefinger so that the pressure of the caliper will not be affected.

5. Do not place the skinfold caliper too far into the skinfold or too far away on the tip of the skinfold.

6. Read the dial 1 to 2 seconds after releasing your grip. Take a minimum of two measurements at each site. Allow at least 15 seconds between measurements to permit the skinfold site to return to normal. If the repeated measurement varies by more than 1 millimeter, take another measurement until there is consistency.

7. Do not take measurements when the skin is moist, because dampness makes it easier to grasp the extra skin and thus obtain larger values. Do not take measurements immediately after exercise because exercise makes the skin moist.

8. Be sure to grasp the same size of skinfold consistently at the same location every time. This requires practice.

Results

Men	
Chest	mm
Abdomen	mm
Thigh	mm
Total of measurements	mm

Women	
Triceps	mm
Suprailium	mm
Thigh	mm
Total of measurements	mm

Determining Body Fat Percent

Add the measurements of your three skinfolds, and then find the body fat percent corresponding to your total in Table 9.A5 for men or Table 9.A6 for women.

Your body fat percent = _____ %

Use Tables 9.A5 and 9.A6 to analyze your results.

Table 9.A5 Percent Fat Estimates for Men: Sum of Chest, Abdominal, and Thigh Skinfolds

Sum of skinfolds (mm)	Age to the last year								
	Under 22	23–27	28–32	33–37	38–42	43–47	48–52	53–57	Over 58
8–10	1.3	1.8	2.3	2.9	3.4	3.9	4.5	5.0	5.5
11–13	2.2	2.8	3.3	3.9	4.4	4.9	5.5	6.0	6.5
14–16	3.2	3.8	4.3	4.8	5.4	5.9	6.4	7.0	7.5
17–19	4.2	4.7	5.3	5.8	6.3	6.9	7.4	8.0	8.5
20–22	5.1	5.7	6.2	6.8	7.3	7.9	8.4	8.9	9.5
23–25	6.1	6.6	7.2	7.7	8.3	8.8	9.4	9.9	10.5
26–28	7.0	7.6	8.1	8.7	9.2	9.8	10.3	10.9	11.4
29–31	8.0	8.5	9.1	9.6	10.2	10.7	11.3	11.8	12.4
32–34	8.9	9.4	10.0	10.5	11.1	11.6	12.2	12.8	13.3
35–37	9.8	10.4	10.9	11.5	12.0	12.6	13.1	13.7	14.3
38–40	10.7	11.3	11.8	12.4	12.9	13.5	14.1	14.6	15.2
41–43	11.6	12.2	12.7	13.3	13.8	14.4	15.0	15.5	16.1
44–46	12.5	13.1	13.6	14.2	14.7	15.3	15.9	16.4	17.0
47–49	13.4	13.9	14.5	15.1	15.6	16.2	16.8	17.3	17.9
50–52	14.3	14.8	15.4	15.9	16.5	17.1	17.6	18.2	18.8
53–55	15.1	15.7	16.2	16.8	17.4	17.9	18.5	18.1	19.7
56–58	16.0	16.5	17.1	17.7	18.2	18.8	19.4	20.0	20.5
59–61	16.9	17.4	17.9	18.5	19.1	19.7	20.2	20.8	21.4
62–64	17.6	18.2	18.8	19.4	19.9	20.5	21.1	21.7	22.2
65–67	18.5	19.0	19.6	20.2	20.8	21.3	21.9	22.5	23.1
68–70	19.3	19.9	20.4	21.0	21.6	22.2	22.7	23.3	23.9
71–73	20.1	20.7	21.2	21.8	22.4	23.0	23.6	24.1	24.7
74–76	20.9	21.5	22.0	22.6	23.2	23.8	24.4	25.0	25.5
77–79	21.7	22.2	22.8	23.4	24.0	24.6	25.2	25.8	26.3
80–82	22.4	23.0	23.6	24.2	24.8	25.4	25.9	26.5	27.1
83–85	23.2	23.8	24.4	25.0	25.5	26.1	26.7	27.3	27.9
86–88	24.0	24.5	25.1	25.7	26.3	26.9	27.5	28.1	28.7
89–91	24.7	25.3	25.9	25.5	27.1	27.6	28.2	28.8	29.4
92–94	25.4	26.0	26.6	27.2	27.8	28.4	29.0	29.6	30.2
95–97	26.1	16.7	27.3	27.9	28.5	29.1	29.7	30.3	30.9
98–100	26.9	27.4	28.0	28.6	29.2	29.8	30.4	31.0	31.6
101–103	27.5	28.1	28.7	29.3	29.9	30.5	31.1	31.7	32.3
104–106	28.2	28.8	29.4	30.0	30.6	31.2	31.8	32.4	33.0
107–109	28.9	29.5	30.1	30.7	31.3	31.9	32.5	33.1	33.7
110–112	29.6	30.2	30.8	31.4	32.0	32.6	33.2	33.8	34.4
113–115	30.2	30.8	31.4	32.0	32.6	33.2	33.8	34.5	35.1
116–118	30.9	31.5	32.1	32.7	33.3	33.9	34.5	35.1	35.7
119–121	31.5	32.1	32.7	33.3	33.9	34.5	35.1	35.7	36.4
122–124	32.1	32.7	33.3	33.9	34.5	35.1	35.8	36.4	37.0
125–127	32.7	33.3	33.9	34.5	35.1	35.8	36.4	37.0	37.6

Percent fat calculated by the formula by Siri: Percent fat = $[(4.95/BD) - 4.5] \times 100$, where BD = body density.

Source: Reproduced from Pollock M. L., Schmidt D. H., and Jackson A. S. Measurement of cardiorespiratory fitness and body composition in the clinical setting. *Comprehensive Therapy* 1980; 6(9):12–27. Reprinted with kind permission of Springer Science and Business Media.

Table 9.A6 Percent Fat Estimates for Women: Sum of Triceps, Iliac Crest, and Thigh Skinfolds

Sum of skinfolds (mm)	Age to the last year								
	Under 22	23–27	28–32	33–37	38–42	43–47	48–52	53–57	Over 58
23–25	9.7	9.9	10.2	10.4	10.7	10.9	11.2	11.4	11.7
26–28	11.0	11.2	11.5	11.7	12.0	12.3	12.5	12.7	13.0
29–31	12.3	12.5	12.8	13.0	13.3	13.5	13.8	14.0	14.3
32–34	13.6	13.8	14.0	14.3	14.5	14.8	15.0	15.3	15.5
35–37	14.8	15.0	15.3	15.5	15.8	16.0	16.3	16.5	16.8
38–40	16.0	16.3	16.5	16.7	17.0	17.2	17.5	17.7	18.0
41–43	17.2	17.4	17.7	17.9	18.2	18.4	18.7	18.9	19.2
44–46	18.3	18.6	18.8	19.1	19.3	19.6	19.8	20.1	20.3
47–49	19.5	19.7	20.0	20.2	20.5	20.7	21.0	21.2	21.5
50–52	20.6	20.8	21.1	21.3	21.6	21.8	22.1	22.3	22.6
53–55	21.7	21.9	22.1	22.4	22.6	22.9	23.1	23.4	23.6
56–58	22.7	23.0	23.2	23.4	23.7	23.9	24.2	24.4	24.7
59–61	23.7	24.0	24.2	24.5	24.7	25.0	25.2	25.5	25.7
62–64	24.7	25.0	25.2	25.5	35.7	26.0	26.7	26.4	26.7
65–67	25.7	25.9	26.2	26.4	26.7	26.9	27.2	27.4	27.7
68–70	26.6	26.9	27.1	27.4	27.6	27.9	28.1	28.4	28.6
71–73	27.5	27.8	28.0	28.3	28.5	28.8	28.0	29.3	29.5
74–76	28.4	28.7	28.9	29.2	29.4	29.7	29.9	30.2	30.4
77–79	29.3	29.5	39.8	30.0	30.3	30.5	30.8	31.0	31.3
80–82	30.1	30.4	30.6	30.9	31.1	31.4	31.6	31.9	32.1
83–85	30.9	31.2	31.4	31.7	31.9	32.2	32.4	32.7	32.9
86–88	31.7	32.0	32.2	32.5	32.7	32.9	33.2	33.4	33.7
89–91	32.5	32.7	33.0	33.2	33.5	33.7	33.9	34.2	34.4
92–94	33.2	33.4	33.7	33.9	34.2	34.4	34.7	34.9	35.2
95–97	33.9	34.1	34.4	34.6	34.9	35.1	35.4	35.6	35.9
98–100	34.6	34.8	35.1	35.3	35.5	35.8	36.0	36.3	36.5
101–103	35.3	35.4	35.7	35.9	36.2	36.4	36.7	36.9	37.2
104–106	35.8	36.1	36.3	36.6	36.8	37.1	37.3	37.5	37.8
107–109	36.4	36.7	36.9	37.1	37.4	37.6	37.9	38.1	38.4
110–112	37.0	37.2	37.5	37.7	38.0	38.2	38.5	38.7	38.9
113–115	37.5	37.8	38.0	38.2	38.5	38.7	39.0	39.2	39.5
116–118	38.0	38.3	38.5	38.8	39.0	39.3	39.5	39.7	40.0
119–121	38.5	38.7	39.0	39.2	39.5	39.7	40.0	40.2	40.5
122–124	39.0	39.2	39.4	39.7	39.9	40.2	40.4	40.7	40.9
125–127	39.4	39.6	39.9	40.1	40.4	40.6	40.9	41.1	41.4
128–130	39.8	40.0	40.3	40.5	40.8	41.0	41.3	41.5	41.8

Percent fat calculated by the formula by Siri. Percent fat = $[(4.95/BD) - 4.5] \times 100$, where BD = body density.

Source: Reproduced from Pollock M.L., Schmidt D.H., and Jackson A.S. Measurement of cardiorespiratory fitness and body composition in the clinical setting. *Comprehensive Therapy* 1980; 6(9):12–27. Reprinted with kind permission of Springer Science and Business Media.

Name _____ Section _____ Date _____

Assess Your Total Daily Energy Needs

Use the following activity to estimate your daily caloric needs.

A. Estimating energy needs for metabolism

1. Convert your body weight to kilograms. Because each kilogram equals about 2.2 pounds, divide your weight in pounds by 2.2 to obtain your weight in kilograms.

   _____ weight in pounds ÷ 2.2 = _____ kilograms (kg)

2. To sustain its metabolic needs, the body needs about 1.0 calorie per kilogram of body weight per hour (men) or 0.9 calorie per kilogram of body weight per hour (women). To estimate the amount of calories you need for metabolism in an hour, multiply your body weight (kg) by 1.0 if you are male or by 0.9 if you are female.

   _____ body weight (kg) × 1.0 or 0.9 = _____ calories per hour

3. To estimate the amount of calories you need for metabolism in a day, multiply the amount of calories you obtained in Step 2 by 24 (hours in a day).

   _____ calories per hour × 24 hours = _____ calories per day (metabolism)

B. Estimating energy needs for physical activity

4. To determine your energy needs for physical activity, you can keep records of every activity you perform during the day and the time spent engaging in each activity. An easier, but less precise way to estimate your energy expenditures for physical activity is to use the following "rule of thumb." Choose the category of physical activity in Table 9.A7 that best describes your usual physical activity level. For example, if you spend most of your day sitting while taking classes, studying, and watching TV, you probably have a sedentary level of activity. If you sit some of the time but move around while working, you might rate your level of physical activity as light. If you are on your feet most of the time and engage in strenuous work such as lifting heavy objects, you are probably expending energy at the heavy level of intensity.

   My activity level is _____.

5. Note the activity factor in Table 9.A7 for your level of intensity and gender. For example, if you are male and you consider your overall physical activity pattern to be in the moderate range, your activity factor is 1.7.

   The activity factor for my gender and level of physical activity intensity is _____.

6. Multiply your metabolic energy needs (the number of calories per day estimated in Step 3) by the activity factor (Step 5).

   _____ calories for metabolism × _____ activity factor = _____ calories for physical activity

7. To estimate the number of calories you expend each day for the thermic effect of food (TEF), multiply the number of calories determined in Step 6 by 0.10.

_____ calories × 0.10 = _____ calories for TEF

8. To estimate your total energy needs for a day, add the number of calories determined in Steps 6 and 7.

_____ calories for metabolism and physical activity

+ _____ calories for TEF

= _____ total calories

This is an estimation of the total number of calories you use each day. If you take in more calories than needed, they may be converted to body fat.

9. If you completed the assessment in Lab 9-2, you were able to determine an average number of calories that you consumed during the 3-day recordkeeping period. Is your average caloric intake about the same, greater than, or less than the total number of calories that you need for a day?

_____ about the same _____ greater than _____ less than

10. If you continue to consume this average amount of calories, explain what may happen to your body weight.

_____

_____

_____

_____

_____

_____

Table 9.A7 Determining Your Physical Activity Intensity Factor

Intensity	Physical activity	Activity factor	
		Men	Women
Very light	Standing, sitting, driving, typing, sewing, cooking, playing cards or a musical instrument	1.3	1.3
Light	Walking on a level surface at 2.5 to 3.0 mph, carpentry, child care, golf, sailing, table tennis	1.6	1.5
Moderate	Walking 3.5 to 4.0 mph, gardening, carrying a load, cycling, skiing, tennis, dancing	1.7	1.6
Heavy	Walking uphill carrying a load; digging by hand; playing basketball, football, or soccer; climbing	2.1	1.9
Exceptionally heavy	Athletic training or participation in professional or world-class events	2.4	2.2

Source: Reprinted with permission from Subcommittee on the Tenth Edition of the *Recommended Dietary Allowances*, Food and Nutrition Board, Commission on Life Sciences, and National Research Council, Recommended Dietary Allowances, Tenth edition. National Academies Press, 1989.

© 2013 Jones & Bartlett Learning, LLC

Name _____ Section _____ Date _____

Tracking Your Body Composition

Test 1 Date: _____

Assessment technique	Value	Classification
Waist circumference	inches	Exceeds standards? Yes No
Waist-to-hip ratio	ratio	Exceeds standards? Yes No
BMI		
Waist-to-height ratio		
Skinfold measurements	% body fat	

Test 2 Date: _____

Assessment technique	Value	Classification
Waist circumference	inches	Exceeds standards? Yes No
Waist-to-hip ratio	ratio	Exceeds standards? Yes No
BMI		
Waist-to-height ratio		
Skinfold measurements	% body fat	

Test 3 Date: _____

Assessment technique	Value	Classification
Waist circumference	inches	Exceeds standards? Yes No
Waist-to-hip ratio	ratio	Exceeds standards? Yes No
BMI		
Waist-to-height ratio		
Skinfold measurements	% body fat	

Test 4 Date: _____

Assessment technique	Value	Classification
Waist circumference	inches	Exceeds standards? Yes No
Waist-to-hip ratio	ratio	Exceeds standards? Yes No
BMI		
Waist-to-height ratio		
Skinfold measurements	% body fat	

Name _____ Section _____ Date _____

How Much Stress Have You Had Lately?

Activity 1: The College Life-Stress Scale

To estimate the amount of stress that you have endured recently, indicate the number of occasions (to a maximum of four) that you have experienced the following events in the past year.

Event	Number of Occasions	Points	Total
1. Death of a spouse	____	87	____
2. Marriage	____	77	____
3. Death of a close relative	____	77	____
4. Divorce	____	76	____
5. Marital separation	____	74	____
6. Pregnancy, or fathered a pregnancy	____	64	____
7. Death of a close friend	____	68	____
8. Personal injury or illness	____	65	____
9. Loss of your job	____	62	____
10. Breakup of a marital engagement or a steady relationship	____	60	____
11. Sexual difficulties	____	58	____
12. Marital reconciliation	____	58	____
13. Major change in self-concept	____	57	____
14. Major change in health or behavior of a family member	____	56	____
15. Engagement to be married	____	54	____
16. Major change in financial status	____	53	____
17. Major change in the use of drugs (other than alcohol)	____	52	____
18. Mortgage or loan of less than $10,000	____	52	____
19. Entered college	____	50	____
20. A new family member	____	50	____
21. A conflict or change in values	____	50	____
22. Change to a different line of work	____	50	____
23. A major change in the number of arguments with spouse	____	50	____
24. Change to a new school	____	50	____
25. A major change in amount of independence and responsibility	____	49	____
26. A major change in responsibilities at work	____	47	____
27. A major change in the use of alcohol	____	46	____

Event	Number of Occasions	Points	Total
28. Revised personal habits	____	45	____
29. Being in trouble with school administration	____	44	____
30. A major change in social activities	____	43	____
31. Holding a job while attending school	____	43	____
32. Change of residence or living conditions	____	42	____
33. A major change in working hours or conditions	____	42	____
34. Trouble with in-laws	____	42	____
35. Your spouse beginning or stopping work outside the home	____	41	____
36. Change in dating habits	____	41	____
37. A change involving your major field of study	____	41	____
38. An outstanding personal achievement	____	40	____
39. Trouble with your boss	____	38	____
40. A major change in amount of participation in school activities	____	38	____
41. A major change in type and/or amount of recreation	____	37	____
42. A major change in religious activities	____	36	____
43. A major change in sleeping habits	____	34	____
44. A trip or vacation	____	33	____
45. A major change in eating habits	____	30	____
46. A major change in number of family get-togethers	____	26	____
47. Found guilty of minor violations of the law	____	22	____

Multiply the number of occasions times the point value for each event.
Add the scores.

TOTAL POINTS _____

Your degree of stress is low if your score is lower than 347. If your score is higher than 1435, you are under a high degree of stress.

Source: Adapted from Marx M., et al. The influence of recent life experience on the health of college freshmen. *Journal of Psychosomatic Research* 1975; 19(1):87–98.

Activity 2: The Inventory of College Students' Recent Life Experiences

The Inventory of College Students' Recent Life Experiences (ICSRLE) identifies individual exposure to sources of hassles and stress experienced over the past month. The ICSRLE was developed uniquely for college students. Student stress can be unique and different from other settings.

Directions

For each experience, estimate how much it has been a part of your life over the past month. Mark your answers according to the following guide:

Intensity of Experience over the Past Month

0 = not at all part of my life

1 = only slightly part of my life

2 = distinctly part of my life

3 = very much part of my life

_____ 1. Conflicts with boyfriend's/girlfriend's/spouse's family

_____ 2. Being let down or disappointed by friends

_____ 3. Conflict with professor(s)

_____ 4. Social rejection

_____ 5. Too many things to do at once

_____ 6. Being taken for granted

_____ 7. Financial conflicts with family members

_____ 8. Having your trust betrayed by a friend

_____ 9. Separation from people you care about

_____10. Having your contributions overlooked

_____11. Struggling to meet your own academic standards

_____12. Being taken advantage of

_____13. Not enough leisure time

_____14. Struggling to meet the academic standards of others

_____15. A lot of responsibilities

_____16. Dissatisfaction with school

_____17. Decisions about intimate relationship(s)

_____18. Not enough time to meet your obligations

_____19. Dissatisfaction with your mathematical ability

_____20. Important decisions about your future career

_____21. Financial burdens

_____22. Dissatisfaction with your reading ability

_____23. Important decisions about your education

_____24. Loneliness

_____25. Lower grades than you hoped for

_____26. Conflict with teaching assistant(s)

_____27. Not enough time for sleep

_____28. Conflicts with your family

_____29. Heavy demands from extracurricular activities

_____30. Finding courses too demanding

_____31. Conflicts with friends

_____32. Hard effort to get ahead

_____33. Poor health of a friend

_____34. Disliking your studies

_____35. Getting "ripped off" or cheated in the purchase of services

_____36. Social conflicts over smoking

_____37. Difficulties with transportation

_____38. Disliking fellow student(s)

_____39. Conflicts with boyfriend/girlfriend/spouse

_____40. Dissatisfaction with your ability at written expression

_____41. Interruptions of your schoolwork

_____42. Social isolation

_____43. Long waits to get service (e.g., at banks, stores)

_____44. Being ignored

_____45. Dissatisfaction with your physical appearance

_____46. Finding course(s) uninteresting

_____47. Gossip concerning someone you care about

_____48. Failing to get expected job

_____49. Dissatisfaction with your athletic skills

Add your total points: _____

Your score on the ICSRLE can range from 0 to 147. Higher scores indicate higher levels of exposure to experiences involving stress. Focus on two key outcomes from your results. First, you can determine your current level of stress by adding your score for each hassle and getting a total. Second, you can discover which of the hassles play a greater part in your life. Scored items rated with a 3 indicate those stressors are more of an issue for you.

Source: With kind permission from Springer Science and Business Media. Kohn, P. M., Lafreniere, K., and Gurevich, M. The Inventory of College Students' Recent Life Experiences: a decontaminated hassles scale for a special population. *Journal of Behavioral Medicine* 1990; 13(6):619–630.

Name _____ Section _____ Date _____

Time Management

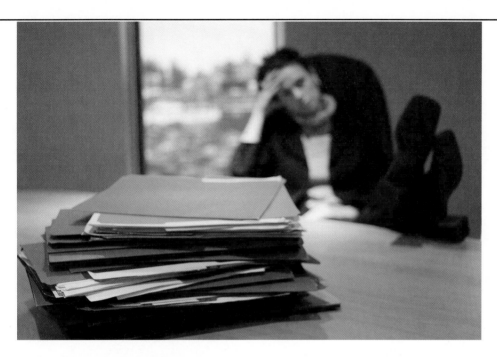

Activity 1: Ranking Tasks

Step 1: Write down all the things you need to get done today with no regard to order of importance.

1. _____ 6. _____
2. _____ 7. _____
3. _____ 8. _____
4. _____ 9. _____
5. _____ 10. _____

Step 2: In column A, list all the things that must get done as soon as possible. In column C, list all the things you would like to do, but that are not essential. In column B, put everything else.

A	B	C
_____	_____	_____
_____	_____	_____
_____	_____	_____
_____	_____	_____

Activity 2: Scheduling

After completing Activity 1: Ranking Tasks, and you have determined what needs to get done, complete your schedule.

7:00 A.M. _____

7:30 A.M. _____

8:00 A.M. _____

8:30 A.M. _____

9:00 A.M. _____

9:30 A.M. _____

10:00 A.M. _____

10:30 A.M. _____

11:00 A.M. _____

11:30 A.M. _____

12:00 P.M. _____

12:30 P.M. _____

1:00 P.M. _____

1:30 P.M. _____

2:00 P.M. _____

2:30 P.M. _____

3:00 P.M. _____

3:30 P.M. _____

4:00 P.M. _____

4:30 P.M. _____

5:00 P.M. _____

5:30 P.M. _____

6:00 P.M. _____

6:30 P.M. _____

7:00 P.M. _____

7:30 P.M. _____

8:00 P.M. _____

8:30 P.M. _____

9:00 P.M. _____

9:30 P.M. _____

10:00 P.M. _____

10:30 P.M. _____

11:00 P.M. _____

Name _____ Section _____ Date _____

Relaxation Techniques

Activity 1: Progressive Muscle Relaxation

Muscle tension is the most common symptom of stress. But where each of us feels it varies. One woman might have a tight neck and shoulders, while another feels an iron band digging into her forehead. It is not always easy to locate and relax the muscles responsible.

Progressive muscle relaxation (PMR) teaches you to isolate specific sets of muscles, tense them briefly, and then relax them. This exercise is especially helpful if your mind is racing, making it hard to settle down to other techniques.

Follow the instructions to try PMR. It takes only about 10 minutes to exercise all the major body areas. There are several sequences. You can start with the hand muscles, progressing to others; begin at the top, moving from head to toe; or reverse the direction, going from bottom to top as explained.

PMR Procedure

Find a comfortable position. Perform the steps while either sitting or lying down, preferably in a quiet, soothing environment.

Breathe deeply, allowing your stomach to rise as you inhale and fall as you exhale. Breathe this way for a few minutes before starting.

For each of the body areas, perform three contractions:

• First contraction: 100% intensity for 5 to 10 seconds

  - Release and relax (exhale)

  - Compare relaxation to contraction

• Second contraction: 50% intensity for 5 to 10 seconds

  - Release and relax (exhale)

  - Compare relaxation to contraction

• Third contraction: 5% to 10% intensity for 5 to 10 seconds

  - Release and relax (exhale)

  - Compare relaxation to contraction

Take your time, slowly working through each of these body areas:

1. Curl toes tightly.

2. Flex the feet.

3. Tighten the calves.

4. Tense the thighs.

5. Tighten the buttocks.

6. Tighten the lower back.

7. Tighten the abdomen.

8. Tense the upper chest.

9. Tense the upper back muscles.

10. Clench the fists.

11. Extend the fingers and flex the wrists.

12. Tighten the forearms.

13. Tighten the upper arms.

14. Lift the shoulders gently toward the ears.

15. Wrinkle the forehead.

16. Squeeze your eyes shut.

17. Drop your chin, letting your mouth open wide.

Your whole body should feel completely relaxed and calm. Now lie still and enjoy the feeling of complete relaxation.

Activity 2: Meditation

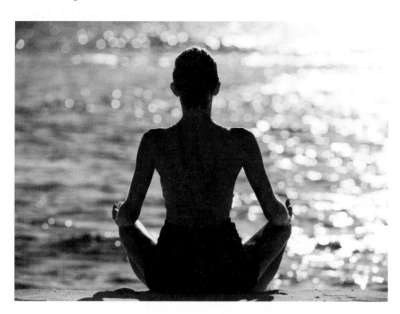

Meditation tends to banish inner stress and exert a calming, healing influence. It not only helps preserve emotional balance in everyday life, but also enhances therapy for a host of illnesses, especially high blood pressure. Herbert Benson developed the following simple, practical procedure for eliciting the relaxation response.

Procedure

1. Select a focus word or brief phrase that has deep meaning for you.

2. Take a comfortable sitting position in a quiet environment.

3. Close your eyes and consciously relax your muscles.

4. Breathe slowly and naturally through your nose while silently repeating your focus word or phrase each time you inhale.

5. Keep your attitude passive; disregard thoughts that drift in.

6. Continue for 10 to 20 minutes once or twice a day.

You can pick almost any focus word or phrase, such as the word *one*. Some meditators find it helpful to focus on the breath—in, out, in, out—rather than on a word or phrase. Others prefer to focus on an object, such as a candle flame. If you want to time your session, peek at a watch or clock occasionally, but don't set a jarring alarm. Getting to your feet immediately after a session can make you feel slightly dizzy, so sit quietly for a few moments first with your eyes closed. The technique works best on an empty stomach, either before a meal or about 2 hours after eating. Avoid those times when you are obviously tired unless you want to fall asleep. Although you will feel refreshed after the first session, it may take a month or more to get noticeable results, such as lower blood pressure.

Activity 3: Track and Record Your Relaxation Technique

After trying the two relaxation techniques in Activities 1 and 2 (progressive muscle relaxation; relaxation response) several times each, which do you prefer?

_____

Why?

_____

_____

Use your preferred relaxation technique daily over a 2-week period of time. Identify for each day your location, approximate length of time taken, and your feelings when finished.

Your preferred method: _____

	Date:	Date:	Date:	Date:	Date:	Date:	Date:
Location							
Length							
Feelings: calm, relaxed, etc.							

	Date:	Date:	Date:	Date:	Date:	Date:	Date:
Location							
Length							
Feelings: calm, relaxed, etc.							

Name _____   Section _____   Date _____

Creative Problem Solving

Activity 1: Scenarios

Directions

Choose one of the following problems. This activity can provide good practice for the times when you will need to apply these skills to real life.

Problem 1: Paul is called into his supervisor's office and told that the company must lay off some employees. Paul will be laid off in 2 months. He is married and has two small children. He has a mortgage payment on his home and a car payment each month.

Problem 2: You are upset after having an argument with your junior high school–aged son about the trouble he is getting into at school.

Problem 3: Maria has four final exams and only 2 days left to study for them. She is anxious because she doesn't think she will have enough time to study for the exams.

Which of the problems did you choose? _____

1. Define the problem.

_____

_____

_____

2. List the facts.

_____

_____

_____

3. List possible solutions (at least four).

A. _____

_____

B. _____

_____

C. _____

_____

D. _____

_____

4. Analyze and evaluate the possible solutions.

_____

_____

_____

5. Select one solution to implement.

_____

_____

_____

6. Evaluate the results (for this assignment, give ways you would evaluate).

_____

_____

_____

Activity 2: Problem-Solving Steps

Write a problem that was or is stressing you. Go through the problem-solving steps.
Write the problem:

_____

_____

_____

1. Define the problem.

_____

_____

_____

2. List the facts.

_____

_____

_____

3. List possible solutions (at least four).

    A. _____

       _____

    B. _____

       _____

    C. _____

       _____

    D. _____

       _____

4. Analyze and evaluate the possible solutions.

_____

_____

_____

5. Select one solution to implement.

_____

_____

_____

6. Evaluate the results (for this assignment, give ways you would evaluate).

_____

_____

_____

Creative Problem Solving

Name _____ Section _____ Date _____

Decision Making: Paired Comparison Analysis

Paired comparison analysis can be used whenever making decisions about almost anything. It provides a framework for comparing your choices or options, and then selecting the best.

Directions

1. What decision are you making? _____

2. Criteria for judging the options should be established before making decisions (e.g., financial, effectiveness, availability). List the criteria you are using here:

   _____

   _____

   _____

3. Write in the options about which you are making a decision in the following Option Table. You may have fewer options than eight.

4. Beginning at the top of each column in the Matrix, compare each pair listed in the Option Table, while asking yourself, "If I could choose only one, which would it be?" Use the criteria listed in Step 2. Circle the number corresponding to your choice.

5. Continuing down each column, compare and choose one of the two options.

6. Count the number of times each number was circled on the Matrix, and fill in the blanks next to the corresponding number on the Option Table.

Matrix

1–2						
1–3	2–3					
1–4	2–4	3–4				
1–5	2–5	3–5	4–5			
1–6	2–6	3–6	4–6	5–6		
1–7	2–7	3–7	4–7	5–7	6–7	
1–8	2–8	3–8	4–8	5–8	6–8	7–8

Option Table

Option	Number of times selected	Rank
1)		
2)		
3)		
4)		
5)		
6)		
7)		
8)		

Which is the best option? _____

　　　Decision Making: Paired Comparison Analysis

Name _____ Section _____ Date _____

Health Food Store Visit

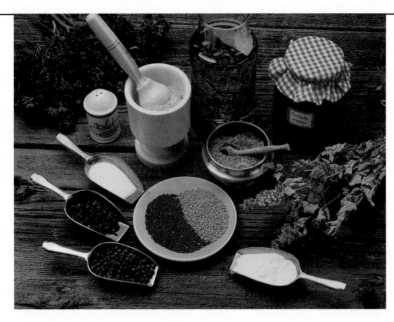

Visit one or more local health food stores. Ask a clerk for a recommendation for a specific ailment, condition, or goal (e.g., cellulite, increase energy, weight reduction).

1. Which condition did you ask about?

_____

_____

_____

2. What did the clerk recommend?

_____

_____

_____

3. What was the cost of the product?

_____

_____

_____

4. Would you use the product if you had the condition or wished to reach a goal? Why or why not?

_____

_____

Name _____ Section _____ Date _____

Fitness Club Visit

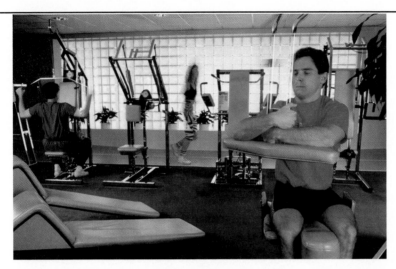

Visit one or more local fitness clubs. Ask about membership fees and request a tour of the facility. Note the type of equipment available and the cleanliness of the facility. Report your findings.

	Club 1	Club 2	Club 3
Membership fees			
Equipment			
Cleanliness			
Staff			
Other			

Based on your survey, which fitness club would you attend? Why?

_____

_____

Name _____ Section _____ Date _____

Shopping for Exercise Equipment

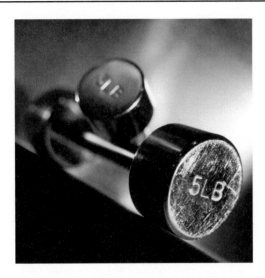

Determine one type of exercise equipment in which you are interested. Contact various sources (e.g., local stores, Internet, classified ads) and report on the following:

- Would you use the equipment if you were to purchase it?

  _____

  _____

- How is it rated in a consumer or fitness magazine?

  _____

  _____

- Is there a warranty?

  _____

  _____

- Total cost (including taxes)

  _____

  _____

- Where can you find the best deal?

  _____

  _____

Index

Photo Credits

© LiquidLibrary; **page 238** © Liquid-Library; **page 239 (top)** © Supri Suharjoto/ShutterStock, Inc.; **page 239 (bottom)** Photographed by Kimberly Potvin

Lab Manual
page 289 © Ablestock; **page 381** © Ablestock; **page 387** © Photodisc; **page 395** © Ablestock; **page 397** © Photos.com; **page 399** © Ablestock

Unless otherwise indicated, all photographs and illustrations are under copyright of Jones & Bartlett Learning. Some images in this book feature models. These models do not necessarily endorse, represent, or participate in the activities represented in the images.